The
Animal Doctor's Answer Book

The
Animal Doctor's

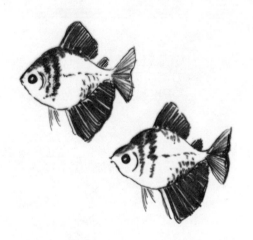

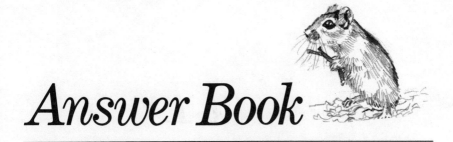

Answer Book

Dr. MICHAEL W. FOX

D.Sc., Ph.D., B.Vet.Med., M.R.C.V.S.

Illustrations by B.J. Lewis

Newmarket Press • New York

Text copyright © 1984 United Feature Syndicate, Inc.

Illustrations copyright © 1984 B. J. Lewis

This book published simultaneously in the United States of America and in Canada

First Edition
1 2 3 4 5 6 7 8 9 0 F/C
1 2 3 4 5 6 7 8 9 0 F/P

Library of Congress Cataloging in Publication Data

Fox, Michael W., 1937—
    The animal doctor's answer book.

    Includes index.
    Summary: Answers more than 1000 questions relative to
the physical and psychological health and behavior of dogs,
cats, and other pets.
    1. Pets—Miscellanea.   2. Pets—Diseases—Miscellanea.
[1. Pets—Miscellanea.   2. Pets—Diseases—Miscellanea.
3. Animals—Miscellanea.   4. Questions and answers]
I. Title.   II. Lewis, Betty J., ill.
SF413.F67   1984   636.08'87   84-6973
ISBN 0-937858-37-4
ISBN 0-937858-38-2 (pbk.)

Quantity Purchases
Companies, professional groups, clubs, and other organizations may qualify for special terms when ordering quantities of this title. For information, contact the Special Sales Department, Newmarket Press, 3 East 48th Street, New York, New York 10017. Phone (212) 832-3575.

By MICHAEL W. FOX

Canine Behavior
Canine Pediatrics
Integrative Development of Brain and Behavior in the Dog
Behavior of Wolves, Dogs, and Related Canids
Understanding Your Dog
Understanding Your Cat
Concepts in Ethology: Animal and Human Behavior
Between Animal and Man: The Key to the Kingdom
The Dog: Its Domestication and Behavior
Understanding Your Pet
Returning to Eden: Animal Rights and Human Responsibility
One Earth, One Mind
The Soul of the Wolf: Observations and Meditations
How to Be Your Pet's Best Friend
The Healing Touch
Love is a Happy Cat

CHILDREN'S BOOKS

The Wolf
Vixie: The Story of a Little Fox
Sundance Coyote
Ramu and Chennai
What Is Your Dog Saying? (with Wende Devlin Gates)
Wild Dogs Three
Whitepaws: A Coyote-dog
Lessons from Nature: Fox's Fables
The Touchlings
The Way of the Dolphin

To all creatures great and small—
my friends and teachers

Contents

Preface

U nderstanding animals' nature has been my lifetime endeavor, and I have learned that no matter what sort of animal you are raising—a puppy, a cat, a parakeet, a tiny gerbil—understanding is the key to its health and well-being. Neither love nor sympathy nor technical expertise is enough; knowledge and informed empathy are also essential.

Understanding animals' basic needs, health care, psychology, and behavior—what was once called animal husbandry—is almost a lost art. In modern "factory"-type animal farming, what is now termed animal production management, the psychology and behavioral needs of animals receive scant attention. But while less than 3 percent of the U.S. population, as farmers, is closely connected with nature and animals today, almost a quarter of the nonfarming population keeps at least one animal as a pet (or, as I prefer to call them, companion animals). Many families have more than one animal, and often enjoy the company of different species. Such mixed menageries are latter-day Noah's Arks; but they are not always the peaceable kingdoms that we would like. This book will help you strengthen your "animal connection" and help preserve the peaceable kingdom in your own home.

What makes a hamster happy or a parakeet so lovesick it pines away? How can you tell when your cat is emotionally upset and not physically sick? Could you have prevented your cat or dog from dying from an epidemic of distemper? Do you know if your dog is neurotic? Could it be your fault? What can you do to make life better for your pet? Here you will find the answers to these and many other questions, both about the medical problems that veterinarians treat and also about the problems that you yourself can prevent or heal through understanding your animal's nature. This is not, however, a book for home doctoring. I deplore pet owners' attempts to diagnose and treat serious animal-health problems themselves. This book will help you avert many problems and will assist you in knowing when your pet needs to be taken to see its own animal doctor. This, I believe, is an animal's right and entitlement, just as a sick child should be taken to a pediatrician.

Wild animals are not discussed much in this book because few, if any, can be domesticated and kept under the right conditions to satisfy their nature. They suffer in domestic circumstances, and, because they are less adaptable, it is more difficult to keep them healthy and to treat them when they are sick. These are some of the many reasons I question the ethics of capturing, breeding, and selling many species of wild animals as pets, and why I vehemently discourage people from keeping them.

It is also important to realize that even though "pet" or domesticated animals are more easily accommodated and cared for because their wildness has been reduced through generations of selective breeding, they have not been changed to such a degree that they have lost their "catness," "dogness," "hamsterness," or whatever their intrinsic nature is. That is why, if we who are their companions, guardians, and foster parents do not make an effort to understand their nature, all kinds of problems—physical, emotional, and social—will erupt.

The Animal Doctor's Answer Book explores a great many of the most common, amusing, annoying, and indeed perplexing problems that have cropped up through years of veterinary consultations and in the thousands of letters I receive for my syndicated newspaper column, "Ask Your Animal Doctor." Most of the questions and answers that have been included here are representative of hundreds (and, in some instances, thousands) of similar queries from pet owners. In reading them, you will be on the way to becoming good "pet shrinks" and healers; and, as a result, your pets will have fewer problems and you will get greater joy and satisfaction. Happier lives all round, in fact; we surely owe our animal companions nothing less.

AN ACKNOWLEDGMENT AND A REQUEST

I would like to express my thanks to Sylvie Reice, who edits my newspaper column and shares with me the burden, bemusement, and enlightenment of an ever-growing volume of mail from all over the United States and from as far away as Guam and Puerto Rico. Thanks also to David Hendin of United Feature Syndicate, who shares my concerns about the welfare and rights of animals and about the earth's ecology, for promoting my "Ask Your Animal Doctor" column.

Without the efforts of my publisher and friend Esther Margolis, her managing editor, Katherine Heintzelman, and other support staff, this book would never have been born or have reached you.

My thanks also go to B. J. Lewis for the wonderful illustrations she has contributed to the book.

And thank you, readers of "Ask Your Animal Doctor," for entertaining and enlightening me with your letters, a stellar selection of which is presented here for the enjoyment of everyone who loves animals.

If you share my affection for and interest in animals as sensitive and responsive beings that enrich our lives in countless ways, and if you share my concern about the billions of animals that are being cruelly and unethically exploited and some driven to extinction each year, then please write to me so that you can learn how to help make this world a better place for all creatures curious, wondrous, and divine.

Just like us, our animal companions can become ill and suffer physically and emotionally. But there are many people who are indifferent to their needs and insensitive to their suffering. There are people who neglect their dogs and leave them on a short chain on their property without shade, shelter, or sufficient food and water. And there are others who experiment unnecessarily on the same animals that we keep as pets—rabbits, guinea pigs, rats, mice, hamsters, gerbils, cats, and dogs—and encourage children to do so through high-school science fairs ("projects" involving blinding sparrows; scalding hamsters; poisoning mice; and electrocuting, starving, and vivisecting rats). One National Science Fair finalist recently used two kittens—family pets—to assess the effects of hair spray on hearing loss. The student actually sprayed gobs of hair spray into the kittens' ears to see if it affected their behavior.

But I recall another student finalist who learned some acupuncture principles from the veterinarian who treated her sick dog with acupuncture. She submitted to the same acupuncture therapy that her dog received, given by a physician, and verified that the treatment had the same effect on her immune system (causing an increase in blood gamma globulins) as it had on her dog.

Clearly, I am not antiscience, nor am I against the legitimate exploitation of animals: otherwise, I would be totally against all pet keeping, which I obviously am not. The Humane Society of the United States shares this view with me, and if you do too then please do write to me for information about how you can help.

Dr. Michael W. Fox
Scientific Director
The Humane Society of the United States
2100 L Street N.W.
Washington, D.C. 20037

Introduction:
Choosing the Pet
That's Right for You

best age for adoption (cats and dogs)

DEAR DR. FOX—I want to adopt a pet. Can you tell me what's the best age to adopt a puppy or kitten?—*L.M.*

DEAR L.M.—Adopt a puppy when it's between six and eight weeks old. This is the age when a puppy most readily develops social attachments—in fact, it is the critical period for socialization. A pup kept with other dogs until it is twelve or so weeks old may become too dog-oriented to make a satisfying pet.

Kittens mature more slowly, and the critical period for them is around eight to ten weeks. If you fall in love with an adult cat or dog, however, there's no reason why you shouldn't adopt it, provided it was socialized properly earlier in life, likes people, and is housebroken.

human/animal age ratio

DEAR DR. FOX—The common belief is that the ratio of a dog's to a human's age is 1 to 7. But I once read that the ratio after maturity (two years of age) is 1 to 4. Which is true? Is our ten-year-old dog seventy or fifty-six?—*MRS. H.S.*

DEAR MRS. H.S.—The notion that one dog year is equivalent to seven years of human age is way off the mark. Dogs are sexually mature by nine to eighteen months, equivalent to a teenager. Dogs age at different rates. Large breeds are old by eight to ten years, while others are middle-aged at this time, equivalent to a forty- to fifty-year-old person. Some aren't close to being septuagenarians until they are twelve or fifteen. If your ten-year-old dog is robust and healthy, he's probably equivalent to an active fifty-five-year-old—but some dogs at this age are on their last legs.

1

DEAR DR. FOX—I know that one human year is equal to seven dog years, but how do I figure it for cats or hamsters? Also, I read your book *The Wolf*, and it's excellent—I love animals. I'm eleven years old.—*L.M.*

DEAR L.M.—I'm glad you enjoyed *The Wolf*. Wolves are maligned and need all the friends they can get. It's true that many people think that one human year is equivalent to seven dog years, but that's not totally accurate. Most dogs are in their teens by six months and can be parents when they are one year old. Irrespective of years or time, all animals and humans go through the same stages of development—infant, juvenile, adolescent, adult, middle age, and old age. A hamster can be a parent at three months and is old at four years. It would take a special mathematician to figure out exact human age equivalents.

DOCTORS PRESCRIBE PETS AS MEDICINE

In Millersburg, Ohio, the Castle Nursing Home gave pet dogs to a number of patients who had isolated themselves from human contact. Therapists at the home reported that after these isolated patients began to relate positively to their pets, their relationship to the other patients and personnel improved.

Dr. Boris Levinson, a professor of psychology at Yeshiva University, claims that the differences in mental and physical well-being can be attributed to "an actual chemical change in the brain" that occurs when there is a pleasant interaction between a pet and its owner.

ABOUT DIFFERENT ANIMALS AND BREEDS

Birds

A FEW WORDS ABOUT A FEW BIRDS

Parakeets are the best-selling birds in America and also the least expensive . . . Finches can sing and are colorful, but they like another bird in their cage . . . Cockatiels are extremely affectionate and establish close bonds with their owners . . . Not all parrots speak, and they range in price from $60 to $5,000. The costlier, the rarer. Best to buy parrots bred in captivity because buying those taken from the wild may accelerate their extinction.

---

how to tell sex (canaries)

DEAR DR. FOX—Please, come to my aid. I bought a canary, thinking that it was a male—the pet store said so. After a year and a half, to my disbelief and humiliation, it laid two eggs. I didn't think males laid eggs! Do they?—*J.K.G.*

DEAR J.K.G.—You're not the first canary owner to be surprised with a present of eggs. It happens to be very difficult to distinguish the sex of canaries by looking at their posterior genital apparatus. It's also difficult to tell what sex they are when they're very young. Experts can tell the difference by listening to the young birds when they endeavor to sing.

Only the male canary sings, and it's on the basis of this that breeders and pet stores give buyers a guarantee that the canary is male and therefore will sing. Adult females, incidentally, do not need to be bred to lay eggs, since egg-laying is part of their natural cycle. However, a male, of course, needs to be present for the eggs to be fertile.

how to tell sex (doves)

DEAR DR. FOX—I have a male dove who does nothing but eat, drink, and sleep. He doesn't even fly as much as my female doves. What's wrong with him? Also, how do you tell a female ring-necked dove from a male ring-necked?— D.T.

DEAR D.T.—Doves, like people, have different temperaments, some being easygoing if not lazy, while others are assertive and active. It's difficult to tell the sex of ring-necked doves (also called Barbary doves), since males and females look identical. Males behave differently, however, and that's how you tell who's who. Males have a louder and longer "coo-coo" call and display a bob-up and bob-down bowing movement of the head and neck in front of females. Female doves are less demonstrative; only the boys show off!

how to tell sex (parakeets)

DEAR DR. FOX—I have two parakeets, one green and one blue. I'd like to mate them, but for all I know, they might be two females. How can I tell the male from the female?—T.M.C.

DEAR T.M.C.—You should know, first of all, that parakeets need a special nest box and proper feeding before it's OK to breed them. And you should really read up on the subject. (My book *Understanding Your Pet* will help.)

But you're right, there's no use planning if you don't have a male and a female. A male parakeet has a blue-colored cere—that fleshy little ridge or crescent at the base or top of the bird's beak. In females, it's creamy pink or brown.

longevity

DEAR DR. FOX—My ring-necked dove is about seventeen years old. When I picked her up from the ground, she was hurt and unable to fly. She has been well cared for all these years. People don't believe she's that old. Is her age unusual for a bird?—E.S.

DEAR E.S.—Certain species of birds can live to a ripe old age. Parrots can attain seventy years and more. Doves, pigeons, and laying hens can make it into the late teens and early twenties. Such longevity is not unusual in birds that are well cared for in captivity, but in the wild their natural life expectancies are considerably shorter because of disease, injury, and predators.

most popular bird

DEAR DR. FOX—I would like to buy a bird for companionship. Do you have any recommendations?—A.E.

DEAR A.E.—Budgies—more often called parakeets—are the No. 1 bird in the country, and no wonder why. They're easy to care for, are not overly noisy, are extremely affectionate and responsive, and can be taught all kinds of tricks, from playing dead to shaking hands to mimicking human speech.

TIPS FOR BUDGIE BUYERS

Buy your budgie—or parakeet, if you prefer to call it that—when it is between the ages of six weeks and three months. At that age it's old enough to care for easily and young enough to tame and train. A young bird's forehead has stripes. These gradually recede, and when the bird reaches maturity, its forehead will be completely white or yellow. Male birds are the best talkers. It may be difficult to distinguish sex in a young bird—ask your pet-store dealer for assistance.

Cats

EVER THINK OF A WATCH-CAT?

Despite their serene nature, cats can serve as excellent burglar alarms, because they are so acutely aware of activity in their surroundings. When cats sense intruders, they will react vocally or physically. Often they signal with eyes and ears simultaneously. Perked-up ears and wide-open eyes may signal impending danger.

---

breeds that shed less

DEAR DR. FOX—Are there any breeds or types of cats that shed less than others? Are there any breeds less suitable for being strictly housecats?—CURIOUS

DEAR CURIOUS—All healthy cats shed their coats regularly, old growth being constantly replaced by new growth so they never wear out. The shorter the coat, the less of a problem and the easier it is for you and your cat to groom out loose fur every day.

All cats adapt well to living indoors provided they are raised inside from the start and don't get a taste of the outdoors. Life can be better for the indoor cat if it has a companion cat of about the same age and of the opposite sex, ideally both being neutered.

DEAR DR. FOX—My husband is severely allergic to cats, even though he has been taking weekly shots for years. I know that a person allergic to dogs can tolerate poodles, but is there any breed of cat a person allergic to cats could own? We both love cats and feel so deprived.—J.L.

DEAR J.L.—Some unfortunate people are allergic to just about any kind of animal that has fur and "dander"—microscopic particles of skin debris that get into the air. Some people cope by getting goldfish as pets or nonshedding breeds of dog, such as poodles, Kerry blues, or Bedlington terriers. Siamese cats cause less of a problem for some cat-sensitive people. You might give this a try. Before investing, however, maybe you could borrow a Siamese for a while to see the effect on your husband. A breeder might agree to such an arrangement. If this works out, vacuum the house daily and keep the pet out of the bedroom, study, or lounge room. A dust precipitator or negative ionizer may also help.

VOX VETERINARIA

There's a cat breeder in California who claims to have created, through modern gene-splicing, a cross between a cat and a skunk, which she calls a honey bear. Many reporters have picked up this nonsense as fact and given it credibility. My office at The Humane Society of the United States is tired of replying to people's queries about the origin of these honey bears. They are nothing but regular cats that this woman has bred. No university has done any gene splicing of cats and skunks.

---

how to tell sex

DEAR DR. FOX—Is there any way to distinguish male kittens from female kittens when they are only a few weeks old?—K.H.

DEAR K.H.—Yes, and it's fairly easy once someone has shown you the difference. Beneath the round anal opening, little girl cats have a slitlike orifice, while tiny toms have a more rounded opening in the same position. This causes some confusion, because a tomcat's penis points directly backwards. Just above and on each side of the penis are the testicles, which can be felt even in small kittens.

longevity

DEAR DR. FOX—We have had many pets—snakes, turtles, fish, hamsters, gerbils, rats, guinea pigs, dogs—you name it. But one outlived them all and that is our cat, Minni, who is twenty-four years old and still going strong. Do you know the age of the longest-living cat?—C.W.

DEAR C.W.—To the best of my knowledge, some of the oldest cats have been twenty-eight to thirty-one years of age. The world record for a cat's age is, I believe, thirty-six years! Such ages are indeed remarkable. Cats on the average live into their mid-teens—generally longer than dogs.

DEAR DR. FOX—We believe our cat has reached an age that would qualify her for some kind of record. The best we can figure is that she is close to nineteen years old. This cat has never really been sick and sleeps in the garage at night, still so strong that she gives the impression she will live forever. Can you tell us the average lifespan of a cat? Do you have any details of the oldest living cat of record?—A.W.

DEAR A.W.—I just had lunch with an elderly couple whose cat recently died at the ripe old age of twenty-three. Yours could last longer than that. The average lifespan of cats is considerably less, and less still for those that are allowed to roam free. (Cars and catfights and infectious diseases contracted from sick strays rob a cat of its nine lives.)

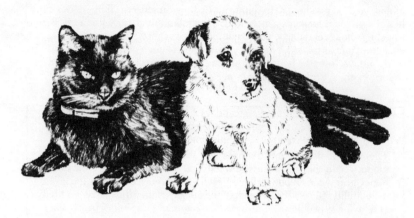

Siamese

DEAR DR. FOX—I have heard that a purebred Siamese cat must have crossed eyes as well as a kink in its tail. Is this true? I'm thinking of buying a Siamese.—*M.R.*

DEAR M.R.—What you describe are undesirable traits in Siamese cats. Unfortunately, we see so many kinky tails and squinty eyes that people are beginning to make them synonymous with purebreds. Inbreeding is the cause of these and even more severe defects that cause sickness and suffering in both cats and dogs. It's best to look for a Siamese cat with big, beautiful eyes and a normal tail.

HAIL THE SACRED CAT!

Cats were part of Egyptian culture as early as 2500 B.C.—depicted in paintings, frescoes, and sculpture. Egyptians used cats to catch rats, but also to hunt, fish, and retrieve wild birds along the Nile river. Later on, cats were revered so much that they became a part of Egyptian's religion, and were represented as a cat-headed goddess named Bastet. One of the reasons the ancient Egyptians believed cats were sacred was that their eyes appear to glow in the dark. The Egyptians worshipped the sun god Ra, and they believed that the cat's eyes magically continued to reflect Ra's rays at night. In truth, the cat's pupil responds rapidly, and at night it dilates to let in as much light as possible.

Dogs

breeds that shed less

DEAR DR. FOX—I recently heard that only the hair of poodles does not affect people who are allergic to dogs' hair. Is this true?—*H.I.D.*

DEAR H.I.D.—Not entirely. Very allergic people can't go near any dog, no matter what the breed. Less sensitive people with pooch allergy seem to be OK with poodles, but the reason is mainly that poodles don't shed and leave their hair all over the place. Other no-shed breeds include the Kerry blue terrier and the schnauzer. For people with mild allergies to pollen, I suggest daily vacuuming when dogs go outdoors and pick up pollen in their coats.

dalmations

DEAR DR. FOX—I would like to buy a dalmation. I just love the way they look. Do you have any advice?—*S.E.*

DEAR S.E.—Dalmations are great dogs if you have plenty of room (or a fire department). They require a lot of exercise. They are bright and playful and make great family dogs. But you must buy only from a responsible breeder. Some dalmations, for instance, are born deaf. And don't buy one from someone who doesn't agree with me that dalmations, being so large, can be (not "are") difficult to handle and should not be owned by an inexperienced person. Make sure you and dalmations are well matched by finding out from the breeder what to expect in the way of temperament.

Dobermans

DEAR DR. FOX—We are planning to retire in the country. The area is somewhat isolated, and we would like to have a dog for companionship and protection. We want a dog that will stand firm, yet not be vicious. I had Dobermans as a child and loved them, but we hear they have nervous temperaments. We would appreciate your opinion.—*B.S.*

DEAR B.S.—If you can find a good Doberman, you will have the kind of dog you desire. Unfortunately, it's difficult to locate good breeders of sound lines of Dobermans and other purebred dogs that have become popular over the years. Pedigree papers don't mean anything any more.

My advice is to find a local breeder and look hard at the temperament of his or her breeding stock. Then have the dog obedience trained. A well-bred, obedience-trained Doberman (please don't have its ears cropped), German shepherd, rottweiler, Airedale, or other large protector-type breed will satisfy your needs. My book *Understanding Your Dog* gives details on how to choose a good pup from the litter.

THE NATURAL HISTORY OF DOGS

The origin of the domestic dog is an enigma and controversial. Many experts believe that humans domesticated the dog as a hunting partner, but there's an equal amount of evidence to disprove this. Dr. Barbara Lawrence of Harvard University found dog remains in North America that were dated 8400 B.C., which at least indicates that the dog was one of the very earliest of humankind's animals. Later, dogs were probably bred for selective abilities, such as hunting, working, etc.

German shepherds

DEAR DR. FOX—I am not sure if my dog is a German shepherd or not. A friend told me that the roof of a German shepherd's mouth is black. Is this true? Also, when should their ears start standing up? (My dog is five months old.) Is it common for some German shepherds to get darker gradually as they get older? My dog started out tan, but now he's more black.—*K.J.*

DEAR *K.J.*—Many breeds of dog have black or pink tongues, roofs of mouth, etc., and it doesn't mean a thing. The only way to be 100 percent sure that your dog's a German shepherd is to know who his parents were. Not all purebred shepherds have upstanding ears, but they should be pointed and "wolfish," even if they flop a little. Shepherd pups, like many other breeds, change color after they shed their puppy coats and grow adult ones. This new coat may again vary in color and texture from season to season.

DEAR DR. FOX—I have two unrelated German shepherds, and one of them has trouble keeping weight on, although he eats more than the other one; at times you can even see his rib cage. I've been to the vet often, and it always seems that he has worms. Would worms affect his weight gain, and if so, why doesn't it affect the other shepherd?—*B.B.*

DEAR *B.B.*—What you are seeing are genetic or constitutional differences in your two shepherds. One has a greater resistance to hookworms and roundworms than the other. Temperament is often linked with susceptibility to stress and disease. Shy, timid, hyperactive, and overreactive dogs, for example, have been shown to be much more susceptible to traumatic injuries and certain infections. This is why it is so important for breeders to select for sound, stable temperaments and the overall health and well-being of dogs—not just for the owner's convenience.

Labradors

DEAR DR. FOX—I would like to get a good short-haired dog, such as a Labrador retriever. While researching this breed I found that they may bark incessantly at noises. I am not fond of this trait. Can the barking be reduced by having this breed fixed?—*J.E.*

DEAR *J.E.*—A good Labrador is a quiet, easygoing dog with a very stable temperament and thus is most likely to be a neurotic barker. But to get a wholesome Lab, you must find a reputable breeder of Labradors and discuss your concern with him or her. Are they noisy and hyperactive or fairly quiet and obedient? Keep looking till you find what you want. Then raise your pup right—which means obedience school for both of you.

MODEL DOG: THE MALAMUTE

Have a lot of space in your backyard? Then consider the malamute as a pet. This wonder dog, hailing from Alaska, is one of the strongest of dogs, yet is a small eater for its large size. And despite movie stereotypes of them as vicious killers, malamutes are friendly by nature and so gentle that the Eskimos used them as babysitters.

Samoyeds

DEAR DR. FOX—We have inherited a six-year-old Samoa. Is she too old to breed? If not, where can we find other dogs of her kind? Can you tell me anything of the history of the Samoa breed?—*V.T.*

DEAR V.T.—There are dingolike village dogs that come from the islands of Samoa, but I doubt you have one of these, since they are quite rare. My bet is your dog is white, fluffy, and bouncy and has pointed ears and a curly tail. If this is so, then you have a *Samoyed*, and the local library should have books on this breed. These are great little dogs once used for draft work in the cold Arctic. Although they are an active working breed, they generally adapt quite well to the more sedentary existence of a household pooch.

DO YOU KNOW YOUR TOP DOGS?

Here's a quiz all dog-lovers will enjoy. Do you know the names of the dogs belonging to the following U.S. presidents? (1) John Kennedy; (2) Franklin D. Roosevelt; (3) Dwight Eisenhower; (4) Richard Nixon; (5) Gerald Ford.*

---

small dogs

DEAR DR. FOX—I am anxious to adopt a small dog like a Yorkshire or poodle. However, I heard that a statistical study showed a connection between small dogs and multiple sclerosis. Is this a real danger?—D.B.

DEAR D.B.—There is no connection between people having multiple sclerosis and possessing small dogs. However, there is a connection—still extremely tentative—between the occurrence of multiple sclerosis in people and dogs who contract distemper. The wise step, therefore, is to have one's dog vaccinated against distemper and given an annual booster vaccination as well. There are several diseases that we can contract from cats and dogs, but this number of diseases is insignificant compared with the number of diseases that we can pick up from other human beings. I therefore feel that being afraid of animals because they might make one sick is an unhealthy zoophobia.

DEAR DR. FOX—I would like some information on teacup- or pocket-sized dogs, since I am interested in getting one. Any advice?—R.J.D.

DEAR R.J.D.—Teacup-sized dogs are dwarf variations of toy breeds, the most prevalent (yet still relatively rare) being the "teacup" poodle. It is true that these creatures only weigh a few ounces, but their survival rate is extremely low.

You may be able to obtain one from a breeder of toy poodles, but since they occur so rarely it may take a lot of time and effort to find one. Even though they are cute, I personally would not encourage you to purchase one because of their poor viability and short life expectancy.

Staffordshire terriers

DEAR DR. FOX—Two days after buying Popsie, a female Staffordshire terrier, another Staffordshire terrier attacked two sisters walking home from the local market, sending the younger girl to the hospital. Ten days later another attack by the same breed occurred in our area against an eight-year-old.

---

*Answers: (1) Pushinka (2) Fala (3) Heidi (4) Checkers (5) Liberty.

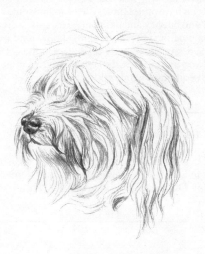

We smack Popsie when she bites and say "No!" She seldom tries any more, but how can we prevent such a tragedy?—*C.R.*

DEAR C.R.—Staffordshire pit-bull terriers have been ruined in this country by many breeders. They have become popular and are bred for fighting (even though pit-bull fights are illegal). Recently, I've heard of several people throughout the country who have been torn up by these dogs, as have dozens of people's pets.

I would not own one unless it came from a good kennel in the United States or the United Kingdom (from Staffordshire), one where the dogs are not bred to be fighters. And I would urge that city ordinances be passed either to prohibit ownership of pit bulls or to insist on owners having at least $50,000 liability insurance. The chance of a mangled child isn't worth keeping such aggressive animals.

DOGS FOR ALL SEASONS

Do you know which dog has no bark but yodels? . . . Which dog is used to retrieve water ducks? . . . Can you name the dog used to hunt badgers? . . . Which dog was owned exclusively by the Japanese Imperial Family? . . . Which dog uses its front paws for bull-baiting?*

Welsh corgis

DEAR DR. FOX—When I bought our dog, I was told it was a Welsh corgi. No one has ever heard of this breed. Have you? I have looked in all my animal books,

*Answers: Basenji, Irish water spaniel, dachshund (also called badger dog), Akita, boxer.

but no luck. He is reddish-blond and long-haired, with a small build, and is very alert.—*M.A.M.*

DEAR *M.A.M.*—Welsh corgis are indeed reddish-blond, with upright ears and a short coat. You can find pictures of this breed in a number of books on purebred dogs: Checks your local library or pet store. Welsh corgis are the favorite of the Queen of England. In Wales, these short, stocky dogs are used for driving cattle. They are active, attentive, and very trainable pets who make great companions for someone who likes a spunky dog.

wolf-dogs

DEAR DR. FOX—I have seen an advertisement selling half-dog, half-wolf pups and am thinking of buying one. Do they need special care?—*S.R.*

DEAR *S.R.*—Don't buy! Some "wogs" (wolf-dog hybrids) have reliable temperaments, but many grow up to be unstable—not savage (wolves aren't savage), but extremely fearful, just like wolves. They don't adapt well to captivity and take experienced handling.

I am opposed to the breeding of such mixed-up mixtures. Read my *Soul of the Wolf* book for the kinds of difficulties you can encounter having a wolf or a "wog" as a pet. If you love wolves, join a conservation society, and if you want a good dog, adopt a mutt—the best of breeds—from your local humane society.

DEAR DR. FOX—We are planning to buy a wolf-dog. Please advise about shots and training and the best age to buy one.—*D.K.*

DEAR *D.K.*—Forget it, please! Wolf-dogs can be very beautiful, and they certainly have an air of mystery and give you a sense of pride and excitement at the thought of owning one. But many, especially those with a lot of wolf blood, grow up to be extremely fearful and unstable animals. I do not advise people to own such hybrids. Let wolves be wolves and dogs be dogs—the two don't mix, and it's sheer selfish indulgence to propagate such mixed-up misfits. Sure, a few turn out OK, but the really wolfish ones don't. Why not get a wolfish-looking dog instead, like a German shepherd or Belgian sheepdog?

Fish

most popular pet

DEAR DR. FOX—Can you tell me which is the most popular household pet? My friend and I have a bet. She says it's cats and I say it's dogs.—*G.T.*

DEAR *G.T.*—Believe it or not, it's fish! Twenty million people are now into fish as a hobby, making it the second most popular hobby in the country. (Photography is first.)

Why? Fish don't take much care; they're beautiful, varied, and inexpensive. The initial investment is small—a ten-gallon aquarium with accessories can cost less than $35 to $40 and a fishbowl adds a decorative touch to any room. Convinced?

Frogs

DEAR DR. FOX—I have two pet tree frogs who stay in a terrarium in my room. All my friends say frogs are disgusting, and their mothers would never let them have one in the house. What is so disgusting about frogs?—*N.F.*

QUESTIONS AND ANSWERS ABOUT FISH

Q: Who first domesticated fish?
A: The Chinese, about a thousand years ago. They developed the common goldfish from carp.
Q: Are goldfish always gold?
A: No. They are pink, red, and even silver.
Q: What's the best fish for a beginner's aquarium?
A: You guessed it—that same goldfish we're talking about. Goldfish are hardy and live long lives.

DEAR N.F.—Hurrah for your good sense, because I don't think there's anything disgusting about frogs either. It is sad how people judge both animals and humans by their color or stripes. Some folks think of frogs as slimy and untouchable, but I think they are exquisite jewels of creation. However, some very pretty frogs do produce a poison that hunters use on their arrow tips in order to kill prey quickly. Don't worry, however, because you won't find the poisonous kind in your pet store.

Geese

DEAR DR. FOX—We would like your opinion on the choice of a pair of domesticated geese as pets for a suburban yard. We have heard that they make good watch animals and family pets. Is this true? However, we do not want pets which will make so much noise that they become a neighborhood nuisance. Also, are there any diseases that might be transmitted by geese?—R.M.
DEAR R.M.—Great idea! Geese are most companionable and very territorial creatures, so they make good pets and excellent "watch geese." But be sure to check about local ordinances. In many cities and townships there are strict laws that prevent one from owning farm animals, and yes, there are some diseases that geese can transmit to people, salmonella (food poisoning) being one of the most common. However, if you buy healthy birds and keep them healthy, you should have no problems except for their honking. Geese can honk and honk—and there's always one neighbor who will complain about noise, even the beautiful sounds of geese. You had better be aware of this possibility before making a goose of yourself in the neighborhood.

Gerbils, Guinea Pigs, Hamsters, and Mice

best choice for child

DEAR DR. FOX—I am thinking of getting my five-year-old son either a hamster, a gerbil, or a guinea pig. Which one of these will be the easiest to care for? We will keep this pet in the house, so I am also wondering about odor. How often will the pet's pen have to be cleaned?—MRS. G.S.

DEAR MRS. G.S.—I recommend the gerbil for your son. Hamsters can be nippy and are a bit smelly, while guinea pigs require experienced handling. Gerbils are one of the most popular of cage pets, and one reason is that they are extremely clean. They were originally desert animals and don't require much liquid or produce much urine. Gerbils are also friendly and gentle and like to be with other gerbils; they have to grow up together, though, because putting strange mature adults into a cage will result in battles.

companion animals (hamsters)

DEAR DR. FOX—Whenever I look into my hamster's cage she gives me a very lonely look. Maybe it's my imagination, but should I get another hamster to keep her company? If so, should I get another female or a male? My friend says that if I put a male into the cage, my hamster will fight with him. How do I go about mating her? Or isn't it advisable?—R.H.

DEAR R.H.—It's your imagination. Hamsters, like many nocturnal animals, have large "appealing" eyes, and it's easy to read emotion into them. Lonely your hamster is not! Hamsters actually prefer to live a solitary life once they are weaned. Your friend is right: put another hamster in your hamster's cage, and whammo—chances are there will be trouble. If you want to get another and hope for them to mate, keep it in a separate cage and let the two hamsters interact occasionally on neutral territory—in a large "play box" or some other safe container.

how to tell sex (gerbils)

DEAR DR. FOX—I would like to know how can I tell a male gerbil from a female gerbil.—J.A.

DEAR J.A.—As with a guinea pig, a mouse, or a young hamster, you "sex" (tell the sex of) a gerbil by holding it in one hand with its tummy facing toward you, and then gently squeezing it and looking toward the hind end. If it's a male, you will see a little bulge on each side of the scrotum where the testicles are. Don't squeeze too hard, of course. With very young animals the testes have not descended, and you will have difficulty sexing them. The reason why sexing rodents is so difficult is that the genital apparatus in both males and females tends to stick out behind in the same position. With a Q-tip, however, you might be able to

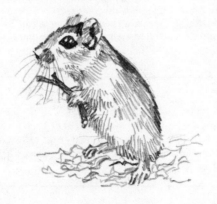

make a gentle investigation and see the difference between a little boy gerbil and a little girl gerbil.

GERBILS ARE GROUPIES

Gerbils are desert animals and don't need much water, so their cages don't need as much cleaning out as those of rats and mice. Consequently, they are relatively odor-free. This, coupled with their docility, makes gerbils excellent pets for youngsters. They like to live in family groups, are very active and enjoy a running wheel in their cage. The more often they are handled, the better pets they will be.

---

longevity (gerbils)

DEAR DR. FOX—Is it true that gerbils only live from nine months to three years? And if so, is three years an old age for them? Because I've had a gerbil for *five* years and I got him when he was one, which would make him six. Right now he can't stand up straight, his tail is crooked, he eats with his eyes closed, and when I put my hand in his cage he doesn't wake up because he doesn't know I'm there. Is he suffering?—C.F.

DEAR C.F.—Six years is surely close to, if not the world record for a gerbil. Congratulations to both of you. Gerbils do tend, like many other animals, to eat with their eyes closed. It surely is a sign of aging when your pet is slow to waken from deep sleep. So long as he's eating well and is still grooming himself, there's no need to consider putting him to sleep. Being old doesn't necessarily mean that a creature is suffering and should be euthanised.

longevity (guinea pigs)

DEAR DR. FOX—I read in a book about guinea pigs that the male guinea pig lives longer than the female. Why is this?—L.M.

DEAR L.M.—Guinea pigs have a lifespan of six to eight years, and according to the references that I have checked, there's no significant difference in the life-span of males (boars) and females (sows). As with most mammals, however, there is a tendency for the males to have a slightly shorter life expectancy. For a variety of reasons, males tend to be the "weaker sex," so to speak. Guinea pigs are social, herd-living creatures, so it is probably wrong to keep one alone and apart from its own kind.

HEALTH REMINDER

Gerbils, hamsters, and mice make excellent first pets for children aged five or six. But it is wiser not to keep the animal's cage in the child's bedroom. It is not very common, but some children can be allergic to the dust particles that come from the cage or bark.

Horses

longevity

DEAR DR. FOX—Your advice is great, but even greater is your genuine love for animals. To have animals' love is almost as great as having the love of people. As you can guess, I am a pet owner. I'm really writing to ask, how old is the oldest horse you've heard of? Is it possible to get our horse in the *Guinness Book of World Records?* She is thirty-four or thirty-five years old and in perfect health. I think it's all the good care and love we gave her that got her this far. Do you agree? Also, how do you calculate an animal's age in human years?—D.C.

DEAR D.C.—Having a horse that is around thirty-five years old is a wonderful achievement for both horse and owner. Yes, it does take good care and love to keep a horse alive and well that long. Most horses, even thoroughbreds, are finished much, much earlier. However, thirty-five is no world record, since there are some retired workhorses and even Welsh pit-ponies that push into the forties before they push up the daisies. Other pets, such as parrots and turtles, will even outlive their owners. There's no easy scale of equivalents to match an animal's age with that of a human being. Age periods or stages are better indicators—infant, juvenile, adolescent, adult, middle-aged, and old, and on the basis of these stages one can make some approximation.

Rabbits

good environment

DEAR DR. FOX—I strongly disagree with you regarding rabbits being good house pets. Rabbits chew electrical cords, shoes, wood, and paperboard walls. Outside, they chew plant leaves, bark, and trunks of plants, dig holes under fences, and, if they're not too large, slip under links of chain-link fences. Otherwise yes—they are intelligent, beautiful, playful, quiet creatures and can easily be housebroken. But they love to run and play outside, and to keep them in a cage seems sinful. In all fairness to both rabbits and prospective owners, you should mention these facts.—B.A.

DEAR B.A.—Thank you for mentioning that no pet is perfect and that we must understand their ways and appropriately cater to their wants. Regarding rabbits, outdoors or indoors, either place must be made safe. A good place for a rabbit is a well-screened-in porch with a double door. But while you're protecting your rabbit from its instincts you must, at the same time, provide satisfaction for its instincts. As pet birds must fly—but not into the fire or a cat's jaws—so rabbits must chew—not electrical cords, but carrots and hunks of wood. And dig they must—not in the garden or your best rug, but in an earth- or paper-filled box. Withal, rabbits make great pets!

longevity

DEAR DR. FOX—When our neighbors brought over a baby cottontail rabbit that the cats had got at, I took her in and nursed her back to health. She has lived with me for seven months. I checked the ASPCA, and they said rabbits live in the wild for only six months. I think she would live longer and be better off with me than to let her live only six months in the wild. Don't you agree?—M.C.

DEAR M.C.—Cottontail rabbits are difficult to raise. Only too often, in spite of the best care, they fade away. The older they are, the better their chances of

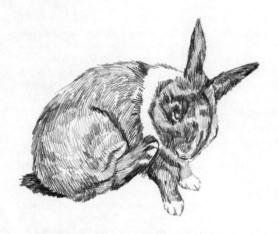

survival seem to be. Since your rabbit is now tame and presumably has no fear of humans, you obviously shouldn't set her free. Rabbits live many years in the wild provided a predator doesn't get them. The ASPCA was just giving you their average lifespan. Life in the wild is hard. That's why bunnies have so many babies—only a few survive.

A PUREBRED ANIMAL OR A "MUTT"?

adopting from a shelter

DEAR DR. FOX—You're always recommending that people adopt mongrel dogs and cats from the animal shelter. But isn't it true that these animals are rejects and are frequently sick?—A.R.

DEAR A.R.—Some of the best pets come from adoption centers such as the local humane society. I do not agree that adopted pets have greater medical requirements than purebred dogs from a breeder. All need vaccinations and checking for worms. The better humane societies have sufficient space to quarantine newcomers and sick animals, so infectious diseases—with the exception perhaps of kennel cough—can be controlled. You are likely to have *more* problems with some purebred dogs, since mongrels are generally more resistant to disease and have fewer inherited and congenital defects and other problems arising from inbreeding.

responsible breeders

DEAR DR. FOX—It seems to me from reading your column over the years that you are prejudiced against purebred dogs and favor mongrels. Why do you have an axe to grind? I love my purebred poodle, and if I were buying another dog, it would be the same—a purebred poodle.—A.L.

DEAR A.L.—I do have an axe to grind, but it's not against purebreds so much as about their well-being and future. Many breeds, especially more popular ones such as the Doberman, German shepherd, border collie, and, yes—poodle—are riddled with genetic (inherited) defects in structure, physiology, and temperament. Unethical breeders and large commercial "puppy mills" are helping to ruin the breeds so that purebreds are an endangered species. There is no quality control. People need educating. So A.L., and readers, don't buy without first looking at the parents and seeing if they are healthy and of a good disposition. Also, buy only from a responsible breeder. If you're going to buy blindly, then I advise mutts. They're healthier and don't suffer from inbreeding, which is at the root of most disorders in purebred dogs.

DEAR DR. FOX—I belong to a purebred-dog club and many of the members are angry at you for saying publicly that purebred dogs have many genetic problems. So who is right?—*A.D.*

DEAR A.D.—Because of my critical stance, many dog clubs think I'm against *all* purebred dogs and breeders, and that they're all against me. Not true! There are also breeders who want me to tell all, since the more informed people are before they buy a dog, the more they will demand genetically sound animals. Good breeders want that, since the dog world can well do without puppy mills and unethical quick-buck breeders who couldn't care less about breed quality.

PET SHOPPING HAZARD

When buying a purebred animal, it's essential to get a health guarantee as well as a certificate of parentage. Inbreeding has, unfortunately, produced a number of genetic problems. Even though these problems generally develop late in the life of a purebred, a responsible and honest breeder will work out some acceptable arrangement with a purchaser. But a health guarantee in hand is a safety measure.

ENCOUNTERS WITH WILD ANIMALS

DO NOT TOUCH!

Children should not handle any wild baby animal that they find. Its parents may later reject it because they smell your child's odor on it.

Also, a wild skunk, fox cub, or other animal may be rabid.

In many states it is mandatory to have a permit to own any wild animal, young or mature.

---

opossums

DEAR DR. FOX—Every evening a 'possum comes up to our porch to eat the food we put out for our cat. At first, I was frightened and screamed until it ran off. Now I consider the animal a kind of pet. He comes and eats each evening. Can I make a real pet of him?—*L.T.*

DEAR L.T.—'Possums are odd-looking critters if you're not used to them; no wonder you screamed when you first saw it. Other people might have attacked it. Likewise, you look odd to a 'possum, and so it might react like a person—fearfully or aggressively—until it gets used to you. Both of you should keep a respectful distance, because either of you could misinterpret the other's intentions and get bitten or scared away for good, as the case may be. Please follow the basic rule—don't make a pet of a wild animal. Touch not, except with gentle voice and appreciative eyes.

WILDLIFE WARNING

With summer approaching, your family will be moving outdoors and quite possibly meeting up with raccoons, skunks, foxes, and 'possums, among others. Some words of warning: cute as these creatures may be, they do not make good pets and may be rabid. When those animals achieve maturity, they can and often do turn unpredictably on the hand that feeds them. They aren't vicious—more likely confused and misunderstood.

---

wolves

DEAR DR. FOX—We have had several incidents with a wolf. This wolf is about six inches taller than our German shepherd. It started when we kept finding our dog's dish in the middle of the pasture. Then, finally, we saw the wolf. It came through the pasture within fifty feet of our trailer. My husband opened the door, and the wolf just stood there and looked at him. My husband shot it with birdshot, and it ran off.

We thought that this was the end, but the wolf has been coming back. Recently, when I came across him, he kept growling and snarling at me. I'm sure that if our dog hadn't been with me, the wolf would have attacked me. How should we handle this when the wolf comes back?—MRS. T.M.

DEAR MRS. T.M.—First, let me say that I believe you did not see a wolf but a large coyote-dog hybrid. In my experience with wolves and from accounts of wolves in the wild, they are extremely shy of humans. No wolf, except perhaps a rabid one, is going to stand and look at you and growl. But why did your husband shoot at it? The fact that the animal carried the dog's dish into the middle of the pasture is no reason for attempting to injure or kill it.

Remember that a domestic animal is more likely to attack a human being than a wild one that has less fear of humans. My suspicion is, therefore, that if this is not a rabid wild animal, it is in fact, tame. So you will have to be careful and keep your dog with you whenever possible.

PART ONE

GOOD HEALTH AND PROPER CARE

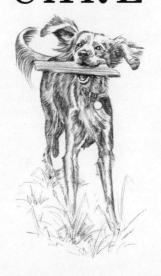

I n the wild, animals take care of themselves; nature gives them the resources and opportunity to satisfy their basic needs. With our domesticated animal companions, we take on the role of Mother Nature, and for them to enjoy good health we must know what the best environment is for them, as well as provide the right food, exercise, and general care. The first part of this book deals with these responsibilities, and more.

In nature, animals get injured and fall sick, and so they frequently live much shorter lives than the animals we keep as companions. We can do a great deal to help our pets enjoy healthier, longer lives, free from many of the burdens of disease and physical suffering. Indeed, some pets such as toy poodles and delicate Persian cats could never exist in the wild, as they need so much extra care and attention. In Part 1 you will learn to recognize many common pet ailments and how to apply the basic principles of preventive medicine and health-care maintenance.

Nature can seem cruel to animals when we discover how many young ones are born each year that do not survive. This is part of nature's economy and wisdom—natural population control. Because our pets are protected from these regulatory forces, pet overpopulation has become a serious problem. Consequently, the social as well as the health benefits of neutering pets will be discussed, along with proper care when pets do become parents.

Good health comes from proper care and understanding, and this covers a large territory. With good care your pet will enjoy a healthy and long life and will need to see the animal doctor only in times of emergency and for routine health-care maintenance. To be taken to its doctor when it needs to go is one of your pet's basic rights, and one of the "commandments" of responsible pet ownership, which I spell out in full below.

THE TEN COMMANDMENTS OF PET OWNERSHIP

1. All companion animals should be treated humanely—with patience, compassion, and understanding.
2. All pets have the right to have certain basic needs satisfied—regular exercise, play, companionship, and grooming. They also have the right to a clean and quiet place to live, rest, eat, and sleep.
3. All pets have the right to receive fresh water and a complete and balanced diet each day. They all have the right to receive proper veterinary treatment if they are ill.
4. Like people, all pets have the right to fulfill their lives within the social constraints of responsible ownership, which may include the curtailment of certain needs and instincts—such as the need to roam free or the instinct to breed—for the ultimate benefit of the animal, of society, and of the environment.
5. A caring owner (or, more accurately, custodian or guardian) understands animals' needs and provides those conditions most conducive to ensuring their physical and psychological well-being.
6. No person has the right to exploit any animal inhumanely for profit, pleasure, or other selfish purpose, without regard for the animal's intrinsic worth, interests, and needs.
7. Understanding owners respect and appreciate animals for themselves, independent of personal bias and selfish wants. Such owners attend and listen to animals, and even when they appear to misbehave endeavor to ascertain what the animals need or are trying to communicate. Animals should not be overindulged ("humanized") to the detriment of their physical or psychological well-being.
8. No owner should physically or psychologically abuse, neglect, or abandon an animal. The ultimate responsibility is to ensure that when the time comes, the pet will die painlessly and with dignity, if euthanasia is required.
9. Before obtaining pets or giving them to other people, all people have the obligation to the animals to assure that they will live in a home that will best satisfy their basic needs and also that their basic rights will be recognized and upheld at all times.
10. All pet owners and those who care for animals have the right and responsibility to share with others, especially children, the ten commandments of pet ownership, and to intercede in defense of any animal when its rights are violated and when it is being treated inhumanely, either through intent or indifference (neglect). The same principles hold true for the custodianship of laboratory, farm, and zoo animals—indeed, all creatures under our dominion, including the wild creatures of the land, skies, and water of our planet.

If you follow these commandments, both you and your pet will enjoy enormous benefits from your life together. These benefits will also strengthen our connection with the animal kingdom, putting love and understanding into our dominion over other creatures where power alone has ruled for too long.

1

Giving
Your Pet a Good Home

UNCOMMON PETS AND OTHERS

chameleons

DEAR DR. FOX—I recently purchased two chameleons at a pet store. Could you please tell me how fast they grow and how large they can get? Also—how often should I feed them? I give them each one live meal worm a day.—*B.L.G.*

DEAR B.L.G.—Your chameleons will probably enjoy a branch to climb on, a plant pot laid on its side to hide in, and a thick layer of sand on the aquarium floor. Given adequate food, and that means as much as they will eat, chameleons grow rapidly. They won't grow well or eat sufficiently if the room they are in gets cold overnight. Avoid temperatures below 65 degrees F. Some chameleons grow up to a foot in length. I advise you to put several meal worms and crickets in the tank and see how many they eat. One meal worm a day isn't enough.

chinchillas

DEAR DR. FOX—I'm planning on buying a chinchilla. Can I keep it in a 19½-by-10-inch aquarium that is 11 inches tall?—*T.R.H.*

DEAR T.R.H.—Chinchillas grow to be quite large, and your aquarium will be too small for it. They need a nest box lined with shredded paper or a tray to bury themselves in. Others enjoy a sandbox to dust-bathe in. The nest box should be about one square foot, opening onto a living area of about one foot by three feet, lined with wood shavings.

Then you give the chinchilla food and water and a stump of wood or piece of

25

boiled beef shank to chew and keep its teeth trim. Instead of wood shavings, you can put a thick wire mesh "rug" on the "living room" floor, with a pan underneath to collect droppings. You can also check your library for a good book on chinchilla care.

doves

DEAR DR. FOX—My husband is a magician, and three months ago we purchased a dove from a magic store. Our problem is that we can't find any books on the care of doves at home. We need to know about their bathing, feeding, and exercise. We take her out of her cage at least once a day, but she can't fly more than two feet without falling.—A.Z.

DEAR A.Z.—Your dove should have a perch, a nest box, a container of grit, cuttlebone (for calcium), and a varied diet of good quality birdseed, toasted whole-wheat bread, and any fresh greens and fruit she may take to. Doves enjoy dry and wet baths, so fix up a shallow pan of water and one of fine sand or powdered clay. Don't force her—she'll bathe when and if she so desires. She may not be much of a flyer because she has had so little experience, and she may be overweight. I hope your husband's magic will not jeopardize her well-being.

frogs

DEAR DR. FOX—We have a pool in our backyard, and every fall we drain half the water and cover the pool. A young frog has been living in our pool about a month. We have become greatly attached to Kermit and are wondering how we can keep him after we drain the pool.—K.V.

DEAR K.V.—So long as your frog has some way of being able to hop or crawl in and out of your pool when it is half full, then all should be well. Some frogs will drown if kept in water all the time; they need to rest on land and find food. Water is primarily a place to escape or hide from predators on land, and, of course, it is where they court and spawn in the early spring. Why don't you allow Kermit the privilege of leaving—just as he came—on his own?

hermit crabs

DEAR DR. FOX—I was recently given two hermit crabs, and I'm frantic to find out what to feed them and what kind of an environment to make for them. I've gone to the library, but I can't seem to find anything on their likes, dislikes, food, or habitat.—S.D.

DEAR S.D.—Prepare yourself for heartbreak—nearly all hermit crabs soon die in captivity. These creatures need fresh shells when they grow and sea water to reproduce in. While they can live for a while on canned pet food and high-protein table scraps, life in captivity is far from ideal. Can't you just return them to the sea, where they belong?

DEAR DR. FOX—I have two hermit crabs, and one morning I awoke to find Boston in Snapper's shell and Snapper in Boston's shell. What should I do?—L.V.

DEAR L.V.—What Boston and Snapper are doing is quite abnormal. When hermit crabs get to a certain size, they have to find themselves a dead snail's shell to crawl into, since their shell gets too tight. Hermit-crab keepers should rise up and protest the sale of these creatures, whose spirit belongs to the ocean. If you can't put yours back where they came from, please get them some snail shells bigger than those they're now occupying.

DEAR DR. FOX—I have an eight-foot common boa constrictor and am at a loss to find any literature on a boa of her size. If you could suggest a book or advise me yourself, I would be most grateful. I need to know about care and feeding, dangers, etc.—*J.R.*

DEAR *J.R.*—Feeding can be a major problem. Some snakes must be force-fed. Others do fine but need live prey (mice, rats, chickens), which is not pleasing for some people. One danger is that the snake may get lost in any cracks and crevices in the room. Remember—the bigger the constrictor, the bigger the squeeze. There are many books on the care of reptiles, and regardless of how big your boa is, a standard text will suffice. Try your local library or the humane society in your area for useful leads.

DEAR DR. FOX—Twenty-six years ago my husband rescued a turtle from the middle of the street. The turtle lives in our basement. We named him Pierre and pampered him. My husband dug worms for him, but he also loves bread, hamburger, and especially bananas and lettuce. We're selling our home and moving to an apartment in a retirement center that has spacious and wooded grounds. Would he survive there?—*MRS. P.O.*

DEAR *MRS. P.O.*—I think your turtle will probably do well in the grounds of your retirement center—if you decide not to keep him inside. Make sure he is in good condition before you release him. He should not feel light and hollow, but heavy—a sign that he has a good store of fat. Then let him go (with a prayer) around mid-April, when there will be plenty of vegetation for him to eat and perhaps even a mate somewhere in the grounds. It's about time he got back to his natural habitat.

DEAR DR. FOX—My son has two box turtles that we keep outside. How do we determine their sex, what they like to eat, any unusual wants, etc?—*A.D.*

DEAR *A.D.*—Box turtles are land turtles. They like an occasional bath and enjoy a habitat that you can set up, including some earth or sand, vegetation (grass), logs, etc. Males have a slightly indented or scooped-out underside on their shells.

Turtles enjoy a variety of fruits and vegetables, earthworms, lean hamburger, and even chopped hardboiled eggs. They also like to bask in the sun. In winter, if not kept warm, they will busy themselves in leaves and hay and go into a state of suspended animation. They should not be allowed to hibernate if they have not been eating well and don't feel heavy and fat to you. I am opposed to people taking turtles from the wild and keeping them as pets. If they don't start to eat after a week in captivity, return them to where they were found or they will probably die.

DEAR DR. FOX—I have a small turtle named Herbie. One Sunday morning I found him floating on his back, but he still was moving. My dad put him in the bathroom sink with a little warm water. But since we put him back in his bowl he stays in the same place. Is it true that turtles hibernate in the winter, or could Herbie be dead?—*K.B.*

DEAR *K.B.*—Most pet turtles come from warm, tropical climates and don't bury into the mud to hibernate, so probably Herbie is dead. However, cold will slow turtles down. Some reptiles and amphibians can be frozen and will thaw out

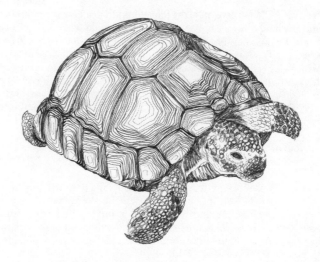

and recover. Most likely, your Herbie developed an infection, possibly aggravated by a nutritional deficiency, since turtles in captivity don't receive the right diet. I do hope Herbie wasn't a land turtle or tortoise. I've heard of people keeping them in aquariums, where they soon drown.

Water turtles or terrapins like to get out of the water frequently to bask in the sun, so a rock or a floating raft is a must. Better luck next time. Keep your turtle warm (65 to 75 degrees F room temperature) and on a complete and balanced diet.

ENVIRONMENT: THE RIGHT STUFF

birdhouses

DEAR DR. FOX—I want to share this experience with other bird-lovers so they won't be disappointed as we were. We purchased a twenty-four-apartment birdhouse, thinking we were going to have a garden of Eden. Little did we realize that if there is one family in the birdhouse, there won't be another at the same time. Some birds sat on a wire watching and watching, but they wouldn't build a nest. I guess they feared for their babies. Was I right?—MRS. P.W.

DEAR MRS. P.W.—You meant well, but you learned that birds have different dwelling habits than people. No—there isn't much point in buying a multiple-tier "high-rise" birdhouse. Birds are territorial, and few would allow other pairs to share their high-rise block, even if there were twenty-three other apartments vacant.

cages (guinea pigs)

DEAR DR. FOX—I'm very busy looking after our family's first guinea pig. The how-to book I bought states that wet behinds are a no-no. I keep my guinea

---

MAKE YOUR CAT A "TREE HOUSE"

Here's an easy-to-make project that will delight your feline. Get a real tree branch—the sturdier the better—and put it in a pot of soil with a little grass. Your cat will love climbing it in your house and will enjoy nibbling the grass too. Both the exercise and the grass are healthful for cats.

---

pig in a large cage on hay. The droppings are supposed to fall through the wire floor onto cedar chips on the tray underneath. However, my little friend always has a wet behind and his white coat is stained yellow. He lets me wash the offending end, but I can't get the stains out. Is there any cure for a wet behind?—*B.H.*

DEAR B.H.—You're talking about one of the most common problems of guinea-pig care. Hay is not the most absorbent of materials and is best used as nesting and play material for cage pets. A wire mesh floor can be quite irritating to a guinea pig's feet, and if the mesh is wide, it can lead to foot injuries—even to broken limbs. I advise you to keep the animal on wood shavings, with a corner box full of hay. Shredded newspaper is a good alternative. The floor should be solid wood; marine plywood is ideal, and it should be scrubbed clean once a week. Clean the cage out daily, and put in fresh litter every day. Use a dropper bottle rather than a water bowl, too, since the latter will spill and wet both the guinea pig and its litter.

cages (hamsters)

DEAR DR. FOX—My hamster keeps getting out of his cage, usually at night. I'm afraid that one of my two cats will eat him or scare him to death. What can I do?—*S.S.*

DEAR S.S.—I suggest you switch from a cage to a glass or plastic fish-tank, all of which are "hamster-proof." Hamsters are well-known escape artists. The reason your pet tries to get out at night is that hamsters are nocturnal creatures who like to play when others like to sleep.

DEAR DR. FOX—I breed teddy-bear hamsters, and I'd like to know where I can get hamster cages cheap.—*C.H.*

DEAR C.H.—First, be well advised and forget about buying cheap cages for your teddy-bear hamsters. Such cages aren't always escape-proof and, if not well built , could be chewed through in no time. A small plastic shoebox-size aquarium is ideal and not too costly.

DEAR DR. FOX—I am an eleven-year-old who loves hamsters and your column. I put my hamster into an aquarium cage with a playhouse, but he climbed on top of the playhouse and got out. Now I've put in a plastic play log instead, but all Chester does is pace up and down and try to climb up my arm to get out. What can I do to make him happier?—*L.M.*

DEAR L.M.—If you don't clip and save my column, give it to Chester to play with. Hamsters love shredding paper and building nests. Buy him an exercise wheel, too; active hamsters like to go for a spin and some get quite addicted. Hamsters are the most active at night, so why not put him in the playhouse for an hour or so and put the playhouse in the bath where he can't escape? Chester will probably also enjoy a tin can or flower pot in his tank to hide in, some sand or wood chips to dig in, and a strip of wood or a thick twig to gnaw on.

DEAR DR. FOX—My father works with wood and often has a lot of wood chips. We were wondering if there would be any harm in using these chips as litter in our hamster cages.—M.W.

DEAR M.W.—Wood chips make fine bedding, but have your father check out whether the wood has been treated with a chemical to stop insects or fungus from damaging it. Such contaminants have been responsible for the death and sickness of many caged animals—especially in research laboratories.

cages (parakeets)

DEAR DR. FOX—Is it safe to put newspaper on the bottom of a parakeet's cage? I am concerned about the ink. Also, do you feel that gravel- or sandpaper perch covers are too rough for a bird's feet?—P.R.

DEAR P.R.—Newspaper print contains so little lead that your bird will not be harmed, unless it starts to eat a *lot* of paper. As for gravel- or sandpaper perches, they are a must for caged birds. The rough surface helps them clean and trim their beaks and also helps keep their claws worn. Beaks and claws still need an occasional trimming, though. Many solitary birds enjoy playing with a mirror and other toys, too. Anything to relieve monotony will help improve a caged bird's overall well-being.

cages (parrots)

DEAR DR. FOX—I have an old parrot cage, and the galvanized bars and water and food containers are beginning to rust. I am tempted to touch them up, but hesitate to do so in case the spray paint contains an ingredient that might harm the parrot. Any suggestions?—O.M.

DEAR O.M.—A little rust on the cage won't harm your bird; it could even be a source of iron when he chews on it. More important than a shiny, new-looking cage is one that is kept clean. A weekly scrubbing is absolutely essential. Simply touch up with a NONTOXIC paint.

DEAR DR. FOX—My parrot likes people when she's out of her cage, but once in it she tries to attack everyone, including me. When she's out, she won't let you hold her, unless the cage is out of sight. Do you understand her strange actions?—M.M.M.

DEAR M.M.M.—I guess your bright bird is telling you in no uncertain terms that she detests her cage. And who wouldn't, unless it's the only refuge against the resident cat? Get your pet a parrot T-bar or gymnasium to perch and live on. She could be feeling helpless when in the cage, and is thus acting defensively—by attacking.

cold weather (gerbils)

DEAR DR. FOX—I'm only twelve, and I have two gerbils. It gets cold where I live and I'm afraid they might die. Can you give me some advice?—J.M.

DEAR J.M.—When hamsters get cold, they hibernate, but when gerbils get

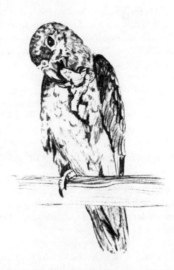

cold, they are more likely to die. Your pets should have a well-insulated little nest box lined with paper and hay (which they will shred up nicely). Don't keep them out on a cold porch, and if your parents won't let you keep them in a warm room, get a heat lamp and put it over their enclosure to keep them warm at night. But be careful not to cook them.

cold weather (older pets)

DEAR DR. FOX—You recently stated in your column that cats won't go outdoors when it's cold. My kitty loves the cold! She rolls in the snow and plays with it, insists on going for a walk in the bitter cold, and sits out on an open porch for hours when the thermometer registers zero.—*CAT LOVER.*

DEAR CAT LOVER—It is surprising how some cats can tolerate the cold, and like dogs, enjoy playing in the snow. Just like children, they are very active and their high metabolism helps them stay warm. Young animals, especially those used to being outside, don't even blink a whisker when it's frigid. But older pets, like older people, slow down and are more susceptible to cold exposure. That's why it's advisable not to allow an old pet out for long in very cold weather.

dog beds

DEAR DR. FOX—For the past six years, my schnauzer-poodle has slept in a bed I made when we got her from the pound. She recently rejected the bed and has been sleeping on the floor. I changed the bedding and gave the box a thorough washing, but she still refuses to use it. Why?—*J.R.*

DEAR J.R.—Maybe the problem is fleas, or the coolness of the floor in hot weather. Some dogs, especially schnauzers, like to stretch out on their bellies with their hind legs stuck out behind. Another possibility—she may like a longer bed now. Heavy breeds should always have some kind of bedding, because on a hard floor they will develop callouses and even bursitis of the elbows.

doghouses

DEAR DR. FOX—Could you please give me some tips on how to help my dog stay warm this winter? Due to my son's allergies my part beagle will be spending his first winter outdoors in a dog house.—*J.C.*

DEAR J.C.—First, don't let him spend long periods indoors, because then he might not get a good winter coat—he might even shed. Next, give him a draft-proof, waterproof, and well-insulated kennel with a good layer of blanket straw or old rug. If it's an especially cold night, bring him indoors. Feed him plenty—he will require more food living outdoors than if he remains indoors. Chances are he'll be healthier in the long run, provided he's always dry and has a warm box or kennel. He may protest the first few nights, but don't give in. Start in the fall so he can get used to it psychologically and physically. If you put him out suddenly when winter is in, he might get ill.

DEAR DR. FOX—My one-year-old chow insists on sleeping on the cement at our back door when he has a choice of the garage or his doghouse—both with rugs. I'm concerned that he might get sick when it turns colder. Would it have an adverse affect on him if in winter he's outside all day but sleeps in the basement at night?—*J.H.*

DEAR J.H.—Some dogs are too dumb or too dependent to seek shelter when they should. I've seen dogs whining, wet, and freezing by their owner's back door because they refuse to use their kennel in the yard. So make up your mind. If he's to stay out all day, he might well be healthier sleeping out all night, and that will require a warm, draft-proof and waterproof kennel. But remember, your dog won't use it if you let him indoors to sleep. Then you're in for trouble, because he'll want in all the time and could well get sick from exposure—moping pitifully at the door for you to let him in.

fish tanks

DEAR DR. FOX—I want to start a tropical fish aquarium. Do you have any tips?—*C.L.*

DEAR C.L.—There are some basic rules for fresh-water tropical-fish-keepers. Don't overstock the tank; too many fish will mean stress and disease. To keep the water clean, you need a water heater, an aerator, and a filter. Overfeeding will foul the water. Keep the tank away from direct sunlight, which can cause over-heating and a green bloom of algae in the water. When introducing new fish, quarantine them first in a separate tank or in a jar kept warm by partial immersion in the tank. If the fish are still healthy after ten days, you may introduce them to the others.

DEAR DR. FOX—I have started keeping fish. The problem is that neither my room nor my tank are heated. Is this bad? Should I get a heater for the tank? And if so, at what temperature do I set it?—*L.E.*

DEAR L.E.—You don't need a heater if you have goldfish or cold-water fish like minnows. But if they are tropical fish, such as guppies, mollies, swordtails, or angelfish, you should get a heater and a water filter.

Don't put the heat on full to begin with, otherwise the fish may succumb to temperature shock. Tropical fish enjoy a temperature range of around 68 to 75 degrees F. It is surprising at what low temperatures they can survive, but this can result in a stunting of their growth and also make them more susceptible to dis-ease.

POSITIONING YOUR TANK

In considering where to place your fish tank, be careful if you're putting it in the living room. If the tank will stand where people will be partying, make sure it's properly covered. Spilling liquor on a piece of furniture may cause damage, but liquor spilled into a tank will cause the fish inside to suffer, and in all probability to die.

DEAR DR. FOX—The water in my fish tank turns green in just a few weeks after it's been cleaned, even though I always keep my filters clean. Can you tell me what I'm doing wrong?—*M.H.*

DEAR M.H.—First, where does your fish tank stand? Too much direct sunlight on the tank can accelerate algal growth. Overfeeding can also contribute to the murky condition, so keep the fish food contained in a floating rubber ring. It is quite difficult to "balance" an aquarium, and the most common reason for algal bloom, other than spoiled feed in the water, is too many fish. Checking out these three factors should clear up your problem.

DEAR DR. FOX—How do I fight the algae that keep showing up in my fish tank? What are algae anyway?—*M.W.*

DEAR M.W.—Algae are plants, but so microscopic that they seem to be a film (green or brown usually). They tend to grow on the inside of the tank and plants and they can do a nasty job of murking and smelling up the water. What to do? First, for a couple of weeks, cut down on the food and the artificial light—you may be overdoing both. Second, clean the tank's sides with a rubber scraper or an old razor blade.

DEAR DR. FOX—I've had a five-gallon aquarium for many years and have always had a few snails in it to help clean the scum that collects at the bottom. Recently, I had to buy a tank heater for my tropical fish, and now I have so many snails I can't even begin to count them.

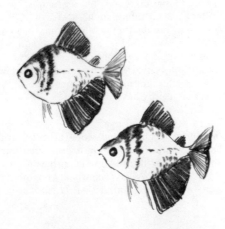

Will this overpopulation of snails harm the natural balance of the aquarium? If so, how do I get rid of them? They match the color of the gravel so well it's difficult (and tedious) to pick them out with a net. Any suggestions?—A.O.C.

DEAR A.O.C.—Since the fish won't eat the snails, and the warmer water is stimulating them to breed, you have an ecologically unbalanced aquarium. Collect all the snails you can and give them to the pet store, which will give them to customers with cold-water tanks. Snails don't really do such a great job of keeping aquarium walls clean.

Many topical-fish-keepers have only a few snails, not as tank cleaners, but more for additional interest. A rubber or razor-blade scraper is better for keeping the glass clear.

THE OWNER'S RESPONSIBILITY

DOG THEFT

Theft of dogs has become a nationwide problem. The dogs are sold for medical research, hunting, breeding, or dog-fighting. Here are some ways to prevent dognapping.

- Don't let a loose dog out of sight.
- Don't leave an unattended dog in a car (locked or not), or in a fenced yard for extended periods.
- Tattoo the dog on the side of its rear flank with its registration number or your social security number. Register the number with the National Dog Registry, 227 Stebbins Road, Carmel, NY 10512.

---

identifying pets

DEAR DR. FOX—I have heard there is an organization that will register a pet and supply the owner with a registration number and tag, as well as a toll-free number to be called if your lost pet is found. The fee for this service is supposedly very reasonable. Do you have any information?—S.C.

DEAR S.C.—What you describe isn't worth a dime. If you really want your dog to be easily identifiable, you must find an organization that will tattoo your pet (usually in the groin). A special tag on the collar can easily be lost or taken off by a dognapper. Pets are still being stolen and sold to dealers who in turn sell animals to research laboratories. Your local humane society or veterinarian may know of a pet identification registry in your area.

leash laws

DEAR DR. FOX—In my neighborhood people permit their dogs (and some are vicious) to run loose, with the result that I have been bitten once and have had several close calls. I love to take walks, and now I may have to give up this healthful exercise. I am eighty years old. When I was a boy, a dog attacked me, and fear has never left me. Don't you think it's unjust?—F.H.M.

DO YOU KNOW YOUR LOCAL ORDINANCES?

Chances are there are laws that state you must get your dog a rabies shot each year and that you must pay a license fee for owning a dog. This is a good plan because your license, no doubt, helps pay for running the local animal shelter.

Is there a local leash law? In many areas dogs aren't allowed out without being on the leash. You could be fined if you don't adhere to the law. Worse, your dog could be hit by a car. Even if the local ordinance doesn't stipulate it, be sure your dog always wears a collar, a rabies tag, and an identity tag just in case it gets lost or picked up by someone who thinks it's a stray.

DEAR F.H.M.—I would like to make it mandatory for *all* dog-owners to read your very important letter. It's indeed unjust that you can't take a walk safely, and it is true that many neighborhoods have free-roaming dogs who are a hazard to children and the elderly. "But my dog is so nice, he wouldn't harm a fly," say many well-intentioned people who let their dogs roam free. Every person who owns a dog should realize that a dog in a pack or patrolling its block is a *very different animal* who may well bite people. In my vicinity, a boy biking in his neighborhood was killed this spring by dogs whose owners thought they wouldn't harm a fly. No dog should ever be off the leash or roam free without its owner. And leash laws should be firmly enforced, if not made even stricter.

neighbors

DEAR DR. FOX—I know about your concern for animals, but may I ask for your concern for people who are *not* bananas over pets, and need to cope with neighbors' "critters"? It's repulsive enough to have to clean the dog droppings from our lawn, but our neighbor's three cats have polluted with urine our lovely open patio.

Is there anything we can use to repel these sneaky cats who wander under our shrubs at all times? I've used pine oil, creosote, hot pepper, cloves, and moth crystals, but so far nothing seems to work. Please help!—*MRS. A.R.*

DEAR MRS. A.R.—You have my sympathy. It is disturbing how indifferent many pet owners are to their neighbors' rights. All your remedies have failed and there really are no others—except responsible neighbors.

All dog owners should pick up after their dogs and curb their dogs to evacuate away from people's property. Dog urine kills lawns. I constantly do my best to convince cat owners to adapt their kittens to indoors (with a walk on a leash every day). This is safest for the cats, too.

Some cat owners think this is cruel confinement, but in truth, they are misguided and irresponsible. No pet should be allowed to roam free, for their sakes, for neighbors' sakes, and for owner's sakes, too, since pets bring some diseases and parasites.

PAYING FOR MISTAKES

In certain states, drivers arrested for moving violations may "work off" their fines by attending driver-legislation classes.

Taking a lead from this wholesome approach, the city of Independence, Mo., gives dog owners who have violated animal-control laws the option of going with their dogs to dog-obedience school. Otherwise, it's pay your fine!

2

Diet and Feeding

NUTRITION AND VARIETY

cockatiels

DEAR DR. FOX—My cockatiel loves gnawing on paper and cardboard. Are these all right for her? How about grilled-cheese sandwiches, ice cream, popcorn, and peanut-butter sandwiches? She does get daily vitamins with her seed. Also, what is that "plastic" that's wrapped around her new feathers?—B.L.L.

DEAR B.L.L.—The "plastic" on your bird's new feathers is natural covering, which, like the tissue at the base of your nails, is a protective sheath that the bird will preen off as its feathers mature. I am concerned about your bird's diet—it should be balanced between commercial birdseed and human food and should also provide her with a variety of fresh fruits and nuts.

The fresher and more balanced the diet, the better her health. Popcorn, grilled-cheese sandwiches, and ice cream should be only occasional tidbits. As for paper and cardboard, such materials provide occupational therapy and are fun to shred and manipulate, but she shouldn't eat them.

lovebirds

DEAR DR. FOX—A peach-faced lovebird came down the chimney and into our home last year. I don't know how long it was in the wild, but it seems quite settled now. Can you tell me why it chews into shreds the paper we put in its cage?

Is there something lacking in its diet? Also, why does it chirp continuously?—*J. O.M.*

DEAR J.O.M.—How nice to have such a pleasant surprise—not everyone has a lovebird come down the chimney. Lovebirds love to chew paper. It's work and play for them—part of their nest-building behavior. Lovebirds with nothing in their cages to play with are indeed being inhumanely deprived. Some lovebirds actually tuck their nesting material, such as straw and paper, into their feathers—a novel way of carrying things. Your bird chirps a lot because it is sociable, and wants plenty of attention. It may well enjoy having a cage-mate of the opposite sex with whom to live, preen, and chirrup. It is, after all, a lovebird, and it takes two to share love.

parakeets

DEAR DR. FOX—My parakeet just loves to eat the leaves of our Boston fern. Are these leaves poisonous?—*K.O.L.O.*

DEAR K.O.L.O.—Since some species of fern are poisonous to animals, I suggest you restrict your bird from eating any more Boston fern. Parakeets do often enjoy eating fresh greens, and a diet of all seeds isn't good, especially when the seeds are old or too rich in oils. Give the bird fresh salad greens, dandelion, fresh sprouted wheat, and millet.

wild birds (how to feed)

DEAR DR. FOX—What started out as a homemade bird-feeder for the birds out back of my house has turned into a minijungle. There are as many as eight to ten squirrels raiding the feeder of its bread and apples. Well, the feeder finally broke and is now on my clothesline, so I can wheel it out to the tree. The squirrels are a treasure to watch, and we'll take care of them through winter. But am I getting in nature's way?—*K.G.*

DEAR K.G.—I like your turn of phrase, "Am I getting in nature's way?" You will be getting in nature's way if you are attracting too many creatures to one spot. This will increase the chances of diseases being spread. And if you provide more than a scattering of food, you may be feeding too many animals, or some species preferentially, which could have negative ecological ramifications.

So put different types of feed out for different species. Read up about what kinds of perches and foods various birds prefer and give the squirrels their own feeding area. Make the birds' feeders squirrel-proof with disks of plastic or tin below and above the feeders.

DEAR DR. FOX—Several years ago, we noticed that a puffed-up sparrow would come into our yard to eat seed that we leave for birds. When it flew in, the other fifty birds eating there would fly away. We made jokes at first, saying it had bad breath or body odor. We have not seen this bird since last spring, and we think it must have died. What do you make of this?—*MRS. D.F.*

DEAR MRS. D.F.—A chubby, puffed-up bird is often sick. It's fluffing its feathers out to keep warm. Birds avoiding sick or maimed birds are following a significant natural survival response. It's most likely that indeed, the sparrow died.

Attracting many birds to one place where food has been left is risky and can increase the spread of contagious diseases. So, even though you mean well, it is advisable that you put out only a little food for a few birds each day.

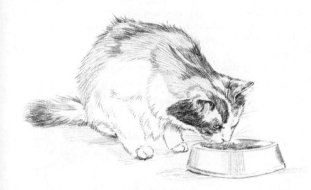

Cats

balanced diet

DEAR DR. FOX—I have read that cats can get kidney problems from an improper diet. My finicky cat eats only canned tuna, lots of dry food, and a little semimoist food. He likes broiled liver, and he gets brewer's yeast once a day. Is that a healthy enough diet?—C.E.H.

DEAR C.E.H.—Your cat's diet is adequate, but be careful not to overdo the tuna, since canned tuna by itself is not a complete and balanced diet. Add some vegetables, peas, and corn, and a little whole-grain rice slowly cooked with an equal quantity of fish or chicken when it's almost cooked. Also, it would be better if you moisten the dry food with warm water. Cats sometimes don't drink enough, and this may cause kidney and bladder problems that some experts think might be aggravated by feeding them only dry food, or food containing too much magnesium salt, commonly termed "ash."

DEAR DR. FOX—My cat has a passion for raw liver. If she had her way, she would forget the canned food and eat liver twenty-four hours a day. Dad gives her only a teaspoon or two at a time, but if anyone comes around she acts like she's starved and begs for more liver. How nutritious is a diet of raw liver?—A.V.Z.

DEAR A.V.Z.—A diet of only raw liver is bad: it is unbalanced, lacking in adequate fiber, carbohydrate, and certain essential minerals, and it may or may not be too low in fat. In fact, a diet of all liver (or all tuna) can cause serious illness due to an excess of vitamin A.

A little raw liver, however, is to be recommended, as is an occasional tidbit of raw or lightly cooked fish, chicken, or lean beef. It is wisest to feed cats a variety of fresh foods and high-quality table scraps in addition to well-balanced top-brand commercial cat foods.

catnip

DEAR DR. FOX—I know my cat's body language and what each meow means. But why does he turn up his nose at catnip? He'll have nothing to do with the mint plant and prefers perfume or shaving lotions.—F.S.

DEAR F.S.—Some cats are quite unimpressed with catnip. People are similarly indifferent or insensitive to certain odors, while others are hypersensitive to them. This is sometimes sex-related in cats or can have a genetic background. Many species of animals will seek out certain plants, fruits, and mushrooms—just like people of all cultures—to alter their states of consciousness.

dry food

DEAR DR. FOX—We have a five-year-old neutered cat. In the last year, he has had two bouts with a blocked bladder. Each time, doctors have inserted a catheter in him, and he takes liquid medicine in a special diet food every day. What can we expect in this case? What causes this?—H.G.

DEAR H.G.—In my experience, it is advisable to take your cat off dry food and feed him only moist food with salt added. Make your cat drink plenty of water (and milk if he will take it). Also feed him about one gram of vitamin C daily to keep the urine acidified, and massage the pelvic region—the lower back and base of the tail.

Some vets think a special diet is unnecessary and that fish is OK, but others disagree. I don't. It is vital that your vet check your cat's anal glands, which may be blocked; this problem seems to be related to the bladder syndrome. Avoid giving your cat any stress—don't leave him at a boarding kennel or for a long weekend alone at home. More research is certainly needed on this complex disorder.

DEAR DR. FOX—Is it true that a dry-food diet can cause bladder problems in cats? My cats were brought up on dry food and will not eat canned food. Also, they are always trying to lick the salad oil off plates. When I give them some olive oil, they act as if they can't get enough. Is this strange behavior for cats?—B.S.W.

DEAR B.S.W.—I always advise raising kittens on a variety of foods so they don't get hooked onto one kind. Dry catfood may not actually cause bladder problems, but once cystitis develops, many veterinarians do advise not feeding dry food unless the cat also drinks plenty of water or milk. A little salt added to the dry food may help make them drink more.

As for the olive oil—give them half a teaspoon daily in their feed. Cats need fats, and natural oils are an essential part of their diet that may be lacking in dry food.

DEAR DR. FOX—I have taken in a stray cat who won't eat dry food unless I give him a tiny pat of butter beforehand. Isn't that strange behavior?—MRS. T.J.

DEAR MRS. T.J.—The question is: How did you come around to making this discovery? Sounds like you have a very intelligent feline who knows how to manipulate you. Some dry catfoods are sprayed with fat and other flavorings to enhance their taste. The butter may help whet his appetite in a similar way and make the dry food easier to swallow. A little melted butter poured on the food may help, too. But don't overdo things or you'll get a fat cat.

farm cats

DEAR DR. FOX—Years ago on our farm, our cat lived to thirty-four years of age. We fed her fresh milk twice a day, sometimes a piece of dry bread. The cats caught mice or whatever. When she died she was blind in one eye and a bit hard of hearing. In those days (1960), farmers never bought catfood.—MRS. B.

DEAR MRS. B.—Your cat is certainly a record-maker. However, many free-roaming farm cats don't live long because of disease and lack of veterinary care.

Of course, good farmers call the vet as needed and also neuter their cats to prevent overpopulation and epidemic diseases.

All farm cats should have rabies shots. They are a source of meat contamination with toxoplasmosis that they pass on to cattle from the infected mice cats eat. Be sure to cook your meat well.

Working cats down on the farm earn their keep by controlling rodents and driving away birds. Fair payment is humane care, but too often they are left to themselves and only the fittest survive. Your ancient cat was certainly one of the fittest.

fish (cravings for)

DEAR DR. FOX—Why do most cats go crazy for fish and other seafood?—H.R.C.

DEAR H.R.C.—This could simply be inborn "nutritional wisdom," since seafood is more nutritious and contains more essential trace elements than regular meats. My theory is that since cats were originally desert-dwelling creatures (where there aren't any fish) and relished eating a variety of reptiles, snakes, and lizards, the flavor of fish evokes an instinctual preference, since reptile meat has a slightly fishy flavor.

Pet-food companies might profitably explore this possibility. "Essence of snakemeat" could be beneficial to encourage convalescent cats to eat and infirm cats to take to special diets.

fish (problems with)

DEAR DR. FOX—Is it so that fish or fish products cause cystitis in cats, especially neutered males?—S.B.

DEAR S.B.—I do not believe that fish, fish products, or dry catfood high in ash content actually cause cystitis in cats. However, I do feel that dry catfood can aggravate this problem once a cat has developed cystitis.

The most important thing is to make sure that the cat is drinking plenty of water. If not, its food should be moist. Dry food is unnatural, and cats, originally desert animals, may have their fluid-regulation mechanism disrupted if they drink little and eat mainly dry food. Furthermore, since they conserve water by concentrating their urine, metabolic byproducts in certain foods present in the urine may actually irritate the urinary system.

food spoilage

DEAR DR. FOX—Do dog and cat foods spoil sitting on the shelf in a store or at home?—G.S.

DEAR G.S.—Canned foods are unaffected, but I suggest you use up your dry commercial pet foods; don't keep them in your cupboard for too long, because they tend to lose their nutritional value. Also, heat and oxidation will destroy many of the vitamins in foods. I suggest you shop in a busy and reliable market where the food doesn't sit on the shelf too long.

DEAR DR. FOX—Can a cat get very sick or die from eating canned food that has spoiled from sitting out too long during the summer months? My cat likes to nibble throughout the day, so the food often stays out for twenty-four hours.—MRS. B.T.

DEAR MRS. B.T.—Canned catfood is heat-sterilized before it is sealed in the can, so the chances of food poisoning are minimal. Many cats prefer unchilled food, so after the can has been opened and partially emptied, put it on a shelf in the kitchen. Cover it well to stop the contents from drying up and losing its palatability and to keep flies away in the summer. Feed the rest later in the day, rather than letting it go stale in the cat's bowl. Unlike dogs, who eat rotting carrion, cats like only fresh food, and yours will probably avoid eating spoiled food. In the summer months, keep the half-used can in the refrigerator until an hour or so before serving.

milk

DEAR DR. FOX—More than a year ago we adopted a very thin, stray black cat badly in need of food. Of course, we took care of that. We fed him plenty of good food and a saucer of milk every day. A month after he arrived, I noticed blood in his stool—every few days, then none for a month or so. This pattern has kept up, but because he has gained weight, has a shiny coat, and is very alert, we have hesitated to take him to a veterinarian, as it often entails x-rays and a lot of expense. But we will comply with whatever you suggest.—C.S.

DEAR C.S.—The saucers of milk may be helping your cat by keeping his stools somewhat loose. Milk has a laxative effect, and the blood in the stools may possibly be due to constipation and straining. Alternatively, a sprinkling of Metamucil or similar gentle laxative may help. But one can't be sure that constipation is the aggravating factor until your cat is examined by a veterinarian. I think the expense is warranted. Only too often, pet owners try to save a few dollars and don't get their animal to the vet soon enough, by which time the problems are worse and the bill bigger. Would you hesitate if it were your child? A dependent creature has a right to health care.

DEAR DR. FOX—My daughter left her cats in my care while she went away for a few months. I tried to give them milk, but they don't like it. Then I tried evaporated milk diluted with water and they love it. Will a saucerful every day (with other foods, of course) bother them?—A.H.

DEAR A.H.—A little raw, pasteurized, or diluted canned milk won't harm any cat. Some are sensitive to the lactic acid in milk that can cause loose stools, but if your daughter's cats are not lactose intolerant, go ahead with the diluted canned milk. Also, provide water. Cats on dry catfood need to drink plenty, and milk, if they like it, will help ensure that they take in adequate fluids. This may help alleviate such problems as feline cystitis, a serious and common bladder disorder in cats, which may be aggravated by an insufficient volume of water each day.

DEAR DR. FOX—Our vet recently said that milk was bad for our cat. But she loves it so and will cry endlessly until we give her some. We've noticed that occasionally it gives her diarrhea, but anything's better than her constant crying. What do you suggest?—B.H.

DEAR B.H.—You can solve the problem by getting your cat lactic-acid-free milk. It won't cause diarrhea because it has been treated with acidophilus. Your cat might also like yoghurt in a little water as an alternative.

As for your cat's crying, you give her milk when she cries, and in this way you reward her constantly and encourage her to cry. Give her a little milk only when she doesn't cry.

FEEDING HAZARD

Recent research has shown that when plastic containers, such as cups and dishes, are filled with water or other liquid consumables, they will gradually dissolve. This could be hazardous to your pet's health and yours. Salamanders developed skin problems and did not reproduce normally when kept in a water-filled plastic, polycarbonate shoebox-type mouse cage. All recovered when put into glass bowls.

So alternate plastic drink-containers with glass. That way they will be cleaned more often, too.

---

variety of foods

DEAR DR. FOX—Do cats get tired of only one flavor of food? My family says that cats aren't like people and can happily eat the same food all the time.—*C.P.*

DEAR C.P.—Most cats enjoy variety, as is certainly evident from the way they eat table scraps and special treats. While it is true that many wild animal species tend to specialize in certain kinds of food, they still consume a considerable variety. Wild cats eat anything from insects and birds to mice and lizards. Cows and deer eat a variety of green foods in addition to grass and leaves.

Although lynx may hunt snowshoe hare, Arctic wolves, and caribou, their prey preference may be determined by a lack of availability of other species. I'm convinced pets do like some variety, since their natural diets in the wild are very varied.

DEAR DR. FOX—My cat will eat only a certain food for two to three weeks, then switch to another for a few weeks. Is this normal?—*M.E.*

DEAR M.E.—Cats often switch brands of food at various intervals of a few weeks to a few months. My guess is that they enjoy a change of diet. Certainly wild cats eat a wide variety of natural foods from season to season.

So, provided your cat doesn't fix on one type of food that isn't a complete and balanced diet (such as an all-tuna catfood), I wouldn't worry. Also, be sure she gets plenty of good-quality table scraps.

vitamin supplements

DEAR DR. FOX—Would it be harmful to give my tortoise-shell cat a high-potency multivitamin/multimineral formula such as Centrum, which is intended for human use? I know there are products made exclusively for cats, but they don't have as many nutrients. I know that my cat lacks vitamin B-12 because she is often sluggish.—*B.H.M.*

DEAR B.H.M.—If your cat is not ill, why do you want to give her a multimineral/multivitamin supplement? If your cat is ill, then she should see a veterinarian and not be subjected to home remedies.

Nutritional supplements are not without value, but far more important is what you feed your cat. If it's just one kind of commercial catfood, that could be the problem. Be sure it is a complete and balanced dietary formula, and offer your cat a variety of good table scraps such as lean meats and vegetables.

DEAR DR. FOX—Our cat's claws are splitting and cracking. He eats a mixture of dry and moist catfoods that are nutritionally balanced, according to the label, but he refuses table scraps or milk. He uses a scratching post, but it's not helping the problem. Why?—D.B.

DEAR D.B.—Individual animals often have slightly different nutritional requirements, so I would suggest you give your cat a multivitamin supplement (which your veterinarian can prescribe), plus a pinch of powdered kelp and yeast and some high-quality protein in the form of cottage cheese or lightly cooked fish or eggs. The claws of cats do split and crack frequently when they live indoors, and they are often shed. There is no cause for alarm, unless the claws become sore or break close to the quick.

Dogs

balanced diet

DEAR DR. FOX—How would you advise me to feed an eight-month-old miniature poodle? He refuses to eat canned dogfood, but he will eat a small amount of Alpo dry kibbles after he has played with it. He always seems to want what we're eating. I tried just feeding him dogfood, but he can go for a week and hardly eat anything.—B.E.G.

DEAR B.E.G.—The value of good commercial dogfood diets is that they are balanced. Most dogs will eventually give in and eat canned food if they are deprived of food, but you obviously have an exception. Your minipoodle will do fine on human food, provided he gets a sufficient variety to make his diet balanced.

In other words, don't overdo the meat. He should have some cereals, a source of carbohydrates, such as cooked whole-grain rice and dry dog biscuits. Cook rice with a little chicken or beef plus fat for flavor, and vary his protein intake with cottage cheese and parboiled egg. Encourage him to eat a few vegetables, if possible. The fresher the food, the better. The main thing is not to let him train you into feeding him just meat.

DEAR DR. FOX—Our beagle never likes dry or canned food, so we put fried liver in it. She picks out the liver and eats nothing else. It is bad for a dog to have the same thing every day? She never tires of it—and it is cheap.—J.Q.

DEAR J.Q.—It is not harmful for a dog to have the same kind of food every day, provided it is a complete and balanced diet. Liver isn't, and some livers are contaminated with drug residues from all those chemicals that are fed to "factory" farm animals. You should gradually wean your dog off the liver by feeding smaller and smaller amounts mixed with a good quality commercial dogfood.

DEAR DR. FOX—How can I get my dog to eat dogfood? He prefers chicken and pork neck bones and our table scraps.—S.B.

DEAR S.B.—Your pooch is a food-fussy fastidious manipulator. He's trained you to feed him just what he likes, and what he likes isn't what's best for him. Chicken meat and pork neck bones is not a complete and balanced diet; furthermore, the bones could cause problems. A hungry dog will eat. So give him regular dogfood of good quality and add a little chicken gravy and meat to make the transition easy. Don't give in. If he goes on a hunger strike have your vet give him a B-12 shot after four or five days to stimulate his appetite.

DEAR DR. FOX—My Shih Tzu likes to eat vegetables and fruits rather than meat. Also, he eats only at night, and even then it's hardly enough for a growing puppy. What do you suggest?—A.R.

DEAR A.R.—You show sense in being concerned. An entirely vegetarian diet for a pup or human infant is inadequate for growth unless you are an expert nutritionist and really know how to prepare a complete and balanced meal. Balance his diet with animal protein in the form of cottage cheese, cheese, egg, and vegetable protein such as beans, lentils, and tofu (soy protein). And be sure to add some bone meal, a little fresh cod-liver oil, and brewer's yeast for B vitamins. Then your pooch will be a lacto-ovo-vegetarian, like many healthy people who are concerned about their health and are trying to cut down on meat.

bone meal

DEAR DR. FOX—I read an article about a woman who was a health food enthusiast and whose death by cancer was connected to the large amounts of ground bone meal she consumed as part of her diet. My dogs eats treats daily that contain ground bone meal. Is this dangerous to their health?—K.B.

DEAR K.B.—I doubt very much that eating large amounts of bone meal is likely to contribute to cancer. More likely it will cause chronic constipation. A tablespoon per day for a thirty-pound dog is a good, nutritious supplement, and safer then giving the dog a bone to chew.

HEALTH REMINDER

Bones can kill dogs. Be sure that you never give your dog any bone that can splinter easily. That rules out chicken, pork, turkey, and lamb. These bones can cause choking or bowel blockage or perforation. The one kind of bone not likely to splinter is a raw (uncooked) beef knuckle or soup bone. Not only will your dog enjoy it, but the right bone will also help keep your pet's teeth clean and gums healthy. So play it safe—and that means keeping your pooch away from bones in the garbage, too.

---

canned food (problems with)

DEAR DR. FOX—I hope you can help with my problem, which involves our bull terrier. He leaves a brown spot wherever he urinates on my lawn. The lawn is beginning to look like a disaster area. Anything we can do? He's a good dog and we love him.—MRS. D.C.

DEAR MRS. D.C.—The high level of ammonia in the urine is probably killing your grass. So you may wish to cut down on the amount of canned meat your dog is eating and give him more dog biscuits or meal. Try adding a little cider vinegar to his food or drinking water, working up gradually to a tablespoon per day.

puppy food

DEAR DR. FOX—What kind of food do you recommend for a puppy? Dry, canned, burger-type, or chunk?—J.J.

DEAR J.J.—Puppies need a diet higher in protein than adult dogs. Pups of smaller breeds require a more concentrated diet, and those of larger breeds need extra minerals and vitamins A and D. Most well-known brands of pet food cater to most pups' requirements, but if you have a toy or giant breed, consult with your veterinarian or the person who bred the pup. Dogs have individual requirements that vary according to age, breed, and temperament. Be sure that at least 25 percent of your pup's diet is fresh rather than processed and preserved commercial food. Add table scraps, scrambled egg, cottage cheese, or a little raw or lightly cooked lean beef or chicken to the commercial diet.

smell and taste sensations

DEAR DR. FOX—I often wonder why I give Sam, my dog, such delicious table scraps. She just bolts them down the same as she does commercial dogfood. Can she taste the difference?—M.G.

DEAR M.G.—What really turns on your dog's appetite is the aroma more than the taste of a food. That's a canine characteristic—their sense of smell is fantastic—way beyond our limited sense of smell. Can they taste the difference? They do differentiate between sweet, sour, and bitter. You should be more concerned with satisfying your pooch's nutrition than her taste.

variety of foods

DEAR DR. FOX—Is it OK to feed our poodle some cheese every day for a treat? Also, would it be safe to buy a flea medicine for our three-pound poodle puppy?—J.V.

DEAR J.V.—A little cheese for your dog each day is quite all right—provided he eats his regular food, wich should be a complete and balanced diet. I would not advise giving your small poodle any medicine without veterinary supervision. Some over-the-counter medications, safe in larger dogs, can be very poisonous to small ones. Does your dog really have fleas? Don't get sucked into "preventive" treatment with worm and flea medications; treat only when and as needed and only under the vet's advice.

DEAR DR. FOX—My miniature poodle is accustomed to eating one-fourth can of Mighty Dog and a small handful of kibble morning and evening (plus a few treat cookies scattered through the day). When we are traveling, would it be bad for her to eat the meat flavors of catfood in the new extra-tiny cans (Fancy Feast), as that way there would be no leftovers? She eats whatever she's given, so that's no problem, but I wouldn't want her to get sick.—J.S.

DEAR J.S.—No problem in giving your dog a little of the commercial catfood you mention. But don't overdo it, since a change in diet could mean digestive upsets (diarrhea, etc.), which is the last thing you want on your vacation. Also, go easy on the between-meal snacks—too many dogs are overweight today, and obesity leads to a host of health problems and a shorter life.

vitamin supplements

DEAR DR. FOX—What do you say to giving a dog a couple of vitamin C tablets every day? Also, when I have meat drippings, I add flour and water and make a gravy and put that over the commercial dry food. Is this good or bad?—D.J.H.

DEAR D.J.H.—Healthy adult dogs do not need vitamin supplements, provided they're given a good balanced diet with occasional high-quality fresh-food table scraps. Dogs are more omnivorous than cats and will enjoy a wider variety of leftover vegetables, cereals, and dairy products.

Your gravy sounds delicious. You really don't need to add flour and water, since there are plenty of carbohydrates in the dry dogfood. Just don't make it too palatable, or he will overeat. Add other table scraps as well as gravy—the more you have left over, the better.

water

DEAR DR. FOX—Who is right? I always thought plenty of water should always be available for one's dog (Buffy is a collie-sized ten-year-old). My veterinarian says that dogs don't need all that much water.—A.B.

DEAR A.B.—A veterinarian who says that an old dog should have a restricted supply of drinking water should be censured and his or her license to practice revoked. Older dogs drink more to compensate for failing kidneys. To restrict drinking can lead to uremic poisoning, sickness, and death. Dogs, especially older ones, should have fresh drinking water available at all times. And more is needed in the summer because much body water is lost when dogs pant to keep cool.

Fish

DEAR DR. FOX—Could you please tell me what to feed Siamese fighting-fish babies? A book I read said to feed them protozoa, paramecia, or rotifers, but we did not know how to get them. As a result, we lost all but ten of the fry.— SHANNON.

DEAR SHANNON—Better pet stores can provide microorganisms called infusoria for feeding Siamese fighting-fish fry. You did well (and the parents did) to raise ten. Some pet-supply catalogs and fish-hobbyist magazines carry advertisements for such live-food preparations. Alternatively, the local zoo or aquarium may be able to help next time. Forewarned is forearmed, so if you plan to breed again, do make your "connection" soon.

Guinea Pigs

DEAR DR. FOX—My albino guinea pig loves to eat greens. Everybody says it is bad for her. Is that true? Also, should she be in the sun?—M.R.

DEAR M.R.—Your guinea pig should have a variety of food to choose from— guinea pig commercial pellets, cereal, toast, fruit, vegetables, and greens. Rather

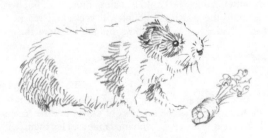

than restricting her to one kind of food, let her choose. Animals possess what is called "nutritional wisdom," but they can't use it if they have limited choice. Guinea pigs, like rabbits, will enjoy basking in the sun, but there should be some shade available.

Hamsters

DEAR DR. FOX—I recently purchased a young hamster, about four or five weeks old, from a neighborhood store. I have been feeding him a mixture of seeds and alfalfa pellets. Is there anything better than this for an all-purpose diet? Does he also need a vitamin supplement in his water?—C.S.

DEAR C.S.—Your hamster's diet is adequate, but I recommend giving your pet a little more variety. Hamsters enjoy whole-wheat bread, granola-type cereal, a small quantity of cheese, fruit, raw vegetables, and even an occasional earthworm. With sufficient variety and the addition of natural foods, you would not need to give him a commercially prepared vitamin supplement.

DEAR DR. FOX—We grow sunflowers in our garden and are wondering if we could pick the seeds and feed them to our hamsters and gerbils. Will fresh seeds hurt them?—CAROL

DEAR CAROL—Let the sunflower seeds ripen and dry naturally. Break them up and let them sun-dry. Don't feed them to your pets if they get moldy. Seeds that aren't dry will mold and will make your pets sick. Don't feed your pets too many or they'll get fat. Seeds are rich in oil as well as protein, and they will give your animals a glossy coat. Try some lightly toasted seeds on your cereal, or bake some rolled oats, almonds, honey, and raisins and make your own cereal. Your pets will love it, too!

Mice

DEAR DR. FOX—My brother and I received two white mice, Claude and Claudet, as pets. Claudet is doing well, but Claude seems overweight. Both diets consist of a laboratory rodent chow, oats, and grains. We have recently got Claude a treadwheel to run in, but his weight still remains over two ounces. Can you help him?—M.M.

DEAR M.M.—Mice, like most animals, naturally regulate their food intake and, even when provided with a lot of food, never overeat. Your Claude sounds like an exception. Provided he is active and enjoys his treadwheel, I wouldn't worry. Putting him on a restricted diet could cause more serious problems. If he's unhappy living with Claudet, he could be eating more than he should; so, as an experiment, separate the two for a couple of weeks and see how his weight changes, if at all. Chances are he's an obese mutant, but none the less lovable for all his fat.

Rabbits

DEAR DR. FOX—Here are some tips from a successful orphan-bunny-raiser. At first, I made the mistake of feeding lots of clover and the rabbit died. The second time, I successfully raised six orphaned rabbits. I fed them (with a dropper)

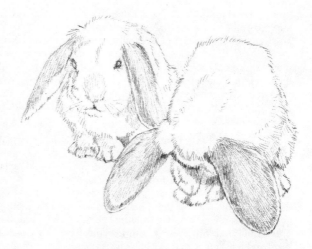

condensed milk diluted with a little water every two hours. When they were big enough to eat, I gave them commercial rabbit chow ground up in the blender and clover. At eight weeks, I released them—lively and healthy. (I had continued to give them milk.) Apparently too much greenery too soon gives them diarrhea.—B.A.M.

DEAR B.A.M.—Congratulations. You're a born rabbit nutritionist. Clover, high in protein, can cause "bloat" and severe indigestion. Baby rabbits lack the bacteria in their intestines to cope with such food materials. In the wild they get inoculated with such bacteria by eating the feces of other rabbits. This is a natural process called "rejection" and is probably one of the reasons why domestic orphan rabbits don't often survive.

DEAR DR. FOX—I would like to change my rabbit's diet. For the last two years he has had only dry rabbit food. Could you prescribe another food for him?—K.J.W.

DEAR K.J.W.—Any change in an animal's diet that is too abrupt can cause digestive problems. So whatever changes you do plan, do it slowly. If your rabbit is healthy, why bother to change from his dry food? Simply continue with his regular feed and add a little variety, such as a half-handful of fresh grass, hay, granola, carrot, parsnip, spinach, or lettuce every few days. Rabbits also enjoy chewing on a block of wood—it helps keep their teeth trim—or an old soup bone or mineral block that most pet stores carry.

Turtles

DEAR DR. FOX—I have a small box turtle about the size of a silver dollar. I put it in a terrarium with dirt and patches of grass at either end. I put fresh pieces of lettuce, apple, tomato, and other fruits and vegetables in for him, but it seems like he never eats. Also, I have a hermit crab. Would it be safe to put them together?—L.B.

DEAR L.B.—Turtles don't eat very much, but some fresh earthworms and moist catfood would be a good addition. Do you have plenty of new, bigger shells for your crab? No, I wouldn't put the turtle and crab together. The trouble with keeping wild creatures such as reptiles, amphibians, and crustaceans (crabs and such), is that they don't always adapt well and slowly starve to death. The care of these is extremely complex. So why don't you let them go free if you really care for them? Hermit crabs belong by the ocean rather than in someone's home. Their right to life is surely greater than our right to keep them for our own amusement. Gerbils, hamsters, and other cage-adapted pets should satisfy your needs, and they aren't likely to fade away and die.

DEAR DR. FOX—I have a very old (seventy-five years) Western box turtle. He only likes to eat hamburger meat. He will not eat vegetables or fruits, or even plants. Is he getting enough nourishment? What should he be eating? And how can I get him to eat other things?—A.S.

DEAR A.S.—Many reptiles enjoy some meat in their diets, but an all-meat diet (in spite of claims to the contrary by some pet-food manufacturers) is bad for any creature. It is deficient in calcium and in certain vitamins and trace minerals. You should feed your ancient turtle lean meat lightly dusted with powdered bone-meal and a little powdered kelp (seaweed) and a crushed multivitamin tablet or emptied-out capsule. Put only a little of this supplement on the meat so he will get used to it slowly. And do try him on some bananas, papayas, and other good fruits and vegetables. Your turtle is an oldie.

DEAR DR. FOX—I have a problem feeding my pet box turtle in the winter when he slows down. The past three winters I've managed by waiting until he yawned and then stuffing pieces of banana or bread into him. He shows little interest in the night crawlers I provide, and he spits out lettuce. I keep him in an aquarium, so he never goes into hibernation, and he's always up in the morning when I turn on the lights.—K.M.

DEAR K.M.—If your turtle is a native box turtle and not a tropical import, it might be best to let him hibernate. Beginning next fall as he starts to slow down, keep him in a hay-lined, well-insulated box in an outdoor shed. Don't put him out if he feels light and hasn't been eating well.

Tortoises put on fat for their winter "sleep." Keeping him up all winter could upset his metabolism, leading to obesity or difficulty in resuming normal eating in spring. If you do plan to keep him up all next winter, continue with the force-feeding. Feed him scrambled eggs or lean ground beef if he refuses to eat meal worms.

SPECIAL FEEDING PROBLEMS

bad breath (cats)

DEAR DR. FOX—One of our housecats has terrible breath odor. She likes to drink milk, while the others don't. Could that be it? What can we give her to help her?—D.P.

DEAR D.P.—Milk won't make her breath foul. Most likely, she has dirty teeth, possibly a buildup of tartar and infected gums. Halitosis is a sure sign of dental problems. Her teeth probably need a thorough cleaning by a veterinarian.

I also advise feeding her some dry food. Try different brands until you find one she likes. A diet of all-moist food tends to collect on the back teeth, while the dry food helps keep the teeth clean and gums healthy. See your vet soon—an unattended bad mouth can lead to serious and distressing oral disease.

bad breath (dogs)

DEAR DR. FOX—We have two beagles, six and seven years old, mother and daughter. The six-year-old has brown, awful-looking stuff on her teeth that's hard to get off. We had her teeth cleaned last summer and again in the fall, even though she chews a special "bone" about once a day. She also has a very bad breath odor. Any advice?—*MRS. B.O.*

DEAR MRS. B.O.—Some dogs, like people, seem to suffer more from bad breath than others in the same house eating the same food. Individual body chemistry and metabolism are at the root of it. You should reduce your dog's intake of canned meat and meat byproducts and give her cottage cheese and vegetable protein instead. This usually helps. As for the brown scale on the teeth, some dogs build up this tartar rapidly. The only solution is to have your vet scrape the dog's teeth clean, then give its teeth a nightly brushing with abrasive toothpaste or powder on a piece of gauze wrapped around one finger, or on a toothbrush.

DEAR DR. FOX—Josie, my minipoodle, has dreadful breath. She is only four and we are careful about diet and teeth cleaning. Our doctor says nothing can be done, but I wonder if there is a chlorophyll product I could give her.— *R.G.*

DEAR R.G.—Chlorophyll tablets do help some cases of halitosis and will even mask the odor of a female dog in heat to keep amorous males away. You can get these from any health store. They are not poisonous, so you can give about one gram per ten-pound body weight daily.

Encourage your pooch to chew on a beef knuckle bone or rawhide strip. Consider brushing her teeth with doggy toothpaste (which pet stores sell), applied each morning and night with either a brush or a gauze-wrapped finger. Sweet kisses from then on, I hope.

demand feeding (dogs)

DEAR DR. FOX—Our vet told us to put our puppy on demand feeding, and to keep her dish filled with dry dogfood at all times. He said that she would eat only when hungry, never become overweight, and never gobble her food. We followed his advice and now our dog is two years old and everything the vet told us came true. Do you endorse this method?—*L.E.H.*

DEAR L.E.H.—Demand feeding, or free-access feeding, is satisfactory for most dogs. Dogfood can even be put in a dispenser that drops the food into the bowl. The method doesn't work for all dogs, however. Some animals seem incapable of self-regulation and end up getting obese. Dogs that are left alone for extended periods seem to do better when they can snack on dry food at their leisure. But again, some will eat excessively, perhaps to alleviate boredom or loneliness. Demand feeding is fine, provided the dog doesn't go hog-wild. I guess it's worth an experiment—one can always return to regular feeding if necessary.

excessive hunger (cats)

DEAR DR. FOX—My cat has a ravenous appetite. I feed her plenty, I assure you, but she's never satisfied and begs constantly for food, winding herself around my legs and/or sitting by her dish and staring at me. She was spayed in September and gets little exercise because she doesn't want to go outside. Is something wrong with her?—*MRS. J.R.B.*

DEAR MRS. J.R.B.—Boredom, reduced activity with being confined indoors, plus hormone imbalance caused by neutering combine to create a hungry cat. She may quickly become a fat cat, who'll eventually turn into a dull, lethargic, and sickly butterball that ages rapidly.

Your only solution is cut back on her food. Give her a little cottage cheese and boiled rice seasoned with a little chicken or fish as a morning snack, plus a little raw liver. Give the same in the evening with a little canned or dry commercial food. No between-meal snacks. Don't give in: her health depends on you.

excessive hunger (dogs)

DEAR DR. FOX—My dog is obsessed with eating! He constantly begs. I feed him plenty, believe me—commercial food as well as dry food in his bowl all the time. He also gets dog biscuits, and some days he'll eat ten of them. Once or twice a week he gets meat scraps from our dinner. If you're carrying food in your hand, he practically knocks you down to get it. Don't ever leave food on the coffee table and walk away! I feel a dog would only act this way if he's hungry. What's up?—*L.B.*

DEAR L.B.—There can be many reasons for constant hunger—a dog may have worms, or he may simply not have enough food because he is so active all the time. But many dogs are food beggars who like to solicit their "pack leaders'" attention and indulgence, and they soon learn how to manipulate their owners effectively at mealtimes. Your dog may be in this category, but to be certain have your vet give him a physical. My bet is that he's a food beggar and needs discipline at the table. So no tidbits. If you give in once, he'll never take no for an answer and will continue to be alert for food.

excessive thirst (cats)

DEAR DR. FOX—Our twelve-year-old cat can't seem to quench his thirst. Our vet ignores the question when we ask him about it.—*P.S.*

DEAR P.S.—Go to another vet. Cats rarely drink much, since they are a desert species. So a cat that is drinking a great deal is most probably sick. Diabetes and kidney disease, for example, are often associated with excessive drinking. After you have taken your cat to another doctor, and if my suspicions are correct, then you should file a complaint about your veterinarian's indifference and negligence (if proven by your cat's sickness) with the state veterinary board and the Better Business Bureau.

excessive thirst (dogs)

DEAR DR. FOX—My large part-German shepherd and part-collie dog wants to drink water all the time. Neither the veterinarian nor the animal hospital could find anything wrong. They said it was a behavior problem and put her on Valium four times a day. This has been going on for one year. She still wants water, but I restrict it. Is there anything at all you could suggest?—*C.K.*

DEAR C.K.—Your dog's condition, polydipsomania, usually has some physical cause, such as pituitary malfunction associated with diabetes insipidus. Sometimes a brain tumor is responsible. However, since your dog checks out physically OK, you should try to pinpoint psychological stress that triggers your pooch's polydipsomania. If she is physically sound and isn't drinking excessively to compensate for kidney failure or liver disfunction (common problems in older dogs), then there should be no reason why her water intake shouldn't be restricted. She may simply want more attention and exercise.

fear of food dish (dogs)

DEAR DR. FOX—We have an unusual problem with our English setter. It started with his being afraid to drink water from a dish. Now he seems to be afraid of the food in his dish. He stands way back and stretches forward and will eat only a small amount at a time. We coax him because he has lost weight, but he still acts afraid.—*J.O.*

DEAR J.O.—A phobic reaction to food and drink is most unusual in my experience of dog behavior problems. I would suspect that your dog may be suffering from progressive blindness, an inherited disease of setters. Have him examined by your veterinarian, and meanwhile try feeding him in a well-illuminated spot.

DEAR DR. FOX—When I read your column regarding the English setter that was afraid to eat or drink from his dish, I decided to share a similar experience with you. My Yorkshire terrier was developing the same problem and got to the point where he would reach out with a front paw very carefully just to tip the dish so he could eat his food off the floor.

It took some close watching before I discovered the problem. My dog wore a metal collar, his dish was stainless steel, and he walked on nylon carpeting. When he walked across the nylon carpet and put his nose into the dish he got a static electric shock. After moving the collar and changing his dish to a ceramic bowl the problem went away, and he is no longer afraid to put his nose in the bowl. Hope this helps some other perplexed pet owner.—*G.B.*

DEAR G.B.—Thank you for sharing a very important observation. You get the First Honorary Award for Insightful Pet-Owner. I am increasingly concerned about the possible effects on pets that live indoors, where contact with synthetic carpeting and upholstery leads to a buildup of static charges. This situation could lead to skin hypersensitivity, excessive grooming, scratching, and allergylike skin disorders. I advise owners to use room humidifiers, which help reduce static, and to avoid wearing synthetic clothes.

gulping food (dogs)

DEAR DR. FOX—How can I keep my St. Bernard pup from gulping down his food like it's going out of style?—*L.J.D.*

DEAR L.J.D.—It is quite normal for dogs to gulp or bolt down their food— that's the way dogs eat. Young dogs should be fed four times a day up to three months, then two or three times a day up to one year. If you're feeding your dog only once a day, he may well eat faster than normal and could get indigestion or even "bloat." Smaller, more frequent meals are advisable.

indigestion (dogs)

DEAR DR. FOX—My adorable poodle has been wonderful company for me after my husband's death. But he doesn't like dogfood and everything he eats turns to gas. The odor is not pleasant, to say the least. How can I help him?—*M.D.*

DEAR M.D.—Many dogs are afflicted with a similar problem, which can be due to a number of factors: gulping down their food and swallowing air (so-called aerophagia); eating overly rich food that's high in cooked-meat content; or having a possible allergic reaction to certain kinds of food. Your veterinarian may be able to suggest a commercially available prescription diet, or you may wish to make up your own formula. Combine one part cooked rice (whole grain), one part egg, chicken, fish, lean meat, or cottage cheese; plus multivitamin drops and a few vegetable or other table scraps. Feed your dog small amounts, breaking up a day's meal into three or four "snacks" to prevent overeating and indigestion.

loss of appetite (cats)

DEAR DR. FOX—I have a beautiful male cat about two-and-a-half years old, with a lot of fluffy fur. Often when he loses his appetite, I give him hairball medicine every day instead of twice a week. Is that safe? Anything else I can do? I get so upset when he stops eating.—B.B.

DEAR B.B.—Some cats are picky eaters, fur balls or no fur balls. One of mine will pick at his food for a few days, then eat with gusto for a week or so, and then switch off again for a while. Keep an eye on your cat's feeding pattern and lay off the fur-ball medicine for a couple of weeks. Groom him well twice a day, not deeply, but just enough to remove loose hair. A healthy cat throws up fur balls regularly every few weeks, depending on its coat type and condition. Other cats never throw up fur balls, but pass the fur out of their system instead. If your cat likes fresh grass (you can sprout some wheat indoors), it works wonders in getting rid of fur balls. In fact, I recommend some grass in every cat's diet.

DEAR DR. FOX—My grandmother's cat has hardly eaten for a month. Will he die? Can you tell me what's wrong with him?—JENNIFER

DEAR JENNIFER—Your grandmother's cat should be taken posthaste to see a veterinarian. One of the first signs of sickness in animals is disinterest in food. The cat could have infected teeth, for example, and respond well to veterinary treatment, or have kidney failure that could be partially alleviated with proper diet and appropriate medication. Some cats do go on "hunger strikes" when they want to hold out for certain foods (usually food that's not ideal for their health). But that's not the case with your grandma's cat. Tell her that the longer she delays seeing a vet, the poorer the chances will be of restoring her cat's health.

loss of appetite (dogs)

DEAR DR. FOX—Now that my collie can't find grass, she hunts and smells everywhere she goes and will not eat. My vet says she's in perfect condition and will eat when she's hungry. Can you tell me how to stimulate her appetite?— MRS. B.S.

DEAR MRS. B.S.—If your dog is otherwise healthy and doesn't seem too keen about eating, perhaps she needs only one meal a day, or more exercise, or less to eat. Dogs and cats often eat grass to stimulate or clean out their digestive system. It's a kind of tonic. My animals do fine all winter without grass but make a beeline for it come spring. One solution is to sprout a little grass indoors. But for a big collie you may need to grow a lawn in your living room. Perhaps you would rather wait till spring!

loss of appetite (guinea pigs)

DEAR DR. FOX—My guinea pig recently stopped eating her pellets and drinking her water; she would only eat her greens and apples. She was also losing weight. I read somewhere to feed her bread and milk, which worked beautifully! The problem now is that's all she'll eat.—*S.W.*

DEAR S.W.—All pet owners should be aware that whenever any pet—be it a guinea pig, a cat, or a parakeet—goes off its food for more than a couple of days and begins to lose weight or lose its fur or shed feathers, it should be taken to a veterinarian. A thorough examination is the only way to find out what the problem is and what the most appropriate treatment should be. All pet owners should avoid home doctoring when the above signs of sickness are evident. One of an animal's basic rights is to see its vet when sick.

SUMMER APPETITE

In extremely warm weather, 90 degrees or more, dogs and cats can become fussy eaters. Don't offer them treats or favorite foods to tempt their appetites. A reduced food intake results from metabolic change triggered by the warm weather.

Regular eating habits will return as the temperature drops. It is helpful to feed your pet early in the morning, before the temperature begins to climb.

---

overweight (birds)

DEAR DR. FOX—In one of your recent columns you said that birds should get exercise out of the cage, because obesity is a cage-bird killer. My problem is that as many times as I've trained them, my birds just fly around the cage frantically. If and when they get out, they run into the walls, doors, and windows. To add to my problems, I have two cats.—*L.S.*

DEAR L.S.—Other than building a flight cage, I suggest you strictly limit your birds' intake of millet and sunflower seeds. These oily seeds make birds very fat. Two birds sharing a cage and stimulating each other will be far more alert and active than if they lived singly. This means they should be healthier overall and less likely to become obese.

overweight (dogs)

DEAR DR. FOX—I live in a retirement center, and I can't keep people from feeding my dog scraps. As a result Babes is overweight. Can you suggest a diet?—*J.G.*

DEAR J.G.—Part of loving is giving, and I'm sure your fellow dwellers can't resist giving Babes something extra as a treat. You could certainly cut out most of her feeding schedule. Adult dogs need only be fed once a day. To keep her from becoming too hungry, break the food up into two small feeds, given first thing in the morning and late in the afternoon.

You might also try a low-calorie dry dogfood with suitable table scraps to make it more palatable, but go easy on the fat content of the diet. Cottage cheese and boiled rice are good fillers and will help the dog reduce weight. Also, consider getting another dog, ideally one of the opposite sex. They will play together and burn off excess calories.

UNUSUAL CRAVINGS AND EATING HABITS

alcohol (dogs)

DEAR DR. FOX—My four-month-old pup seems to have a strong attraction for alcohol. Can you possibly explain why the pup would like booze? I also would like to know what shots the pup needs and if they are mandatory by law.—B.S.

DEAR B.S.—Pups will try anything. But your pup is not attracted by booze per se, but by what you are doing (drinking). He just wants to join in. You might say he's a social drinker. I wouldn't encourage it. Alcohol is poison to young animals even in small amounts. Besides, addictions are hard to keep up.

As for shots, all puppies should have an annual rabies vaccination, which is mandatory under the law. There are other protective shots to help your puppy resist other contagious canine diseases, but your vet should advise you of these.

cantaloupe (cats)

DEAR DR. FOX—My cat, Snowball, loves cantaloupe. Is this unusual? Sometimes he also eats the rind. Is that OK?—A.R.

DEAR A.R.—Many cats love cantaloupe. Just don't let your cat eat the rind unless you know it's free of pesticides. A friend of mine has two cats. When she puts pieces of melon in the food dish, the dominant one grabs a piece first and carries it into the living room.

The subordinate cat follows closely, whereupon the dominant one growls and moves further away. Then the subordinate one runs back to the kitchen and eats up all the rest of the melon. Greedy cats are often dominant over food, but not always the most intelligent.

grass (cats and dogs)

DEAR DR. FOX—My husband and I have a standing argument about why dogs and cats eat grass. I say they like the taste and eat it to make them feel better. He says that they eat it as just another food—not knowing the difference—and that it promptly makes them sick. Once and for all—who is right?—MRS. A.L.

DEAR MRS. A.L.—Your husband's interpretation doesn't hold water. When an animal gets sick soon after eating a particular food, it normally will not eat that food again. Grass acts as a tonic for cats and dogs, helping stimulate secretion of gastric and bile juices that may be vomited or voided in the feces. By eating grass, sick animals or those afflicted with worms will sometimes stimulate vomiting. Seeking certain plant remedies to balance their bodies and maintain good physical condition may be part of the animal's natural yoga.

DEAR DR. FOX—Our three cats have an intense craving for grass. Although they're usually kept indoors, the minute they're let out they will race for the nearest bit of fresh or dry grass and chew to their heart's content. They'll also nibble at the straw broom and outer husks of corn. Is there some specific nutrient in fresh or dried grass that is essential for the well-being of cats?—W.G.

DEAR W.G.—A sick cat or dog will eat grass in order to vomit and clean out its system. Healthy animals also relish fresh grass, especially after being kept indoors for a long period. Their system obviously needs it, but just what they are taking in, we don't know. Many people who live in city apartments will grow a little grass for their indoor cats. This is certainly a good idea, better than having the cat nibble away at their plants. I trust the cat's own "nutritional wisdom"—grass is undoubtedly a tonic. If you live in the country, let your cat nibble happily on the lawn (on a leash; please!).

DEAR DR. FOX—I would like to grow some grass greens indoors for my cats. Is there a "best" kind?—T.F.

DEAR T.F.—My cats enjoy a typical lawn seed mix primarily of fescue. Some cats relish sprouted wheat or rye, which you too can enjoy on sandwiches (it's more nutritious than a slice of processed meat). Growing your own grass for your cat is one way of keeping the cat from chewing on your house plants, too. Incidentally, many cats also enjoy other vegetables—peas, asparagus, corn on the cob—so give yours a taste test.

DEAR DR. FOX—Each year, on Palm Sunday, when we come home from Mass, we put the palms on our counter top. My cat, Snowflake, likes to jump up onto the top of the counter and chew on the ends of the palms. Then she pushes the palms away and rolls around on the counter top as if she's drunk. This lasts for about five to ten minutes. Is this normal?—D.A.

DEAR D.A.—Cats roll as though drunk as a sign of pleasure. Plant odors and sunlight can trigger such rapturous rolling. It's quite normal. Let your cat have some fresh greens occasionally—try sprouting some wheat or lawn grass indoors.

She may occasionally enjoy a little catnip. You can grow your own outdoors or buy it direct from health-food or pet stores. There are many other mild herbs your cat may enjoy. See what she likes—but always in moderation, please.

DEAR DR. FOX—You've said it's good for cats to eat grass, but recently my vet had to anesthetize my cat in order to take out a large blade of grass, most of which had gone up her nasal passage. I'm afraid to let her eat grass. What do you think?—M.J.A.

DEAR M.J.A.—It's most unusual for a cat to get a blade of grass stuck in its nasal passage. It most likely happened when the cat was retching up the grass it had just swallowed. But people sometimes choke eating meat—and that risk is no reason to stop eating meat. Let your cat continue to enjoy her fresh grass and allay your anxiety with the realization that the chances are one in a million that this accident will happen again.

lettuce (dogs)

DEAR DR. FOX—Our little dog is crazy about eating lettuce. Wouldn't this take the place of grass, which you often say is good for dogs?—M.

DEAR M.—I encourage all pet owners to try out various vegetables and fruits on their cats and dogs. One of my cats loves peas and corn, and my dog relishes a mild vegetarian curry. Variety is not only the spice of life: a varied diet helps ensure that an animal gets all the nutrients it needs. Commercial pet food formulations and nutritional standards are based on the average animal's requirements, but some require more of certain nutrients than others. It's the same for people, too. However, I also believe that grass has a very specific effect in cleansing out the animal system, unlike other greens and vegetables, so do let your dog eat grass whenever it wants to.

manure (dogs)

DEAR DR. FOX—My dog likes to go over to the neighbor's barn and eat horse manure. What can I do?—T.F.

DEAR T.F.—Your dog's predilection for horse manure is common. Many dogs relish these simple equine offerings. Some roll in the material first because they seem to enjoy the odor. Equine excrement contains B vitamins and other nutrients from bacterial action, and certain molds or fungus spores that dogs enjoy. My pets love to dig up raunchy bones to chew on—perhaps bacteria and molds produce certain nutrients that are good for animals whose natural wisdom guides them to such seemingly worthless material.

milk (dogs)

DEAR DR. FOX—My three-year-old St. Bernard is just crazy about milk. After my son falls asleep and I take the bottle of milk to the kitchen, my dog follows me so I can give her the remaining milk. Could milk harm her in any way?—F.Q.

DEAR F.Q.—A small amount of milk or baby formula won't have any adverse effects on your St. Bernard. In fact, not giving her the remaining milk after you have fed your child could have an adverse effect. Your dog is obviously very much in need of attention and jealous of the baby. Giving her the baby's milk is very reassuring. I just hope you won't have difficulties weaning the dog after your baby gives up the bottle.

mint (cats)

DEAR DR. FOX—My part-Siamese cat goes crazy over minty things. She will dig her way into unguarded purses to get at menthol cigarettes, and tries to get at my toothbrush while I brush my teeth with a mint toothpaste. Can you explain this?—K.M.

DEAR K.M.—Give your cat an occasional treat of fresh mint, catnip, coriander, or other herbs. Just like people, some cats really enjoy certain odors and tastes. Keep her off the menthol cigarettes—she might get hooked on nicotine next! Dogs and cats do get hooked on nicotine and will chew and suck on filter-tip butts. Make sure to keep cupboards closed and containers tightly sealed; your cat may be turned on by something minty that has a dangerous chemical in it.

okra (dogs)

DEAR DR. FOX—My eight-year-old miniature schnauzer has a most unusual craving. He always ignored our vegetable garden until we planted okra. When the okra pods are just about an inch long, he barks at them, jumps up and pulls one off, or puts his front feet up as high on the stalk as he can. He then trots off with the okra in his mouth and sits down to feast. What gets him so excited about okra?—MRS. R.V.

DEAR MRS. R.V.—Your dog is a sensible vegetarian. Dogs are omnivorous, and many of their wild cousins like the fox and coyote enjoy eating various wild fruits and other plant foods. I have no idea what it is specifically about okra that he finds so exciting. It's intriguing that he waits until they have grown a bit. Perhaps odor has something to do with his craving. No doubt he learned from you after observing you pick vegetables.

olives (cats)

DEAR DR. FOX—Our cat is crazy about olives. He'll even try to steal them from our salads. After consuming one, he falls on his back licking his legs and rolling from side to side in a playful manner. Have we discovered a "new catnip"?—R.C.

DEAR R.C.—Many cats seem to enjoy olives. A few (no more than four a day) will be good for them, especially if they are in oil. Cats need unsaturated fats, a deficiency that can make them less able to withstand stress and disease. Rolling after eating an olive is a sure sign of consummate enjoyment. A wolf will roll in its dinner (say, a haunch of deer) before feasting. Cats will also roll, for example, as a signal for play.

raisins, rawhide (dogs)

DEAR DR. FOX—My dog loves to eat raisins and chew rawhide bones. Are these good for her?—*P.M.*

DEAR P.M.—They're fine. Raisins are nutritious and rich in iron. But go easy on the rawhide. Some dogs will bite off and swallow hunks of hide, which can cause intestinal problems. If your dog just gnaws on the hide and swallows only shredded fragments, there's no cause for alarm. It will keep him occupied, satisfy his oral craving to chew, and help keep his teeth clean of tartar and his gums healthy.

running tap water (cats)

DEAR DR. FOX—My cat Felix never drinks from his water bowl. He prefers to drink out of the sink or the bathtub. One day I put some rocks in his bowl, and then he drank out of it. When I removed the rocks, he went back to drinking from the sink. Isn't this unusual?—*B.M.*

DEAR B.M.—Putting rocks in the cat's water bowl is an intriguing idea. Your cat may like the flavor of leached minerals. Water that has been standing for a while does get stale, but there is less chlorine in it then. Running water does have a different taste and physical properties than water that is standing.

Perhaps our cats, in their natural wisdom, are telling us something when they lick up drops coming from the faucet. Various minerals and animal byproducts in the soap and shampoo scum in the bathtub may also be attractive to some cats.

soap (cats and dogs)

DEAR DR. FOX—My cat has a strange habit—she wants to drink water coming from the washing machine, which has soap and bleach in it, even though I always have clean water around for her. She also likes to lick the top of my cleanser can. Can you help me with this?—*M.A.*

DEAR M.A.—Cats are often attracted to various household chemicals, such as bleach, disinfectants, deodorants, and detergents. This is why, just as with infants, one must keep all such chemicals carefully shut away in a cupboard. Do not encourage your cat to continue to drink dirty laundry water. Try enticing her instead with a little milk, soda, seltzer water, or regular water acidified with a vitamin C tablet. Because they were desert creatures originally, cats need little water. As they get older and more prone to kidney failure, it is advisable to encourage them to drink whatever fluids they will—except those containing common household chemicals!

DEAR DR. FOX—My pit bull-and-leopard hound is active and in good health. The problem is that he likes to eat soap. Does that mean he needs a food supplement?—*J.R.W.*

DEAR J.R.W.—Cravings in animals (and people) do sometimes mean that there is something lacking in their diet that they are trying to correct. Soap contains tallow, a rendered fatty product from slaughterhouses that is put into animal feed or into soap.

My guess is that your dog probably needs more fat in his diet, especially since he is active, and more so if he has a dry coat. Since some vitamins are fat soluble (vitamins A, D, and E), he may need some vitamin supplementation too.

Discuss those probabilities with your vet, or give your dog one teaspoon per fifteen pounds body weight of vegetable oil plus some lightly cooked or raw liver and fat from beef or chicken.

3

Play and Exercise

dangerous game (dogs)

DEAR DR. FOX—Could you please explain to me why our German shepherd eats bees? All we have to do is say "Bee" and she jumps up and catches one right out of the air and eats it. You would think that she'd get stung every time, but she doesn't. Once she did get stung, but all she did was lie down and rub her face on the ground. Then she went right back to her hobby.—A.B.

DEAR A.B.—Bees do more good than harm, and without them flowers would not get pollinated and our orchards would bear little fruit. Also, you must be careful, because in time your dog could become hypersensitive to bee venom, and hyperreaction could mean death. Why not get some substitute toys for your dog to snap at? My mutt Benji tries to snap and eat bees too—it's a game to chase a pollen-laden bee, but I don't encourage it, nor should you.

excessive exercise (cats and dogs)

DEAR DR. FOX—My dog and I have been jogging together for the past ten years. We run three miles in twenty-five minutes every day except Sunday, when we run seven miles (which takes an hour). Am I running my dog too much or too hard? She is eleven years old.—W.G.F.

DEAR W.G.F.—You may indeed be pushing your dog too hard—she's not a youngster anymore. Some dogs will run themselves into the ground just to please their owners, and they may really be too old or too sick to be running. Just as any human would-be jogger should have a checkup, jogging dogs should see their vets. Meanwhile, take it easy as the weather gets hotter and more humid, and never run your dog after she's had a lot to drink or eat.

61

DEAR DR. FOX—Our dog Snoopy has a heart condition and gets medicine to slow his heart. Lately he's been getting very perky and wants to play. Do you think we should play with him, or would this affect his heart?—*L.T.*

DEAR L.T.—A little play and exercise will do your dog more good than harm, as long as you don't overdo it. No wild chasing, leaping, or retrieving. A few minutes of a little wrestling, tug-of-war, and catch-the-ball (rather than run-and-retrieve) should be fine. Stop at once if your dog starts to show labored breathing, and avoid any strenuous activity during hot weather.

HEALTH REMINDER—HOT WEATHER EXERCISE

During hot weather, it's important to cut back on your pet's exercise. Too much exercise in the hot sun can cause heat stroke. The best times to exercise your pet are early morning or late evening.

Joggers who like to take their pets along, make special note of this caution.

DEAR DR. FOX—My Persian cat and I often play ball. But I notice that after two throws and retrieves, his breathing is unsteady. Could you please tell me if the excitement of playing can hurt him in any way?—*D.F.*

DEAR D.F.—Persian cats have normally pushed-in faces, and this could cause some breathing difficulties, especially when the cat has to carry a ball in his mouth. My advice is to let him catch his breath between pitches. But if after that he also seems to get dizzy and disoriented or has other difficulty in playing for any length of time, take him to your vet. Possibly there could be a problem with his heart or circulation that is reducing his exercise tolerance.

flying (parakeets)

DEAR DR. FOX—I have read that parakeets need exercise or they get bored. However, our parakeets don't come out when they're free to fly. And when they're finally taken out, they fly into the walls and bite my hand when I try to pick them up. What do you suggest?—*L.S.*

DEAR L.S.—Yes, parakeets and most other cage birds will get bored if confined all day in a small cage. And they get obese, too, which can eventually kill them. So a large flight-cage or a safe room for a daily flight is a must. Your birds will protest both being picked up and being put back into the cage, so do it at other times to break the negative association, and give them some special treat when you put them back into the cage. They will fly into walls, but only until they get used to the room. Give them some perches near the walls, too.

DEAR DR. FOX—I bought a parakeet about a year ago, and when I let her out of her cage she banged into the walls. I thought she would grow out of it, but she didn't. I had her wings clipped, but she can still fly. I'm afraid she'll hurt herself one of these days. What should I do?—*T.O.*

DEAR T.O.—Some parakeets get too excited or scared when they're out of their cages and injure themselves. That's why it's good to get a young bird so it can grow up accustomed to flying free indoors. You'll have to use patience in getting your bird used to freedom.

First, draw the curtains to cover the windows—many birds try to fly through a closed window. Next, place the cage on the floor or a table so the bird can get back in if she wants. Finally, put out some perches—tree branches or a clothes-dryer rack—so she has somewhere to perch. Don't give up.

importance of play and exercise (cats and dogs)

DEAR DR. FOX—Recently you suggested that if your cat bites you, you should give him a wool ball to play with. So I made my cat a wool ball and threw it to him. Since then, my cat brings back the ball to me, carrying it in his mouth just like a dog. He puts it in my hand and waits for me to throw it again. Could my cat be gifted?—*S.R.*

DEAR S.R.—Yes, your cat is gifted, as are most cats, only their owners haven't the gift of understanding to make this discovery. How many people never play with their cats? Half of all cat owners perhaps? What a terrible deprivation for both, since when playful relations are established, a new level of trust and understanding is attained and a new avenue for expressing affection opens up.

Keep on throwing that ball of wool. You can also next buy a cat-mobile, which I describe along with other games in my book *How to Be Your Pet's Best Friend*. Remember, those who play together are together also in heart.

DEAR DR. FOX—My brother owns three beagles. He uses them for hunting rabbits. He tells me that it's wrong to play with these dogs because they are hunting dogs, and it's impossible for a dog to be both a pet and a hunting dog. Do you agree?—*J.S.C.*

DEAR J.S.C.—Your brother is off the mark. Many hunters keep their dogs in a kennel or outdoor pen where they have little contact with the family, and these dogs often don't perform well in the field or live as long as those given plenty of human contact.

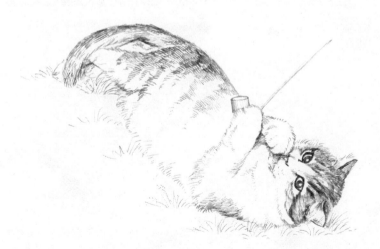

Play is an excellent way of exercising dogs, and it results in better physical condition for dogs than always cooping them up in a pen. It also establishes a bond of trust and affection between owner and dog. The more play the better, I say.

DEAR DR. FOX—My son keeps his Irish setter tied up most the time. When let loose, the dog races around and around the back yard until she's exhausted. Can you tell me why? She's a pedigreed dog and we expect her to be a real pal for the children, but she acts so crazy. Any advice?—MRS. R.G.

DEAR MRS. R.G.—Any dog who is kept tied up for prolonged periods is going to "blow its mind" when released. All that pent-up, frustrated energy combined with lack of regular attention, exercise, and companionship, will turn a dog into a hyperactive pest. Of course her situation could be aggravated if she is a product of bad breeding—in other words, a basically hyperactive dog to begin with—but she might improve with proper care. Let her blow off steam and then get on with obedience training, games, and regular attention, and you may make a good pal out of her. Being shackled is no life for any critter.

DEAR DR. FOX—The man next door is divorced and works five days a week. He keeps his poor dog penned in the backyard, and when he gets home he hardly ever plays with him. I often hear the dog crying, and occasionally I go out to pet him through the fence. When I do, he licks my hand as if he's glad to see someone. He just breaks my heart. What can I do?—L.E.

DEAR L.E.—I really appreciate and respect your concern for your neighbor's dog. Perhaps your neighbor is too tired after a day's work to spend much time with the poor dog. So why don't you go over and volunteer to exercise and groom the dog when his master is away? I'm sure he'll welcome your help. If he didn't love the dog, he would have dumped him long ago.

love of the outdoors (cats and dogs)

DEAR DR. FOX—My eleven-month-old Alaskan malamute has a mind of his own. I wish there were a way to keep him at home. I take him on long walks and give him affection, but he doesn't want to learn tricks. When he wants to go

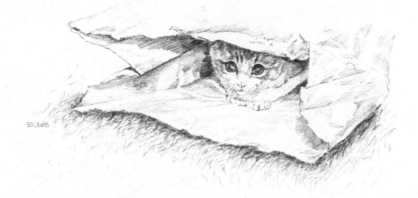

off somewhere, he just leaves; when I call him, he doesn't come half the time. I need to know how to rehabilitate this kind of dog. Can you please tell me more about Alaskan malamutes?—*D.W.*

DEAR *D.W.*—It sounds like your pet has a taste for the outdoors. If he were my dog, I'd have him neutered, and then he wouldn't want to roam so much. I would also build a dog run, or put him on a running line—a wire "clothesline" with a light chain toggled on it and attached to his collar. If you want a dog to be really attached to you, it's best to buy a pup that's around six to eight weeks old. Good luck!

DEAR DR. FOX—Our Siamese has the curiosity of a cat—he wants to go outside, cries at all the outside doors, and sneaks out whenever possible. We immediately retrieve him and bring him back into the house, which makes him very unhappy. We want to protect our beautiful kitty from the outside dangers and wish him to be only a house pet. But should we take a chance and let him have some freedom?—*M.S.*

DEAR *M.S.*—Siamese cats are very trainable, so buy a harness and leash and take your cat for walks. If your yard is absolutely dog-proof, you could attach the harness to a swivel-toggle tied onto a nylon cord that is attached to an overhead clothesline or length of wire. Keep it away from the fence so the cat doesn't hang himself. Alternatively, construct an outdoor pen of chicken wire; a tree stump to climb on, a sunning platform, and a box for shelter in the pen would be enjoyable fixtures.

toys (cats)

DEAR DR. FOX—Every time my kitten sees my rubber-bottomed thong shoes, he sniffs, rubs, attacks, plays, licks, and then sleeps on them. Can you tell me why?—*W.H.*

DEAR *W.H.*—Your cat wants to have some fun. Cats will get into all manner of things around the house, such as certain shampoos, rinses, leather shoes, thongs, and belts. These items all contain animal protein, whose taste and odor are enjoyable to many cats. You could probably design some fun cat toys from mousetail-like leather thongs with fake-fur bodies, or strips of leather tied onto little cloth sacks containing catnip, an herb that excites many cats. Try hanging some of these toys from a doorknob or even from the ceiling, with a coil spring or rubber band attachment to make it recoil when the cat leaps at it.

toys (dogs)

DEAR DR. FOX—I'm a five-month-old Chihuahua terrier, and I love to eat peaches, carrots, candy, wood, and dirt. I also have a habit of digging in the grass and sticking my nose in the ground like a pig. This is all making me sick, so how can I stop it?—*CHICO*

DEAR *CHICO*—You're still young, and you'll just have to learn that dirt and sticks will make you sick. Your owner should give you safe toys, an old shoe or a strip of rawhide to chew on. Things that break and get swallowed can cause you serious internal injury. Enjoy your digging, but not in someone else's lawn. It's a good idea to have a hookworm and regular worm checkup soon, since you can easily pick parasites up from the ground where other infested dogs have been. P.S. Lay off too much candy; fruit, vegetables, and nutritious table scraps will be much better for your diet—and your figure.

DEAR DR. FOX—My cockapoo has many toys but plays only with one, a small, soft, squeaky tiger. Can you explain this preference? Also, how often does a dog come into heat?—B.A.

DEAR B.A.—It's not unusual for a dog to develop a preference for one specific toy. The animal may simply like the way it squeaks or feels. Your cockapoo may think her squeak toy is alive; in her mind, it's a puppy or small prey. Female dogs sometimes have false pregnancies and will covet a favorite toy or even a sock and use it as a puppy substitute, carrying it around, curling up with it, and even growling protectively over it. Dogs usually have two heats a year.

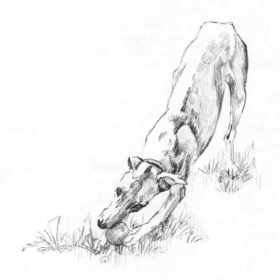

4

Grooming

DEAR DR. FOX—After being scratched and clawed, I give up. So tell me, how does one give a cat a bath without a fight?—A.B.

DEAR A.B.—I'll give you a question in return: Why would you want to bathe a cat in the first place? Many people have the idea that cats should be bathed regularly, like children. This is nonsense! Cats are desert animals; they groom themselves with their own saliva and keep themselves very, very clean that way.

Only a sick cat or one with a serious flea infestation should be dipped or bathed. Then, rather than immersing the cat, it's preferable to have someone gently hold it while you sponge it with warm water containing the antiflea medication or a mild shampoo. After that, rinse it off with warm water. You may dry the cat with a towel, or, if it's not afraid of the noise, with a hair dryer.

bathing and shampooing (dogs)

DEAR DR. FOX—I would like to know how often a short-haired beagle should have a bath. He is an indoor dog and is rarely in the woods or fields.—C.E.H.

DEAR C.E.H.—Some indoor dogs need to be bathed every couple of weeks, others every few months. This wide variable is due to the fact that some dogs secrete more "doggy-smell" oils than others, so one has to gauge things more by one's nose and personal tolerance level than any set rule. However, for outdoor dogs regular bathing is questionable, since the oils in the skin help keep the coat slick and waterproof. For very smelly dogs and sensitive owner-noses, every few days a "dry bath" with baby powder or cornstarch rubbed into the fur for a few minutes and then brushed out is very effective.

DEAR DR. FOX—We have a fifteen-year-old border collie. She is awfully dirty, and her hair is oily. We are scared to give her a bath because she might catch cold. Would an instant shampoo be too harsh for her skin? Any suggestions?—L.B.

DEAR L.B.—Old dogs tend to get rather smelly whether they live indoors or out. An outdoor dog shouldn't be bathed very often because, unlike an indoor dog, it needs to have the protective oils in its coat, which a shampoo would remove. So I would suggest a shampoo no oftener than once a month. Dry your dog well, and brush her daily to stimulate the skin and help bring up the natural oils. Use baby powder to eliminate some of the doggy odor. Rub it into your dog's coat (outdoors) every week or so as needed. Let it stay in for a few minutes, then brush out vigorously.

DEAR DR. FOX—My sister bathes her dog in people shampoo. Is this OK, or could it be harmful? The dog has a real "doggy odor."—J.T.

DEAR J.T.—Regular shampooing with any kind of human shampoo is bad for a dog. Healthy cats never need to be bathed. A good grooming is best for both cats and dogs. Bathe a dog as infrequently as possible. If you must shampoo your dog, use a mild shampoo.

bathing and shampooing (parakeets)

DEAR DR. FOX—My parakeets like to take baths but don't seem to like it when I spray their feathers. Is it OK to put some bath spray into the bathwater?—R.B.

DEAR R.M.—Detergents of any kind will remove the natural oils from your birds' feathers, so I advise fresh water for a bath. Some bird fanciers like to give their birds a dish of powdered soil or fine sand to dust-bathe in. Wild birds generally dust-bathe themselves and rid themselves of mites and lice.

body odor (dogs)

DEAR DR. FOX—Over the years I have noticed that right after we begin giving our dog heartworm preventives, she emits an offensive odor. It stops in the fall when medication is discontinued. We bathe her, but the odor returns immediately.—J.M.

DEAR J.M.—Heartworm and certain other medicines can and do cause a change in an animal's odor, especially when the drug is on the animal's breath—like garlic! But better to live with a dog who smells "off" for a while than risk contracting heartworm. Dog owners, when summer approaches, please have your dogs checked for heartworm, and give preventive medicine if and when your vet indicates it is needed. Heartworm is a common canine killer.

DEAR DR. FOX—We bathe our cocker spaniel every Saturday and brush him every day. He has no fleas and no worms and is healthy and friendly. Our only problem is his smell. When you step in the house, it hits you.—E.G.F.

DEAR E.G.F.—"Doggy odor" is a common problem, but especially with certain breeds. First, get some room-deodorizing dispensers. Then check your dog's ears as a possible source of "D.O." As usual, give your dog its weekly outdoor rub with baby powder.

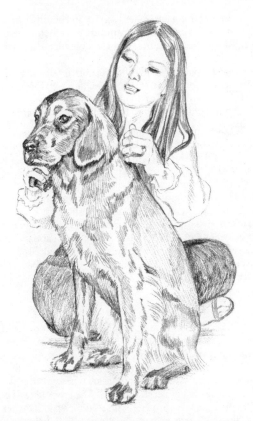

DEAR DR. FOX—We have a Chinese pug who has a foul odor we can't eliminate or control. I can bathe him in the morning and he will smell clean, but before nightfall the odor is back. His breath is also foul. Since Pug is strictly a house dog, his problem keeps the house polluted. We need your advice.—R.E.W.

DEAR R.E.W.—Smelly dogs, no matter how lovable, are certainly a problem. Body odor can come from various parts of the dog's body—from dirty, tartar-covered teeth, infected gums, ears, feet, and glands, or excessively oily skin. A bath with mild shampoo every other week and a daily grooming with a powdering of baby powder into the coat first (well rubbed in) will certainly help.

I would give him more fresh-cooked vegetables, hamburger, and cottage cheese. Canned meat and meat byproducts can also contribute to body odor.

brushing (cats)

DEAR DR. FOX—I have to spend about an hour a day brushing my cat. I work so hard to remove hairballs and snarls, but by morning she has just as many as the night before. My vet wants to shave her, but I hate the thought. The hairdresser has solutions that keep hair from snarling. Would they hurt her?—B.L.

DEAR B.L.—Static cling causes the laundry in the dryer to cling together. The same with your cat—when she runs around on synthetic nylon and polyester carpets and upholstery, she builds up a static charge that is aggravated each time you brush her.

A moist brush may help, but a good thinning out (not shaving) by a pet groomer is the answer. In fact, a good groomer will make life easier for you and your knotted cat. Be careful of all antistatic and anti-hair snarl chemicals. When your cat grooms herself, she might ingest some, to the detriment of her health.

DEAR DR. FOX—I cannot keep up with the tangles in my cat's hair, which is about three inches long on various parts of her body. I've had to take her to the vet on three occasions, and since we live on a fixed income, this is a hardship. Any advice?—MRS. R.H.

DEAR MRS. R.H.—First, you should realize that cats were never meant to have long hair. That is a product of human intervention with cats' genetics. I suggest a daily grooming or combing (a moist brush will cause less static tangle) and a careful trimming to thin out the long fur and remove underfur matting.

A trip to the groomer would be worthwhile. A good cat handler can do wonders. Too many vets give too many tranquilizers to fur-matted cats whose owners don't put in a daily grooming. Once your cat's coat has been cleaned, make grooming a daily routine.

brushing (dogs)

DEAR DR. FOX—We comb our Lhasa apso puppy every day. Do you think that is too much? I think a brush would do a better job, but she does not like it, no matter what kind I try. Any ideas?—B.L.H.

DEAR B.L.H.—Lhasa apsos need a daily grooming because their coats tangle so easily. I would advise a visit to the groomer, who will trim your dog's long "feathers" and make the coat easier to manage. The groomer will be able to suggest the ideal brush. Fine wire brushes with a rubber-pad base act rather like a comb, and your dog may prefer that to a bristle brush. To help the coat develop a nice sheen, put a teaspoon of vegetable oil in the food each day, plus a pinch of brewer's yeast or a crushed yeast tablet.

ear cropping (dogs)

DEAR DR. FOX—Our Great Dane puppy bitch is allergic to the adhesive tape used in wrapping cropped ears. The cropped edges quickly get irritated. Since neither we nor our vet could come up with any alternatives, we stopped wrapping. Is there any cosmetic surgery that could be performed to make her ears stand? Could it be done at the same time she's being spayed?—L.L.

DEAR L.L.—Why would you or your veterinarian even consider cropping your dog's ears? This is a barbaric practice done for show purposes and has absolutely no benefit to the dog. Vets who do this unnecessary mutilation, and owners who insist it be done, should have their heads examined.

Your dog is probably too old now to make her cropped ears stand up by themselves. The mutilation is best done around eight weeks of age. Some vets put plastic inserts into the dog's ears after they're cropped to make them stick up when they won't by themselves. Why make your dog suffer from your vanity? The ears are one of the most sensitive parts of a dog's anatomy. Have a heart!

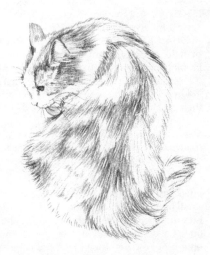

DEAR DR. FOX—I bought my Doberman when he was three months old and had his ears cropped shortly thereafter. He can hold his left ear up when he's out playing or when he's around a lot of people, but otherwise it flops. My vet says the muscles in his ear are not strong enough to hold the ear upright, but my intuition says he may grow out of it. Could you please comment?—H.W.

DEAR H.W.—My first reaction to your letter was, "Poor puppy! Having to have the most sensitive part of his body—his ears—cut up at three months of age!" And why? To live up to some brutal, ridiculous standard of certain people in this country who think it's OK to crop dogs' ears. (It's outlawed in England.) In my opinion, vets, breeders, and show people who have their dogs so mutilated should be boycotted. And I have little respect for show judges who still accept ear-cropped dogs and do nothing to eliminate this inhumane practice from the show ring.

As for your pet, nothing can be done, so let it be a lesson to all who ask what's wrong with your dog.

fur balls (cats)

DEAR DR. FOX—What can I do so that my cat won't shed her fur so badly, especially in winter months? I brush her about once a day, but that doesn't seem to help. She vomits and has fur balls about once a month. Is that something to worry about?—R.C.B.

DEAR R.C.B.—Keep up the brushing, since some cats shed all the time. Don't get upset about the fur balls. They are messy, but it's quite natural for a cat to throw up fur balls every few days or weeks. Not all cats do this; some pass the fur out in their stools instead. Fur is swallowed normally as part of self-grooming. Giving your cat some roughage like dry food or fresh grass can help the passage of fur balls and reduce the buildup of large balls of fur, which will cause digestive problems and loss of condition.

hair trimming (dogs)

DEAR DR. FOX—My husband insists that we should cut our old English sheepdog's hair from around his brown eyes and under his chin because he dribbles so much. I thought you weren't supposed to cut a sheepdog's hair in order to protect his eyes.—MRS. H.A.

DEAR MRS. H.A.—Old English sheepdogs were bred to have faces covered by hair to protect them from getting their eyes injured while running through brambles and thornbushes when rounding up lost sheep. It is a myth that clipping their heads so they can see will make them go blind.

On the contrary, chronic eye infections are common in this breed, because their eyes are being constantly irritated by long hair. So let your dog see and enjoy the light of day, and trim his "beard," too, so he doesn't soak you with it. Sheepdogs who have had their eyes covered for years will be more sensitive to light when their eyes are cleared. So after such a "facelift," keep the dog indoors for a few days out of direct sunlight, and all should be well.

DEAR DR. FOX—I usually groom my minischnauzer with an Oster clipper, but occasionally I take her for a professional grooming. In the beginning I noticed small bumps on her back after each clipping. I rubbed them with sulfadene, and they disappeared. Now, after clipping, she develops red spots with white centers on her abdomen, pants, and becomes very restless. On one occasion she kept me up most of the night, and I did not know how to relieve her. The vet gave her a cortisone shot. It took about six hours for her to settle down. Why does this happen and what can I do about it?—B.G.

DEAR B.G.—Your dog probably developed a hypersensitive "clipper burn" reaction. Try lubricating the head of the clippers with a different kind of oil, and make sure the clippers are sharp and properly aligned. Neosporin cream should be put on accidental "burn" areas to prevent secondary bacterial infection. Dogs with very sensitive skins should be clipped and snipped by hand; electric clippers may be just too rough on them.

SUMMER HEALTH REMINDER

Do not shave your dog all the way down to the skin. Dogs may sunburn, and their fur actually insulates them from heat and insect bites. A trim is sufficient.

In addition, daily brushing is necessary to remove the heavy undercoat. Take the precaution at the same time of checking for external parasites—ticks and fleas. Pay special attention to between the toes, in and behind the ears, under the front legs, and the head area.

DEAR DR. FOX—When my mixed breed eats or drinks, her long ears (she is part cocker) get in the dish, and the fur gets matted together. Bathing will not take out this matting. Can you help? I'd like to do this by myself, because I am a senior citizen and the vet wants $25 to help.—A.K.

DEAR A.K.—Poor cocker spaniels, bred to have such long ears that they get in the way all the time, get matted with food and dirt, and become infected. The idea, I'm told, behind this man-made abnormality was that long ears would help the dog scent and track better by dragging on the ground and stirring up the trail. It certainly would benefit cockers if breeders selected for shorter ears. The best you can do is to trim the long "feathers" off the ends of your pooch's auditory appendages and buy a small, narrow, deep food bowl (a no-spill water bowl would be ideal) so that her ears fall on each side of the bowl outside the rim.

DEAR DR. FOX—A veterinarian has told my friend not to trim the hair in front of her Lhasa apso's eyes because they are too sensitive to sunlight. Is this correct?—*S.A.*

DEAR S.A.—It is a common myth that dogs with long hair over the eyes need it to protect their eyes from sunlight. Of course, when you lift the hair the dog will blink, and you will see that its eyes are reddened from irritation by the hair. Your friend will be doing her Lhasa a favor if she trims the dog's bangs or ties them on top of its head with a ribbon.

GROOMING TIP

Do not use turpentine or paint remover, which can burn the pet's skin, to remove tar or paint from an animal's coat. Instead, simply cut out the patch of affected hair. It will grow back soon enough.

---

nail clipping (cats)

DEAR DR. FOX—Our cat, Mandy, seems to have her claws out so that even when she's just walking around the house they catch in the carpet. Also, we have found small pieces of claw around the place. Are we supposed to clip our cat's nails? Is she just clawing on purpose? Is something lacking in her diet that causes her nails to become brittle and break?—*M.I.*

DEAR M.I.—No, there's nothing lacking in your cat's diet. It is quite natural for old claws to shed and new nails to grow. Very often the claws of indoor cats and, to a far greater degree, indoor dogs require trimming. Since indoor pets walk on a soft carpet surface most of the time the nails don't wear down naturally. When you trim the claws, have someone hold the cat, then squeeze the paw to extrude the claw and snip the end with nail clippers—tip only, or it will hurt and bleed.

DEAR DR. FOX—Since I have kept my previously outdoor cat indoors, her claws have grown longer. How long should they be, and how often should a veterinarian clip them?—*E.V.*

DEAR E.V.—Get your cat either a scratching post made of tough carpet material tacked onto a vertical board or a tree stump with bark on it. This will help your cat adapt to life indoors and keep her claws down. Your vet can show you how to snip your cat's nails with clippers. It's a painless job and easy, provided you hold your cat correctly and she's not afraid.

DEAR DR. FOX—My three-year-old cat will not let me brush or cut her nails. When I try, she scratches and bites me. Another problem I have with her is that lately she has started to scratch the rug on the stairs. No matter what I do, I can't break her of this habit.—*M.B.*

DEAR M.B.—Many cats object violently to having their claws trimmed and even to being groomed. Fortunately, cats can and do groom themselves well, so unless you have an especially unkempt cat, let her be and don't force the issue.

Have you tried giving your cat a carpet-covered, catnip-spiced scratching post? It may really turn her on so that she prefers it to your stair rug. But if she were my cat and were only clawing a small area of the rug, I'd live with it. One can't have too perfect and immaculate a house with a healthy and active cat in residence—and it's worth the tradeoff every time.

nail clipping (guinea pigs)

DEAR DR. FOX—My three-year-old guinea pig's nails are very long, and I would like to trim them. How far back do they have to be cut, and can I use dog clippers?—L.C.

DEAR L.C.—Dog clippers or even nail clippers will do very well for this job. But you'll need another person's help—someone to hold the guinea pig gently but firmly. Then extend its leg and hold the claw up to the light. You should see a red or pinkish quick toward the base of the claw. Cut a short distance away from this to avoid bleeding. The process is painless, unless you accidentally snip this sensitive quick. If your pet struggles, it's not because it hurts, but because it's afraid and doesn't understand what's going on. Good luck!

5

Ailments
and Preventive Medicine

THE LOOK OF HEALTH

anatomical questions (hamsters)

DEAR DR. FOX—I'm thirteen years old and planning to be a vet when I get older, because I love animals. I have a question about one of my hamsters. Every night (it goes away during the day) I notice a blue dot in his right eye. Sometimes it covers almost all his eye, and other times it is very small.—ANIMAL LOVER

DEAR ANIMAL LOVER—If what you describe as a blue dot seems to grow out of the inside corner of your hamster's eye, then it is his third eyelid—a protective membrane that covers the eye when an animal sleeps but also shows when the eye is infected. If there's no discharge from the eye in the morning, don't worry. But if there is a discharge or if your hamster is pawing his eye, have a veterinarian look at it. Good luck in your future career as a veterinarian—it's hard work getting your DVM degree, but it's worth it, I think.

anatomical questions (pigs)

DEAR DR. FOX—A friend of mine says that pigs don't have veins. Several people agreed with her. I couldn't find anything in the encyclopedia. It may be a crazy question, but please answer it.—L.P.

DEAR L.P.—Pigs do have veins, as do all animals that have hearts, and that not only includes mammals like us, but also birds, reptiles, and amphibians. Pigs have large veins in their ears that are easily located for injecting anesthetics when they need surgery. I can't imagine why your friends should believe otherwise.

75

Pigs, like other mammals, are more similar to us—anatomically, physiologically, and emotionally—than they are different. Perhaps your friends don't like that idea.

anatomical questions (rabbits)

DEAR DR. FOX—My rabbit has this ball in her neck. My friend says it's her milk glands, so I thought that she was pregnant, only there are no signs of babies. What is happening?—CONFUSED

DEAR CONFUSED—Your friend certainly has confused you. A rabbit's milk glands are not under its neck but in the usual place—on the belly, as in a cat or dog. What your rabbit has is a dewlap, a large fold of skin with fatty tissue beneath. This is an indicator of maturity and a sign of status among rabbits. It may be quite an impressive display—like the hump on a Brahma bull, the beard on a goat or a man, and naturally padded hips in women.

animals in pain

DEAR DR. FOX—How can you tell if an animal is in pain? I know that when you have surgery you are in pain afterwards. How come pets are not always given painkillers after surgery?—P.T.

DEAR P.T.—Some animals in severe pain act very depressed, not wanting to move or eat, in contrast to other pets—and people—who cry and act up a great deal. This pain depression often leads to the erroneous impression that the animal isn't suffering, when in fact it should be given an analgesic. However, painkillers must be given judiciously, as they can interfere with recovery. Some pain helps protect an injured leg from being walked on, for example. Horse racers know this, hence they give powerful painkillers so a lame horse can race and earn its keep—a national atrocity, being fought by The Humane Society of the United States.

beak growth (parakeets)

DEAR DR. FOX—I give my parakeet cuttlebone, and he has gravel and a sanded perch in his cage, but his beak keeps growing! Is that normal?—R.Z.

DEAR R.Z.—What are you worring about? It's very common in caged birds. Check to see if the beak is scaly—that might indicate mites. Is it soft? That could mean a deficiency of vitamins. Otherwise, it's a natural condition; own a bird and be a beak-barber.

dandruff (cats)

DEAR DR. FOX—My cat has a problem that I haven't seen discussed in your column. She has dandruff. My vet gave me some pills for it, but the results were nil.—J.B.

DEAR J.B.—Dandruff in animals can mean many things. Lack of polyunsaturated fats and too much carbohydrate in the diet is sometimes implicated, so a teaspoonful of safflower oil in your cat's food each day may help. Some cats develop dandruff after they have been neutered and eventually begin to lose hair.

Treatment and hormones are indicated in such instances. I would recommend a thorough clinical workup, including a thyroid-function test. It's possible that nothing is wrong and that it's just one of those things, but to be sure, further tests are needed.

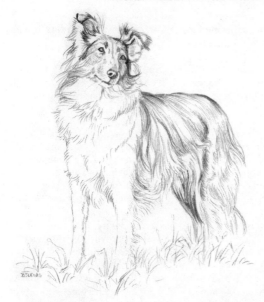

dandruff (dogs)

DEAR DR. FOX—Our dog has a problem with dandruff. Is there some ointment or shampoo I can get for him?—*R.W.*

DEAR R.W.—Dry, scurfy coats are often associated with too much carbohydrate in a diet and not enough unsaturated fats. Some dandruff is natural, since the skin is being constantly renewed and sloughed. Regular grooming will help; so will approximately one tablespoonful of vegetable oil daily in the food per thirty pounds of body weight. A little brewer's yeast is also said to be good for the coat—half a teaspoon per day is sufficient for the average-sized dog.

feather loss (parakeets)

DEAR DR. FOX—My parakeet is molting. He flaps his wings as if flying while in the cage, and small feathers fly everywhere. What can it be and how should I stop it? He also chews on a hanging perch (wood).—*D.B.*

DEAR D.B.—First, you must keep your bird warm (70–80 degrees F) and provided with additional good-quality food, vitamin supplements, and cuttle-fish bone for calcium. Feather loss means tremendous heat loss, because the bird has impaired insulation. Without such care your bird may never regain condition to grow back his feathers.

There are many reasons for feather loss. One is feather lice, which bite through the feathers. So have your vet examine your bird and come up with a cure.

DEAR DR. FOX—I have a blue parakeet that I bought about three years ago. I feed him correctly, and his cage is perfectly equipped. At six weeks of age he started to molt. This year he is going through a bad molting period. He sits quietly all day, as if he is feeling ill. What could be wrong?—*M.W.*

DEAR M.W.—Molting in birds sometimes seems to bring on a general depression or listlessness. Prolonged molting, or poor regrowth of feathers, along with these behavior changes is a sign of illness. But since your bird has molting at six weeks of age, he may be suffering from French molt, which is linked with overbreeding and possibly poor nutrition.

There is no cure. Such birds chill easily and succumb to infection, especially respiratory diseases. So if you decide not to have him put to sleep, keep him warm at all times and fortify his diet with vitamin A, B complex, and iodine. If he will take a little flaked or powdered kelp (seaweed) plus multivitamin drops on his seed, so much the better.

feather loss (parrots)

DEAR DR. FOX—I turned a ten-by-twelve-foot cage into an aviary for my parrot. The aviary maintains an even temperature and contains a large, always open cage, high and low perches, and window sills. He gets a diet of seed, apples, raw peanuts in the shell, and occasionally a little meat and cookies. But even with this care, he molts all the time and is getting bare patches. What am I doing wrong?—F.P.W.

DEAR F.P.W.—It sounds like your bird has a nice aviary. However, not all exotic birds—and that includes parrots—adapt well to captivity. Molting can be due to a variety of factors, including dietary imbalance or insufficiency, feather mites, drafts, lack of sunlight or warmth, and emotional stress, including boredom, when the bird may scratch and mutilate itself. Be sure the seed you give is fresh. Add vitamin drops (A and D), and provide your bird with a greater variety of fresh fruits, including grapes and bananas. He may enjoy an infrared heat lamp and do better under a strip light that emits some ultraviolet. Have your vet also check for feather lice or mites.

fur changing color (cats)

DEAR DR. FOX—Cherokee, my six-year-old solid-black cat, turned 50 percent gray a few months ago. I assumed it was because of his age. But over a period of about two months, he turned totally black again. He is on daily medication for urinary problems. Could the medicine have caused the sudden appearance, then disappearance, of grayness?—K.H.

DEAR K.H.—Ever hear the popular saying about stress turning someone's hair gray overnight? It's not simply a myth; there are actual cases on record of human beings, mules, cats, and dogs turning gray after some serious physical or psychological stress. I would suggest that your cat's change in coat was related to some form of stress and not his medication. And if it were due to aging, your cat would stay gray and not grow a normal coat again. Most likely the physical and emotional distress of his urinary problem is to blame, although social stress in the home could also be at the root of his troubles.

DEAR DR. FOX—One summer when we went on vacation and left our dear Siamese with a neighbor, we had a frightening experience. The cat we found on our return was a different color—nearly all cream-white, with the black markings gone. We learned she had refused to eat and was constantly mourning our absence. Have you ever heard of this strange hair-change phenomenon?—E.B.

DEAR E.B.—Your account illustrates dramatically how animals can and do suffer emotionally. Color change, even turning gray all over, has been described in humans and animals under emotional stress, but not, to my knowledge, in Siamese. So you have a first.

Siamese cat owners *have* commented on how pale their cats were after a few weeks at a boarding kennel. They usually think it's due to lack of sunlight. Clearly, in the light of your cat's consistent reactions, the conclusion is that loss of dark pigmentation can be a sign of emotional distress, pigment production being closely related to the hormonal system that is activated under stress. Furthermore, emotional distress does affect the body's physiology and ability to withstand disease.

DEAR DR. FOX—Two years ago, my husband and I adopted a stray adult common alley cat. He was a beautiful solid black color. In the last two months three-quarters of his fur has turned auburn. In the sunshine, parts look bright orange. I have never seen a cat like mine. What causes this?—K.H.

DEAR K.H.—Some cats do change color after basking in sunlight. Even lying by a sunny window can bleach out the coat, bringing a reddish highlight to a black coat.

Siamese, in contrast, turn darker when in a colder environment, since their coat pigmentation is affected by temperature. Orange-red coat color (and hair pigmentation in humans) has been linked with excess copper in drinking water, leached from copper pipes by water acidified with industrial pollution. Some pet-food dyes can have similar effects.

DEAR DR. FOX—My Persian cat is bathed about every six weeks with all the best solutions, but in the last two months she has developed yellow- or brownish-stained paws, especially the front ones. She has been snow white since birth and is in perfect health.—W.A.P.

DEAR W.A.P.—In my experience, yellow-stained paws can relate to food coloring. Many catfoods contain dyes that can turn various parts of the animal's coat a yellowish or brownish color. I suggest that you consider making up a special diet for your cat or try a brand of catfood that contains no coloring.

fur loss (cats)

DEAR DR. FOX—My ten-year old cat grooms all the time and is losing her coat in places. I was told it was probably an allergy. Would brewer's yeast help her fur to come in? I have a flea collar on her, just in case fleas are causing the problem.—MRS. R.Mc.

DEAR MRS. R.Mc.—You'll have to do some detective work to find out if, indeed, your cat has an allergy. First, take the flea collar off; some collars are responsible for *contact dermatitis*, resulting in hair loss and reddening of the skin.

Next, to find out if your cat has fleas, check for flea droppings in her coat. These are shiny black specks, like coal dust, which turn reddish-brown when put on a piece of white paper and moistened with a drop of water. If you find fleas, bathe your cat with a cat shampoo that contains a flea-killing insecticide, and then follow up with a flea dip while the cat is still wet from her bath. As for brewer's yeast, some people claim it repels mosquitos and fleas, but there is no documentary proof.

Instead of an allergy, it is also possible that your cat has a hormonal imbalance. Skin disorders generally require quite involved tests and trial treatments before the best solution can be found. You'll have to be patient with your vet and your cat alike.

DEAR DR. FOX—My cat's fine silky hair comes out all over everything, and she has become the devil to live with. Is there any vitamin or medicine I can give her? She is spayed and is usually no trouble.—E.A.F.

DEAR E.A.F.—Some cats shed almost constantly, while other indoor cats have a more seasonal rhythm. Diet is not usually a factor in a chronic shedder. If your neutered cat is shedding so badly that she's developing bald spots, however, she may need hormone replacement. Meanwhile, try to get your cat used to having her fur vacuumed. Many cats enjoy a daily vacuuming, and this makes it much easier to get rid of loose fur. Using a moist sponge to wipe up fur on rugs and cushions will cut out the static electricity and make cleaning time less of a chore.

DEAR DR. FOX—My cat is healthy, but she is losing all her fur around her tail. She seems to be breaking out there, also. She is terrified of strangers, and getting her to a vet would be very difficult. (She's been once, to be spayed.) Is there anything I can try before going through the ordeal of taking her to the vet? Our vet always has a number of dogs in his office, and she becomes a biting, slashing, terrified animal when I try to take her out of the house. Does she remember being spayed?—MRS. T.Y.

DEAR MRS. T.Y.—Some vets will make house calls, so open up the phone book and do some checking till you find one. Cats have scent glands on their tails, and sometimes these become infected or, because of a hormonal imbalance, function abnormally. That your cat has been spayed may be part of the problem. Make sure she isn't self-mutilating. Tense, anxious cats will literally tear out their fur, so you may need to focus on what might be affecting her emotionally. My guess is that hormone-replacement therapy will correct the problem.

DEAR DR. FOX—My cat, Tiger, has been shedding his winter fur for a couple of months now. Could you tell me how long this will last?—A.W.

DEAR A.W.—Come winter, many cats start to shed just as though it's summertime. The most prevalent reason is because they are resting on a hot radiator or by a hot-air vent much of the day. So groom your cat more frequently—this will help reduce fur-ball problems. Buy a humidifier, which will not only reduce your heat bills but make the atmosphere better for you and your cat.

DEAR DR. FOX—Every summer, my tiger cat gets so skinny his sides sink way in. When fall comes he starts to fill out, and becomes Mr. Five-by-five. Can you solve this mystery?—S.E.A.

DEAR S.E.A.—The same thing happens to one of my animals at home. Come summer, she looks so different that one of my neighbors once accused me of starving her. Another neighbor thought I had adopted another animal. Many cats and dogs look shiny after they've shed down to a light summer coat. Also, it's not unusual for the weather to affect their appetites. Don't you feel less like eating on hot days? If you insist on worrying, then to be on the safe side, take a stool sample to your vet and have it checked for worms.

fur loss (dogs)

DEAR DR. FOX—My cocker spaniel and German shepherd are constantly shedding all over the house. Is there anything I can do, besides brushing, to stop this problem? It gets tiring sweeping the floor three times a day.—K.M.

DEAR K.M.—Dear tired floor-sweeper, I'm afraid that living indoors is part of your dogs' (and most dogs') shedding problem. If they were outside most of the time, their coats would be "in synch" with the seasons. Indoors, with heat, air conditioning, and artificial light, the natural coat cycle can be disrupted. Diet is another factor: lack of natural fats and oils and excess calcium in some pet foods can cause dogs' coats to become dry and shed. Supplement your dogs' food with vegetable oil and nutritional yeast (one teaspoon of each per thirty-pound dog), and get your dogs used to a daily grooming with the vacuum cleaner. Yes—it's quick and easy once your dog accepts it. There is no alternative—we can't let our dogs roam free.

DEAR DR. FOX—Our poodle has lost most of her hair, except on her head. We had her operated on recently, and it was thought that the surgery would stop her hair from coming out, but it didn't. I give her vitamins A, D, and E. What else can I do?—D.K.

DEAR D.K.—Your poodle was probably operated on to see if she had a tumor, most likely around the adrenal glands. The vitamins and oil probably won't do any harm or be of much benefit either. Your vet should explore some hormone-replacement therapy, but that may well be a shot in the dark. Perhaps it's best to get your dog a coat. There are a variety of styles and colors at your local pet store—or you can fashion your own. Many poodles are bald, and don't look at all bad when suitably attired for a walk outdoors.

fur loss (squirrels)

DEAR DR. FOX—We have a family of squirrels living in a tree in our back-yard, and they are losing their fur. Some of the small ones are almost bare except for their tails. I feed these animals, and I wonder if there is something I could give them to help cure their condition.—M.C.

DEAR M.C.—The squirrels most likely have mange, a mite infestation that can cause extensive hair loss. Really, there's nothing that you can do, save catch them in a humane box-trap and give them appropriate medication, which is nei-ther a practical nor an ecologically sound solution.

Diseases do help regulate wildlife populations. The best you can do is to put out a little food for the squirrels, but not too much, otherwise you will be encouraging a population explosion that may lead to more sickness, suffering, and ecological imbalance.

pigment changes (dogs)

DEAR DR. FOX—My Siberian husky is white with one blue eye and one brown eye. Every winter his nose turns from black to pinkish-red. Why does this happen?—D.C.

DEAR D.C.—Loss of pigment on dogs' noses is quite common with changes in season. Less sunlight in winter can mean less skin stimulation of pigment-producing cells called melanophores.

Some dogs like collies have impaired pigment production that can lead to sun-burn and solar-ray hypersensitivity. You have nothing to worry about—like odd-colored eyes, it's just one of those things and probably has a hereditary basis.

pigment changes (goldfish)

DEAR DR. FOX—I have five goldfish living together. I noticed that one of these fish has red eyes, unlike the others, and its underside is white! Does this mean that the fish is an albino? Or is it diseased? We've had this fish for years, and it's a favorite.—A.B.

DEAR A.B.—It's not unusual for healthy goldfish to lose or gain pigment on certain parts of their bodies. Some people believe that feeding them a little raw chopped meat or liver will help them stay a rich color. Actually, goldfish are "gold-plated"—that is, their pigmentation is only scale-deep. Those without any pigment anywhere are true albinos. Yours is piebald, and quite healthy, I'm sure.

DEAR DR. FOX—I've had my goldfish for about one year, and I have never changed their feeding time or been irregular in changing the water. One night I noticed red bloodlike streaks through one of my goldfish's tail and all his fins. What's wrong with him?—*G.H.*

DEAR G.H.—There's no simple answer for your fish's exotic illness. If there are no lumps or blemishes on your fish's fins (which would indicate a fungus or bacterial infection), I would suspect a possible nutritional problem. If you are using a dry commercial feed, add a little lean, raw hamburger, liver, or chopped earthworms, plus one tablet (100 mg) of vitamin C dissolved in the water. Prior to changing the dirty water in the fishbowl, always let the water from the tap stand in an open bowl for twenty-four hours. This will help get rid of chlorine, which can make fish sick. It will also prevent sudden chilling; fresh, cold tap water can cause red streaks to appear, a sign of congestion from an abrupt temperature change.

weight loss (cats)

DEAR DR. FOX—My part-calico cat has lost a lot of weight, even though he eats well. He comes home for meals; otherwise he stays out for hours and hours. He's pathetic to look at—skinny and scared, like a drug addict. Are there are vitamins I can get for him? At present I can't afford a vet, but I need help.—*S.N.*

DEAR S.N.—Since your cat wants out all the time, one possibility is that he's a super-"horny" tom and is literally wearing himself out. The best cure is to have him neutered. Your cat could also have internal parasites (such as tapeworms) from killing and eating mice and other wild animals outside. He could even have feline viral leukemia tumors that are draining his strength. A thorough veterinary examination is necessary. Vitamins can't hurt, but neither can they cure. Tell the vet that you are of limited financial means—most vets are understanding and will give you a break.

PHYSICAL IDIOSYNCRACIES

extra toes (cats)

DEAR DR. FOX—About three months ago we adopted an all-white kitten, and recently we have noticed that he has seven toes—four fingers and a thumb that has two little fingers on the side! Is this rare, and will it do any harm to him in the future?—*S.*

DEAR S.—You do have an unusual cat—in England we called them "mittens," and this trait of having supernumerary digits is heritable. I'm not sure what the percentage incidence of this is, but it is lower, I believe, in the pure varieties of cats such as Siamese and Abyssinians, because it is considered an undesirable quality in show cats. People are sometimes born with an extra finger or two also, and in some cultures it's regarded as a sinister or powerful sign. I'm sure it's of little use for mouse-catching, but it won't get in the way of happiness for your feline friend.

odd-colored eyes

DEAR DR. FOX—My family has been farming for more than fifty years. In that time, all our calves were born with dark-brown eyes. A month ago, a calf was born with *blue* eyes. Is this unusual? We want to keep her for show. Do you think her eyes will change to brown as she gets older?—*M.U.*

DEAR M.U.—Calves are sometimes born with one or both eyes lacking the normal brown pigment. Their irises appear blue or pink—pink in true albinism. Animals with blue or pink eyes tend to be more prone to other eye abnormalities. In spite of the temptation to create something unique—such as blue-eyed cattle—it's best not to go against nature. I would advise you not to breed this calf, as you might also be selecting for other genetic defects as well.

"third eyelid" (cats)

DEAR DR. FOX—Three of my five kittens, as well as their mother, have a white film on part of their eyes. Would this be from lack of sleep or what?—M.S.

DEAR M.S.—You could be seeing a large "third eyelid," which is located on the inner corner of each eye. A sick cat will show more third eyelid than a healthy one. But some cats naturally have rather prominent third eyelids. This could be the case with your cat, and her kittens simply inherited their mother's trait. So long as your cats are healthy, you needn't worry.

VETERINARIANS

cost of care

DEAR DR. FOX—Our "boy" cat is the equivalent of ninety human years old and still in excellent health, but Cinderella, his mother, who is the equivalent of a century old, has had three trips to our vet within two months—to the tune of $125. That may be reasonable by today's inflation, except when you're on social security and ends don't meet. The prognosis is not too good—possible liver or kidney impairment. Is there such a thing as special rates for pets belonging to senior citizens? Cindy is a frail nothing now, but she goes along on a two-block walk every day. How valiant can you get?—K.D.

DEAR K.D.—Yours is an important and touching letter. Within the next twenty years, the senior-citizen group will be in the majority in the United States, and what will be needed (and is, in fact, needed now) are pet hospitals for low-income people and pensioners.

For years these have existed in the United Kingdom; in England they're called People's Dispensaries for Sick Animals. These are supported by charity. However, some veterinarians in the United States see this as a form of socialized medicine and a threat to private practice and profit. Some work for local humane societies that may give you a discount, since more and more societies are setting up much-needed, reduced-fee, full-service clinics. Pet health care is another option.

good veterinary care

DEAR DR. FOX—Recently my husband and I adopted a stray cockapoo. The dog is very loving but also very timid. At the vet's he wouldn't sit when the vet tried to look down his throat. She advised me to let go of him so he could get used to her. Then she proceeded to grab him off the table by his neck, shake him, and slap him. She said he was "just one of those spoiled dogs." She probably didn't hurt the dog, but I took my business elsewhere. Is this ethical behavior for a so-called animal-loving vet?—DOG LOVER

DEAR DOG LOVER—The animal doctor could have misread your dog's behavior, but chances are that he had indeed been spoiled as a pup, overindulged, and never given any discipline. A good shake (but no hitting) is necessary to establish dominance, which is all the veterinarian was trying to initiate. She could have been a little more diplomatic and empathetic!

I advise obedience training. Fewer people would be bitten and more dogs would be socially adjusted if their owners would avoid the temptation, especially with cockapoos and other cuddly breeds, of letting them have their own way. Love and discipline make a good dog; love alone can mean a canine delinquent.

DEAR DR. FOX—We've recently had the most aggravating experience. When our horse became ill, we called our vet, a young, sympathetic doctor, but he was out on an emergency, so we called Dr. X, who told my wife to call another vet. Then, the next day, the vet we finally got to treat our horse needed a certain catheter, which only Dr. X had. Reluctantly we called him, and again, he was nasty, saying since he was third in line, he was out of the picture, and he hung up on us. Most vets have compassion toward animals and people, but this guy must have a mental problem. Do you agree?—R.S.

DEAR R.S.—Vets are human, just like you, and some are short-tempered, oversensitive, and very touchy when they feel threatened by younger colleagues. The fact is, your own vet should have called to borrow the catheter for the equine emergency; you should not have been caught in the middle. It is unfortunate that there are some personality types in the vet profession who don't have much time for people. But, conversely, a not-so-bright doctor may have a fantastic reputation simply because he's charming with his clients.

trusting your vet

DEAR DR. FOX—About a year ago our poodle developed a blood condition in which his blood cells manufactured more blood than his body could use. But our vet got the blood count down to normal with medication. In the meantime, our poodle has developed a tumor in his nose, which causes him great difficulty in breathing and also makes him nervous. Our vet says it's inoperable. Should we take him to another vet? We love him dearly and would like to see him more comfortable.—D.S. VON H.

DEAR D.S. VON H.—You raise an important issue for all pet owners. The important element in pet owners' relationship with their animal doctors is trust. If you don't trust your vet, then, yes—go to another one or seek a second opinion. To me, your vet seems to know what he or she is doing, having dealt well with the blood problem. Why not share your uncertainty with your vet? Your vet might suggest another colleague in the area to see for a second opinion. Then you will feel OK about whatever decision is made. Trust in your vet is especially important if and when you have to decide about putting a suffering pet to sleep. Doubt can lead to guilt and self-recrimination over not having done everything possible to save your pet.

when to see a vet

DEAR DR. FOX—My dog has a bone or a stick jammed between her two teeth. We tried to get it out, but it's really stuck. I'm afraid this will lead to infection. Any suggestions?—M.M.

DEAR M.M.—How could you wait for a letter to get to me and then wait until I reply! Too many pet owners want free advice when it's obvious that their pet is in distress and in need of immediate veterinary treatment. A sick or injured animal should not be denied proper veterinary care, and lack of money is no excuse. Most vets and humane societies will give people a break, since their primary concern and responsibility is the alleviation of animal suffering.

As for your dog, you could remove the foreign body in its mouth with a pair of pliers, but then you might break a tooth or tear the dog's mouth. I hope that by now, if your dog is still alive, able to eat, and hasn't a severe infection in her mouth, she has received veterinary first aid.

DEAR DR. FOX—One of my parakeets lived to be seven years old and the other six. Now I don't know whether I should get another one. I cried so much after each one died. The last one spoke in Polish! He ate at the table with us, and the moment I came home he was on my shoulder. I don't know what happened to him. He just swelled up, and store medicine didn't help. I know I should have brought him to a vet. But this probably would have cost more than what I paid for him—$15.—MRS. E.K.

DEAR MRS. E.K.—I don't wish to appear chastising, but we really can't put a monetary value on life—animal or human. Babies don't have a monetary value, yet good parents will go into debt to pay for medical care. You certainly got more than $15 worth of emotional enjoyment from your extraordinary parakeet.

While it might be cheaper to buy a new bird and let a sick one die, don't we have a moral obligation to care for our pets when they're sick? If you buy another bird, please keep in mind that providing pets with adequate veterinary care is one of their rights.

EXAMS, VACCINATIONS, AND MEDICATION

allergic and shock reactions (birds)

DEAR DR. FOX—My cockatiels are fine except for a mild sinus infection, which they each got at different times. Penicillin helped the male, but the female is losing plumage around her earholes and is scratching herself. She's active, but doesn't "sing" very much and has loose stools (from the medication). Is there anything else that I can do to help her?—T.A.H.

DEAR T.A.H.—Your cockatiels should have a culture taken to test antibiotic sensitivity, so the right antibiotic can be prescribed. It is also possible that they have a mite parasite infestation coupled with a secondary bacterial infection. It will help your birds if you keep the area around their cage warm (75–80 degrees F) and draft-free; humidifiers are effective too. Exotic birds can be problem pets because they are not well adapted to living in captivity. Deficiency-related disorders often underlie a number of diseases. I would advise you to give your birds the opportunity to sunbathe in fresh air when it's warm outdoors, and provide them with fresh food—old packaged birdseed from the pet store is inadequate—and multivitamins, especially A and D, which your veterinarian can prescribe.

allergic and shock reactions (dogs)

DEAR DR. FOX—My dog recently had a severe reaction to her first rabies shot. The doctor said it was probably caused by an allergy to the penicillin used as a stabilizer and that by the time she needed another shot, a new vaccine might be available. Meanwhile, can you discuss this reaction as well as any alternate ways to afford protection should it occur?—MRS. M.S. JR.

DEAR MRS. M.S. JR.—Some dogs, just like human beings, develop allergic reactions to vaccines and other drugs. Your dog is most probably allergic to the protein in the vaccine. One should always be on the lookout for the signs of an allergic reaction: distress, panting, difficulty in breathing, hives, and small swellings on the skin that make the hair stick up in tufts. Some pets may even become disoriented and collapse into anaphylactic shock. Treatment with appropriate drugs is usually effective, provided the symptoms are quickly recognized and treatment instigated. Allergic and shock reactions notwithstanding, they are no reason why animals should not be given vaccinations, since the chances of getting viral disease are far greater and the consequences usually even worse.

DEAR DR. FOX—Do older dogs die from distemper shots? Our eight-year-old poodle died ninety minutes after he got a booster shot for distemper. The vet said the poodle died from respiratory failure (he'd been treating the dog for sinus infection for six months). Is it more dangerous not having a distemper shot than having one? I'm worried about our other poodle, who got sick from his booster shot.—*H.L.G.*

DEAR H.L.G.—It is most unusual for a dog to get sick and extremely rare for one to die after being vaccinated, or after a "booster" shot against distemper. I would suspect an acute allergic reaction, and if you are worried, you should leave your other poodle with the vet, who will give it emergency treatment if such a thing were to happen again—which I sincerely doubt.

No animal (or person) should be given any vaccination if it is sick at the time. Only healthy animals should be vaccinated, hence the need for a thorough veterinary checkup before your pet receives its shots.

DEAR DR. FOX—What can you tell me about the parvovirus vaccine? My spaniel had three shots and never had a bad reaction. But from this last shot, he got really sick for a week, unable to jump with his hind legs. I'm worried because he's always been so peppy. Three of my neighbor's dogs have the same problem. What do you think?—*MRS. F.Y.*

DEAR MRS. F.Y.—You should immediately inform your veterinarian about your dog's reaction. Tell him also about your neighbor's experiences with their dogs. The vet will inform the manufacturers, since they are not only liable for damages, but are no doubt also concerned that there might be a bad batch of vaccine. That's not usual, but it can happen.

booster shots

DEAR DR. FOX—Is it true that older cats do not need yearly booster vaccinations? My cats are aged nine, eight, and five, stay indoors, and have always received yearly three-in-one vaccinations. If older cats should not get annual shots, at what age should they be discontinued?—*K.McC.*

DEAR K.McC.—To the best of my knowledge, no vaccination for the diseases that pets need protection from gives permanent immunity. Because the virulence or strength of contagious viral diseases can vary from year to year, it is advisable to give annual boosters, just in case a very lethal strain of virus were to develop in the neighborhood. This should be no chore, since all pets should go to the vet every six months or so for a routine health check, during which time shots can be given when and as needed. There is really no way to ensure that a housecat never gets exposed to infection—you could carry it home yourself. Hence, I advise annual booster shots for all cats—and dogs too.

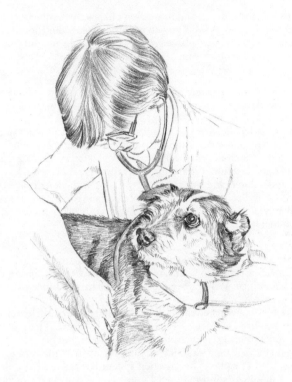

cortisone

DEAR DR. FOX—My vet is very cautious about giving more cortisone to our English sheepdog. He says it could have the opposite effect from what he wants. What does he mean? I thought cortisone was a wonder drug—*MRS. A.J.*

DEAR MRS. A.J.—It *was* a wonder drug—stick with the past tense. Doctors are realizing that good medical practice means cautious use of drugs, and that there has been an overdependence on using drugs, which, in the long run, can sometimes cause more harm than good. Your veterinarian is right—cortisone-type drugs in particular should be used sparingly and with great care. Any such hormones can lead to an impairment of the internal hormone-producing glands and cause all kind of complications. Such drug-created, or iatrogenic, disorders are a great concern today among both animal and human doctors.

DEAR DR. FOX—When our dog started to limp, x-rays showed he had a small growth on the first joint. The vet gave us some cortisone pills for the pain, but cautioned us not to give them to him too often because they could affect his liver and kidneys. Now I am afraid to give him any. Why take a chance? What is your opinion?—*G.H.H.*

DEAR G.H.H.—Your veterinarian gave you fair warning that excessive, prolonged use of cortisone will have adverse effects on your dog. But your vet did not say not to use them. Please, don't get paranoid about negative side effects and worry yourself silly.

Follow the doctor's advice, and if you aren't happy, remember you are free to see another veterinarian. A small growth on the first joint could be arthritis, but it could also be bone cancer, so please get your facts straight and put your mind at rest by seeing or telephoning your veterinarian.

frequency of exams

DEAR DR. FOX—Do dogs who go for regular rabies vaccinations and heartworm checkups need regular examinations too? And what about cats?—C.H.

DEAR C.H.—Ideally, every six months and at least once a year cats and dogs should be "vetted" and given a thorough clinical examination. Why? Because owners often miss such things as a buildup of dental tartar, early signs of an ear infection, obesity, or a tumor. Early diagnosis and treatment means less suffering for the pet and a faster cure. It's also less expensive in the long run. Often, just chatting with your doctor during the examination of your pet can bring to light some problem that needs attention. (And don't forget to take your pet's stool sample along so that it can be checked for parasites.)

pressure syringes

DEAR DR. FOX—In a recent article you mentioned a pressurized, needleless syringe for injecting pets. Our veterinarian and his supplier don't have any knowledge of such a syringe. Where does one find it? We have a thirteen-year-old diabetic poodle.—M.S.

DEAR M.S.—I have received many letters about these needleless pressure syringes (like the ones Dr. McCoy used on TV's Star Trek). These syringes are relatively painless and also reduce chances of infection, but they are very costly. For this reason they are used for giving multiple injections to many patients at one time or to a herd of cattle. The injection system has to be filled with a lot of insulin, far more than you would need to inject one dog, so it wouldn't really work for a pet at home. One would hope minisystems will be developed if there is sufficient market demand, since this is a most humane device.

rabies vaccines

DEAR DR. FOX—My friends and I have several questions about rabies. Is the animal vaccine for rabies truly effective? Surely, some of those animals who contract it have been inoculated, since some are people's pets. Isn't it necessary to be bitten, or scratched, by a sick animal to get the disease? We hear lately that even being near the animal is dangerous. How can we safeguard ourselves? If a pet is vaccinated and kept indoors, can it still contract rabies?—D.H.

DEAR D.H.—The vaccine for rabies is supposedly guaranteed to give an animal complete protection from the disease. Batches of vaccine that are produced by laboratories have to be tested at intervals for their effectiveness. It is very unlikely, therefore, that a properly and recently vaccinated animal will not be protected from this disease. But it is important to remember that the immunity given by the vaccine does not last forever. This is why pets need regular booster shots.

The virus is transmitted especially in the saliva of an animal when it bites a person or licks a person's open wound. It is not true that if you are anywhere near the animal, you will pick up the disease. However, in confined environments, such as caves, it is possible to pick up this virus in the air from infected bats. Out in the open, you are safe. If you see a wild animal behaving in an odd, disoriented way, or if it trots fearlessly toward you, avoid contact with it. If it does bite you, kill it, but be careful not to shoot it or hit it in the brain, because the brain must be intact to be examined for presence of negribodies, which indicate that the animal was rabid.

A pet that is regularly vaccinated against this disease and is not allowed to roam free and unsupervised is unlikely to pick up rabies from an infected animal. This is another important reason that every pet owner should make sure his or her cat or dog receives a regular shot against rabies and is not allowed to roam the neighborhood—especially in rural areas, where it may come in contact with a rabid animal.

DEAR DR. FOX—It's mandatory to give dogs, but not cats, rabies vaccinations in our country. That doesn't seem right to me, since cats can contract rabies from infected wild animals just as easily as dogs. Your opinion, please.—*A.D.*

DEAR A.D.—I agree with you. Any and all cat owners who allow their cats to roam free, especially farmers who have "working" cats in their barns to keep rodents down and birds away from animal feed, should have their cats given a regular vaccination against rabies.

According to the Centers for Disease Control in Atlanta, rabies is on the increase. In 1982, cats had 32 percent greater incidence of confirmed rabies than dogs. Rabies is fatal to humans and is one of the worst ways to die.

sick animals in vet's waiting room

DEAR DR. FOX—When we took our kitten to the veterinarian for her second shot against distemper, there were two kittens in the waiting room who were put to sleep because of this disease. What are the chances of my kitten becoming infected after this type of exposure?—*VERY WORRIED*

DEAR VERY WORRIED—There is always a risk involved in taking a kitten to the veterinarian to be vaccinated when there are sick cats in the waiting room. Fortunately, the first shot probably gave your kitten some protection. In order to reduce such risks of unvaccinated kittens picking up disease on the veterinarian's premises, some vets will do house calls or schedule a specific time to see young animals so as to avoid contact with others in the waiting room. A well-ventilated and regularly disinfected waiting room is also a must. These are factors to check out before selecting a vet.

DENTAL CARE

cleaning teeth (cats and dogs)

DEAR DR. FOX—Do cats need to have their teeth cleaned, and if so, how often? Should we take them to the vet for it? My cat seems to have black scum on her teeth. What causes this?—*K.M.*

DEAR K.M.—Cats do need to have their teeth cleaned regularly as they get older, especially those who eat mainly moist or semimoist cat food. Encourage your cat to eat some dry food. This will stop the buildup of dental tartar, which irritates the gums and causes bad breath and eventually extensive infection. Check the back upper molar teeth especially, since these are the first to build up brown scale. Cats with neglected teeth live a miserable life, and a regular checkup at the vet can help rectify this all-too-common problem.

DEAR DR. FOX—When my elkhound was a puppy, my vet said that her teeth should be cleaned, but that the dog should be tranquilized and that the cleaning should not be done unless Hawkeye was "put out" for another reason. That was five years ago and Hawkeye has never needed to be "put out." Should a dog's teeth be cleaned, either at home or professionally?—R.S.

DEAR R.S.—With the right diet (including hard foods to chew on and keep gums healthy and teeth free of tartar) and good tooth alignment, dogs and cats will naturally keep their teeth clean. However, buildup of tartar, brown scaly calculi, often develops on the upper back molar teeth, check your pets' mouths. Such material should be removed and can often be done in tractable animals without an anesthetic. Toy breeds especially need regular dental checkups, and a daily brushing with toothpaste is the only way to save some dogs' teeth. And yes—this vet's advice was good—whenever an animal has to be "put out" for some reason, the opportunity should be used to clean its teeth.

loose teeth (dogs)

DEAR DR. FOX—I have noticed that a couple of my puppy's front teeth are loose. Are they supposed to be that way?—M.G.

DEAR M.G.—Yes. Puppies, just like children, have "milk teeth" that eventually become loose to make way for the permanent teeth. This means that puppies, just like babies, can suffer from teething problems.

So it is advisable to give them safe chew-toys and to keep them away from satisfying their oral cravings on anything that may splinter or may be easily swallowed and cause internal injury. Look out especially for electrical cords, since puppies can chew through them and get severely burned or killed.

new teeth growth (dogs)

DEAR DR. FOX—Heidi, my eleven-year-old half-corgi half-Pomeranian, lost all her bottom teeth during the last seven months. But about a month later she began cutting a whole new set, and now they are large enough for her to eat almost anything. It is unusual for a dog her age to cut a new set of teeth?—V.B.F.

DEAR V.B.F.—It is indeed unusual for a dog of that age suddenly to develop an entirely new set of teeth. Unfortunately, she's too old to be bred now, because it would be worthwhile to study the inheritance of her extraordinary tooth regenerative ability. You may wish to contact the department of clinical studies at the school of veterinary medicine nearest to you. I'm sure they would like to examine your unique dog.

trimming teeth (gerbils)

DEAR DR. FOX—I'm having trouble with my gerbils. I keep them in a big tank, and they climb up the water bottle and chew on the wire that's on it. Why?—A.G.

DEAR A.G.—Do your gerbils have anything else to gnaw on and play with in their tank? They need a hunk of wood to keep their teeth trimmed down, otherwise their teeth could get too long and need cutting. If not corrected, overgrown teeth interfere with eating and can even kill the gerbil. Gerbils are very curious and playful and enjoy things they can crawl into, around, and over, so "enrich" their tank with some suitable toys, such as an unopened tin can, a small flower pot, and an exercise wheel.

trimming teeth (hamsters)

DEAR DR. FOX—I am a twelve-year-old with a hamster of my own. He is always biting his cage. Is there anything I can do to stop him? Will he get lead poisoning?—M.M.

DEAR M.M.—You ask a very important question. Yes, your hamster could get lead poisoning if the cage has been painted with an old lead-based paint. Hamsters need to chew on hard things to wear down their teeth, which grow constantly and sometimes need trimming. Help your hamster; give him a hunk of wood and a tree branch to gnaw on. Be sure the wood is natural and hasn't been treated with chemicals to repel rot and wood-boring insects. Pet owners who use cages, be advised—the same holds true for sawdust and wood chips.

DEAR DR. FOX—My hamster's top two teeth are growing backwards toward the roof of his mouth. I try to keep them short by clipping them, but it's very hard to keep him still. I keep blocks of wood and salt licks in his cage, but he doesn't seem to use them. I'm scared his teeth are going to grow through his head. What can I do?—P.G.

DEAR P.G.—No orthodontists in nature, unfortunately. All you can do is keep trimming your hamster's teeth. You're right, they could grow into his head and kill him. This does happen to wild rodents whose teeth are misaligned. Without your help your pet would be helpless and would eventually starve to death. Isn't it nice to be needed?

trimming teeth (rabbits)

DEAR DR. FOX—Last November, my son bought a dwarf white rabbit. He recently noticed that Bugs's lower teeth were growing long and almost touching his nose. The top teeth were also growing long and turning up.

We took him to the vet, who said his teeth had to be cut down. We had this done. However, about three weeks later, the same thing happened. This time the vet said the only alternatives were to have the teeth cut or to put him to sleep. Do you know of any other solution?—J.R.

DEAR J.R.—Put a block of soft pine-wood on the floor or a mineral block (from a pet store) for your bunny to chew on. They will help keep his teeth trim.. Also, have your vet show you how to trim his teeth. It's easy and painless with the right snippers, just like cuting your toenails. I would not advise you to breed your rabbit, since misalignment of teeth is a genetic-developmental defect.

worn or broken teeth (dogs)

DEAR DR. FOX—My five-year-old poodle has four broken bottom teeth. What can we do for her?—B.S.

DEAR B.S.—You've probably neglected your dog's teeth. Take her off foods high in sugar and give her teeth a nightly brushing with toothpaste and a brush. If you simply follow the same rules for your dog's teeth as you do for your own, she'll be in good shape. That, of course, includes regular dental checkups at the vet.

DEAR DR. FOX—My dog will soon be ten years old, and her teeth are all worn down. Should I feed her hard or soft dogfood?—S.McB.

DEAR S.McB.—Dry dogfood won't wear your dog's teeth down. But I bet your dog is a rock chewer, and that's why her teeth are worn. All dogs should be discouraged from chewing and carrying rocks. Dry food will help keep a dog's gums and teeth healthy, so you should go easy on the soft moist food. The alternative is to brush your dog's teeth—this is almost essential now for toy breeds whose teeth usually degenerate rapidly, rocks or no rocks.

worn or broken teeth (gerbils)

DEAR DR. FOX—My pet gerbil has a life-or-death problem. Every month or two, her front incisors break or fall off. I have kept her in good health the last year and a half by feeding her soft grains, vegetables, seeds, and peanut butter. Do you think the roots in her teeth are damaged?—HOPEFUL

DEAR HOPEFUL—Your gerbil may require more calcium in her diet. Cereals are high in phosphorus and may not have the right calcium-phosphorus ratio for your particular pet. Rodents in the wild will avidly chew on the bones of dead animals. Put a piece of boiled soup bone in your gerbil's cage for her to gnaw on to her heart's content.

Some pets will break their teeth by chewing and levering on the sides and edges of the cage. This could be another reason for smashed teeth. Rodents are lucky that, just like our fingernails, their teeth grow all the time. I wish *my* teeth did.

DISEASE AND PHYSICAL DISORDERS: SYMPTOMS AND TREATMENT

acupuncture (for disc problem)

DEAR DR. FOX—Our long-haired dachshund developed a "dachsie malady"—the disc syndrome—and was paralyzed in the hindquarters. Before we let her undergo surgery, we explored other avenues, and came up with a vet who specializes in acupuncture. We feel we have accomplished the same end results with this method. I would like to know what you think of acupuncture.—B.M.

DEAR B.M.—Acupuncture is a useful tool in its own right and is based on theoretical principles of holistic medicine. It enlarges the horizons of traditional veterinary and human medicine. There is a recognized professional association of veterinary acupuncture, and this treatment can be an option for many petowners. However, I must emphasize that acupuncture is not a cure-all.

anemia, infectious (cats)

DEAR DR. FOX—What can I do to help my cats when they get infectious anemia? I have lost seven cats in the past four years. They were given shots to no avail. Blood tests verified the sickness as infectious anemia. Now, my four-year-old cat (one of eight) is showing the same symptoms. Help!—V.H.B.

DEAR V.H.B.—There is no cure, no vaccine, and no magic drug to treat feline infectious anemia. My advice is to obtain no more cats until the last of yours has gone. Unfortunately, veterinary research in the field of feline diseases has been poorly funded by granting agencies. I wish more cat clubs and cat lovers would do some fund-raising to support veterinary research centers so that cats and other companion animals can live healthier and happier lives.

anemia, infectious (horses)

DEAR DR. FOX—I have a seven-year-old gelding and would like to know what swamp fever is. Also, do you know a good cure for muck itch? The medicine I'm using now isn't working.—K.S.

DEAR K.S.—Equine infectious anemia, commonly known as swamp fever, is a highly contagious disease of horses that can cause severe debility and death. Since horses can be carriers and so can infect others with this disease, the policy is to test and destroy all carriers of the disease. Your vet can have a test done on your horse to put your mind at rest. Even if it does come up positive, you may not have to destroy the animal, if it NEVER comes into contact with other horses and is otherwise healthy.

Muck itch is a general term for a variety of fungal and other skin problems in horses. If your horse is not responding to medication, don't continue to experiment with home doctoring. See your vet before things get worse.

arthritis (cats)

DEAR DR. FOX—My wife and I read your column religiously because of its useful information, and now we have a personal problem. Our cat has arthritis in her two back hip joints. She is twenty years old, active, bright, and loving, but has difficulty walking. Is there something we can do to help her?—*G.A.K.*

DEAR G.A.K.—Considering your cat's age, I wouldn't give her cortisone, the usual steroid medication, for her arthritis. One should always consider what species the animal is and how old it is before trying any medication. Aspirin can kill cats, and cortisone has serious side effects, especially in older animals. Keep your cat on a high-protein, low-calorie diet, and give her regular massages around the lower back and hip region—especially in the morning. It's amazing how a good massage will help older pets in general and be especially appreciated by those with arthritis.

bites, infected (cats)

DEAR DR. FOX—My young cat, Queenie, stayed out all night and was beaten up by the neighborhood cats. You could tell she'd been bitten, because the hairs were parted and stuck together. When she coughs now, it sounds as if she's sneezing and gargling up something in her mouth. I'm worried about her. What should I do?—*Q.T.*

DEAR Q.T.—From the stress and injuries your cat experienced on her night out, she probably has infected bites, which will cause fever and may also form abscesses that require veterinary treatment. She may also have picked up a virus infection from exposure to other cats. All cats need protective vaccinations just in case they slip out like yours did, and also for protection when they visit the vet, where they're exposed to other sick cats. Your experience is a warning to all cat owners—if you love your cat, be sure it gets regular shots and is never let out to roam free.

DEAR DR. FOX—For some time now my cat has had sores on her back and neck and under her chin. They come and go every month or so. My vet says not to worry, that they could be from scratches or falls or rough playing with the other cats. He offers no medication nor any other explanation. But I am worried. Any suggestions?—*I.F.*

DEAR I.F.—Your cat may indeed have scratches or bites, but these same bites could become abscesses and make your cat quite ill. Other possibilities include parasitic or infectious dermatitis—flea-allergy dermatitis and allergy to a flea collar. If I were you, I'd seek another opinion since I doubt very much that a cat is likely to be bitten and scratched so extensively along its back and neck and under its chin without developing at least one serious bite-abscess.

biting (dogs)

DEAR DR. FOX—My dog keeps biting his hind legs and thighs and chasing his tail like there's something in his rectum that is bothering him. One vet said he had worms, so we had him dewormed, but it hasn't helped. Any advice?—MRS. E.D.

DEAR MRS. E.D.—Chasing and biting the tail and hindquarters sometimes means blocked, painful, or infected anal glands. All dogs who show such behavior should be checked out accordingly. I've never heard of worms causing this problem. Fleas at the base of the tail could be to blame.

Some dogs develop this behavior as a neurotic vice. Discipline (even a squirt with a water pistol), distracting games, plenty of exercise, or light tranquilization for a short period may help if this is a purely behavioral problem.

bladder infection (dogs)

DEAR DR. FOX—My dog has frequent bladder infections. Our vet says to put salt in her food, and that otherwise there is nothing to prevent this condition. What causes bladder infections? Also, is there really nothing else to help prevent infections? It's getting very expensive to take her to the vet each time this occurs.—J.O.

DEAR J.O.—Bladder infections are difficult to treat. Your vet should isolate the bacteria that are causing the trouble and run a sensitivity test to find the best drug to use. Also, find out if there is a pattern to your dog's illnesses, because relapses can be triggered by stresses, such as being left alone for the weekend, a sojourn in a boarding kennel, or a rough time at the grooming parlor. With some infections, acidifying the urine with vitamin C may help. Also, your vet should explore herbal remedies—they're preferable to adding salt to your dog's diet to make her drink frequently and flush out her system.

bladder stones (dogs)

DEAR DR. FOX—Our eight-year-old schnauzer has had three operations for bladder stones, but our veterinarian cannot come up with the cause. Do you have any suggestions about a change in diet? Is there a recommended medicine?— R.D.L.

DEAR R.D.L.—The addition of chemicals to either acidify or make more alkaline the dog's urine does help in pets afflicted with bladder stones. But first, the chemical composition of the stone has to be ascertained. Has your veterinarian considered this? Some animal doctors practicing what is called holistic medicine have found that a radical change in diet may help such problems as those afflicting your dog.

I would suggest that you explore the possibility of shifting your dog's diet away from a high percentage of canned processed meats and meat byproducts to one consisting of more whole-grain rice, vegetables, and a little chicken or fish.

blindness and cataracts (cats and dogs)

DEAR DR. FOX—We have just had the vet confirm that our Persian cat, Poppy, is blind. We noticed that when he was excited he ran straight into walls or furniture. Now he is so affectionate! All he wants to do is cuddle with us, and he has taken to sleeping with us all night because he feels insecure, frightened, and confused, I guess. We are concerned about his becoming too sedentary, fearful, or depressed. Can you give us any suggestions for making his life happier?—J.N.

DEAR J.N.—Blindness must surely cause an animal great anxiety, but, just as with a human, a nurturing environment makes all the difference in the world. From the tone of your letter, I know you will supply it abundantly! It is remarkable how animals adapt to blindness—a wild pelican, blind for years, was fed by its flock-mates. Keep your furniture in the same place, remove any breakables, and put up a "tree" or rug-covered post with carpeted resting shelves at various heights. A blind cat will enjoy this with a little coaxing. Also, try him on a leash and a harness—he may like a stroll and a roll outdoors. And give him a pinch of catnip at times for a "high."

DEAR DR. FOX—I have a miniature gray male poodle, now about nine years old. I have just been told by the vet that he has cataracts, and he shows signs of losing sight. I have tried to learn what can be done about cataracts, but have gotten little response, not even from the vet. Can you offer some good suggestions?—*J.T.C.*

DEAR J.T.C.—Some forms of ocular cataract can be surgically corrected. Sometimes, however, there are additional complications such as glaucoma or retinal atrophy. Have a veterinary ophthalmologist examine your dog. However, do keep in mind that dogs do adapt quite well to gradual blindness, and because of their superior sense of smell, they cope better than we do when they lose sight.

DEAR DR. FOX—Our poodle is the love of our life, and we have spent a bundle on him. The vet now says he has leukemia. He also has cataracts and is completely blind. (The vet says he is a borderline diabetic.) But you'd never believe he is sick or blind. We'd like to have him operated on for the cataracts. Do you think if would be safe?—*E.F.*

DEAR E.F.—I believe it would be risky to subject an aging, borderline diabetic dog to major surgery. While a skilled veterinary eye-surgeon can do much to improve a dog's vision by removing the lenses in the eyes, which become cloudy with age, it is quite possible that such surgery would not help because the retina (the back of the dog's eye) is no longer functional. Have a veterinary ophthalmologist check your dog. But remember, the loss of sight is not as traumatic if the dog is kept indoors in a protected environment.

blood in urine (cats and dogs)

DEAR DR. FOX—I have a cat—a stray—who decided to stay (and when a cat decides to stay, you may just as well relax and accept it). Now the problem: She needs a vet, but I can't get her to his office. I can't hold her for longer than a minute, and she goes wild in a box. She has blood in her urine and uses the litter box about every fifteen minutes. She also has a great deal of trouble with bowel movement. Please help.—*W.M.H.*

DEAR W.M.H.—Your cat is obviously in urgent need of veterinary attention, so call around and find a vet who makes house calls, or one who has an assistant who can come and transport your cat in a sturdy carrier. Alternatively, you could ask the vet for a tranquilizer pill and give it to your pet before you put her in a carrier, which your vet can loan to you. Please don't delay; your cat needs help.

DEAR DR. FOX—For the past year, our dachshund has had a problem off and on with blood in her urine. The vet gave her urinary-acidifier pills, but it hasn't stopped the problem. Do you have any suggestions?—*D.M.*

DEAR D.M.—Two of the most likely reasons why your dog is passing blood are that she has a recurrent infection of the bladder and possibly stones or calculi in the bladder. An x-ray examination will detect the latter. For the former, your veterinarian should examine your dog's urine for bacteria and should run a culture and antibiotic sensitivity test. This way, the most effective antibiotic can be decided on, and your dog's chances of recovery greatly enhanced.

breast infection (dogs)

DEAR DR. FOX—Our dog (registered hound) weaned her puppies, twelve of them, approximately three months ago. One breast has remained large, with knots in it and the surrounding glands. She does not seem sensitive in the area, and there is no resultant discharge. My husband is unemployed and we can't afford a veterinarian. (He charged us $280 for initial shots.) Can you help us? Is this condition serious?—G.C.G.

DEAR G.C.G.—Your dog may have had a mild localized breast infection—mastitis—which will slowly subside. However, she could be developing tumors, which could turn malignant and if not removed spread to her lungs and liver and kill her. Your dog should see a vet if the breast gets larger. Veterinary fees are high, but so are the veterinarian's costs. However, many animal doctors are flexible with their fees, and you might be able to get an extended payment plan. In some areas, full-service hospitals are being set up by local humane societies for pet owners who can't pay for a private veterinarian. This "socialized" animal medicine is highly controversial but is surely not inconsistent with the principles of social democracy.

colds (transmitting them to your pet)

DEAR DR. FOX—I haven't had hamsters very long, and so I've been reading books about them. One book said that a hamster can catch cold from its human keeper, but another book said that only mice and rats catch human colds. Which is right?—C.E.S.

DEAR C.E.S.—While most human viruses will not affect hamsters, there are some so-called orphan viruses that can affect various species. So it's not impossible for you to transmit an infection to your hamster and vice-versa. Some kinds of human flu, for example, originate from pigs and ducks that serve as a reservoir for certain strains of influenza virus. All you can do is make sure that your pets are healthy and see a doctor or veterinarian when you or they are sick.

coughing (cats and dogs)

DEAR DR. FOX—Blacky, my cat, is coughing and sneezing severely. What can I do to cure him? We can't take Blacky to the vet because we don't have the money, especially with pups on the way.—S.L.

DEAR S.L.—Cats are prone to upper respiratory infections and can even develop chronic sinusitis. Coughing, gagging, and vomiting can mean fur balls—pieces of fur that get swallowed and are later thrown up. No need to be too concerned if this is your cat's problem. But constant sneezing, wheezing, and discharge from the nose and eyes require veterinary treatment. Sorry, there are no cheap home remedies. The sooner your cat is examined by an animal doctor, the better and the cheaper it will be in the long run.

DEAR DR. FOX—Recently my three cats caught what my vet said was a cold. Since the temperature was dropping to around 20 degrees F at night in the garage where they stay, I began to let them in the house at night and out during the day when it got warmer. Their colds got worse, and they began to cough and wheeze badly. The vet said to keep them always in or always out, since switching is bad for them. I kept them outside (with access to the garage), but their colds did not go away, and the antibiotics haven't done any good. Your advice?—*M.S.*

DEAR M.S.—Your vet was right. The same rule holds for dogs. It is stressful to pets to allow them outside for a length of time and then inside, since extremes in temperature make them prone to sickness. Likewise, the extreme temperature changes in the fall—some hot days, then others very cold—can bring on stress-related illness.

I advise all pet owners to have their pets examined by their animal doctors in early fall and given booster vaccinations, as needed. This will help protect them when their immune systems are suppressed by thermal stress. I would suggest you inform your vet of your cats' continuing poor health—a step many people fail to take.

DEAR DR. FOX—Each time my wife and I return home, my poodle rushes to the door to greet us and goes into a coughing, wheezing spell. It's pitiful. Is there some remedy for this condition?—*H.M.*

DEAR H.M.—Poodles do suffer from chronic upper respiratory mucous secretion. Some also have very pushed-in faces, which together with a long soft palate can aggravate problems further. Give your dog regular exercise, so that while he runs around he will naturally expectorate. Sedentary beasts do wheeze and cough when they are active only once or twice a day like yours. Don't use any drugs, unless your dog clearly becomes ill. And get a veterinary checkup, to rule out the possibility of infection or a heart problem.

deafness (cats and dogs)

DEAR DR. FOX—For Mother's Day I received a totally deaf Persian kitten. Can there be such a breed?—*V.K.*

DEAR V.K.—No, there isn't a breed of deaf cats. But deafness is genetically linked and is especially prevalent in white, blue-eyed animals. Your kitten will adjust to life quite well, but it's up to you to keep her from obvious dangers. The major problem is that deaf cats should not be allowed out unsupervised, because they are more likely to be run over by cars and/or be suddenly ambushed by other animals.

DEAR DR. FOX—Our one-and-a-half-year-old toy fox terrier, Snoopy, doesn't seem to hear. The vet states that he's probably just ignoring us. We've tried whistles, an accordion, and even clapping hands directly behind his head. These noises don't cause his ears to move or rotate. Calling his name doesn't help either. Because of the vet's comment, we wonder if there is any sure way of telling if Snoopy can hear or not.—*W.P.*

DEAR W.P.—If your fox terrier is a typical fox terrier, he may well be playing it supercool. One of these tough little crackerjacks wouldn't flinch even if a tiger roared in his face—in fact, he might bite back. Fox terriers are good ratters; a rodentlike squeak will get their attention. Get a squeaky rubber mouse, and with your arm very still, squeak it under a rug or pillow so your dog can't see you doing it. If he doesn't respond at once, he's probably deaf. If so, be very careful with him near roads and busy traffic, which can turn a deaf dog into a dead one.

dehydration (gerbils)

DEAR DR. FOX—I have had three gerbils that have all died within one year. I took my first one to the vet when she was sick and he said she was suffering from dehydration. He gave her medicine but she still died. The other two died of the same thing. Could the pet store have been at fault? What causes dehydration?— *E.H.*

DEAR E.H.—You misunderstood your veterinarian. Your gerbil was not sick because she was dehydrated, but rather her dehydration was one of the signs of her being sick. Loss of body fluid can be due to severe enteritis or fever and inability to drink, for example. It is unlikely that the pet store can be held responsible since your pets died some time after you bought them. As for the disease that resulted in dehydration and death, the only sure way to find out would have been to autopsy your pet. This might have helped save the other two.

diabetes (dogs)

DEAR DR. FOX—We have just learned that our dog is diabetic. She gets between 16 and 20 units of insulin daily, and she cries when the insulin injections are given. Would brewer's yeast help? Our dog is thirteen years old.—*W. & J.F.*

DEAR W. & J.F.—Your diabetic dog should first be on a special diet, which I trust your veterinarian has prescribed in addition to the insulin treatment. Canine diabetes, like human diabetes, may well be aggravated by improper diet.

Make sure the pet foods you're buying don't contain much sugar, which is linked with certain forms of diabetes. A high-quality protein diet (fish, chicken, lean beef, cottage cheese) plus a little whole-grain rice will help, together with a teaspoon each of brewer's or nutritional yeast, powdered kelp, and vegetable oil.

Also give your dog a few drops of vitamins A, D, and E and a 500 mg tablet of vitamin C and calcium lactate each day. The nutritional supplements, although not effective in treating diabetes mellitus, are good for older dogs.

diarrhea (dogs)

DEAR DR. FOX—Our cockapoo is a year old now. About once a month she vomits and has diarrhea. Our vet always says it's a virus and gives her a shot and pills. How can it be a virus every month like clockwork?—*MRS. V.R.*

DEAR MRS. V.R.—It's indeed unlikely that your dog simply has a virus infection, considering the recurrent nature of her problem. Overfeeding, emotional stress, a sudden change in diet, or a chronic clinical condition may be at the heart of your dog's problem. I strongly advise you to seek a second opinion, and be sure to take a fresh stool sample in when you take your dog to the veterinarian.

diarrhea (from pets to people)

DEAR DR. FOX—My son has three dogs and a cat. He develops diarrhea every time one of the pets gets diarrhea. Right now, he is constantly feeling very tired and weak. I am wondering if he can possibly have toxoplasmosis.—*W.P.*

DEAR W.P.—From the symptoms you describe, it is unlikely that your son is suffering from toxoplasmosis. It's more likely that one or more of his pets could have salmonellosis, a bacterial disease of the intestines that will occasionally affect people.

There are other possibilities, too. I would certainly encourage your son to have a public health inspector check the water supply. Of course, your son should see a physician.

diarrhea (parakeets)

DEAR DR. FOX—I am very concerned about our six-year-old parakeet. Periodically, he becomes selective in what he eats, gets diarrhea, and seems to prefer gravel more than seeds. When I give him a couple of drops of Pepto-Bismol his droppings become more solid, but it doesn't really help. Is there anything I can give him to stop these spells?—K.T.

DEAR K.T.—There are certain internal parasites and other organisms that cause chronic, recurrent intestinal upsets in parakeets, and Pepto-Bismol will not eliminate them. The infection will cause your bird to go off his feed and to be listless for a while. Selective eating, especially of gravel, is nature's way of curing things, but the cure is only temporary. Appropriate medication in the water or administered by a dropper should prevent further occurrences. But there's no way out of it. Recurrent bouts of diarrhea in cage birds require veterinary examination.

disc problems (dogs)

DEAR DR. FOX—My sister's ten-year-old poodle howled with pain when he scratched himself or did other perfectly normal things, so she took him to a veterinarian. After taking x-rays, the doctor said the dog had a disc problem and put him on medication for ten days. Can a disc problem be cured? What is the prognosis after medication?—M.G.

DEAR M.G.—Disc problems are all too common in certain breeds, cause great distress, and can sometimes also lead to paralysis. A dog that snaps when being petted around the head region or who is afraid of being touched may well have a luxated disc. Frequently, owners don't understand this and punish their dog for behaving aggressively, while in fact the animal is afraid of being petted because it hurts.

The veterinarian is probably giving your sister's dog antispasmodics and analgesics to help alleviate the problem. Surgery can give immediate relief; but medication should be tried first, since the disc problem may resolve itself. I have heard good things about chiropractors correcting disc problems in dogs and would welcome more application of chiropractic principles in veterinary medicine.

DEAR DR. FOX—My dog had a slipped disc and could not negotiate even one step or lower her head to drink from her dish. The dog was put on muscle relaxants by the vet, then she was adjusted once by a chiropractor, and we had immediate improvement. Several days later we had another adjustment with more improvement, and the muscle relaxant was discontinued. The third adjustment a week later completely solved the problem. That was five years ago. I wish you could see her now. She not only chases, she catches rabbits.—J.B.

DEAR J.B.—The best way to treat dogs with "slipped," or more correctly, herniated, discs is a controversial subject. In recurrent cases with severe spinal injury, euthanasia is the most humane solution. However, acute cases respond will to analgesics and muscle relaxants, and an experienced surgeon can operate on afflicted pets and alleviate the problem for good. Veterinary chiropractic is rarely practiced, and I would certainly like to see more work done in this area, since dogs suffer from various back problems similar to humans. If they can gain relief from chiropractic manipulations, so much the better. Your story is heartening.

DEAR DR. FOX—As an owner of four dachshunds, I am familiar with the problem of slipped discs. My veterinarian did research on this "slipped disc" problem and recommended an experimental diet. He claims this increases the muscle strength around the discs, thus preventing them from moving around. Each dog daily receives a special food supplement in addition to his dogfood. He gets 200 mg of vitamin C twice a day, 10 mg of zinc once a day, and one soft-boiled egg yolk on Monday, Wednesday, and Friday; on Tuesday, Thursday, and Saturday, I add two tablespoons of cooking oil. As of now, this diet is working, and my active dachshund has not had a recurring slipped-disc problem for close to one year.— M.F.

DEAR M.F.—Thank you for sharing your veterinarian's successful formula for helping your dog's slipped-disc disorder. To help prevent relapses, a low-calorie diet to keep the dog's weight down is essential, plus regular exercise—trotting, not wild chasing—to build up muscle tone. A disc-prone dog should be discouraged from climbing stairs and jumping on and off furniture. Surgery is effective, but the ultimate answer is sound breeding and regular exercise.

DEAR DR. FOX—My dog has a slipped disc. She can't jump up on the bed or chairs because it hurts so much. The steroids or pills that she has taken make her so thirsty that she continually is drinking and has to go to the bathroom. We don't know what to do. She looks like she's in so much pain! Can you help?—C.H.S.

DEAR C.H.S.—Slipped discs can be so painful and recurrent that the kindest thing to do is to have your pet put to sleep. However, some pets (who know how to manipulate their owners and get extra attention and treats) will act far more distressed than they really are. Ask your vet if your animal is really in such great pain. Meanwhile, your dog should be weaned gradually from the drugs she's on, and probably be put on a diet if she isn't already. Too much weight and too little regular exercise contribute to your dog's all-too-common problem. An occasional aspirin won't hurt, and it's safer and cheaper than cortisone.

DEAR DR. FOX—After having fully recovered from a severe case of pneumonitis, my housecat, Rusty, has developed a ravenous appetite. In fact, she never seems to get enough to eat. The food is not doing her much good, though, as she has extreme dysentery. In spite of this, she is growing, her fur is shiny, and she plays with her toys.—E.W.

DEAR E.W.—Your cat could have liver damage or be suffering from an intestinal infection that resulted from a lowering of her resistance due to the pneumonitis infection. She must be seen by a veterinarian. A change in diet may be needed to help her settle down. Boiled rice, with a little fish, chicken, cottage cheese, and multivitamin drops, for example, is a bland meal that will help, along with whatever appropriate therapy the veterinarian prescribes.

ear infections (dogs)

DEAR DR. FOX—Our English bulldog is in and out of the vet's for an ear infection. Despite medication, it gets worse. The infection drains, it becomes raw, he scratches at it and shakes his head, and you can hear it "rattle." I am sure he is a miserable dog. Please help him.—MRS. H.F.S.

DEAR MRS. H.F.S.—I frequently am filled with anger and sadness at the sight of "puss-headed" bulldogs. Breeding for deep skin folds, plus inbreeding that may adversely affect their ability to withstand infection, may underlie your poor bulldog's problem.

Ear infections that are chronic can be corrected surgically. First, a culture and sensitivity test should be run to find which drugs might best correct the ear disease. I would also have him examined thoroughly for other related problems, such as poor thyroid activity and even a food allergy, which can express itself in the most unexpected ways.

DEAR DR. FOX—Our cocker spaniel is perfect, except for the smell from her ears. None of the medications the doctor suggested has worked. Please help. I hate to invite anyone over because the first thing they say is, "Boy, does she smell!"—N.M.B.

DEAR N.M.B.—Bad ears and cocker spaniels go together like a horse and buggy. With those monstrously abnormal pendulous ears (no offense meant to spaniels—we gave them the ears they have by breeding), they are especially prone to ear infections.

Spaniel owners should check their dog's ears once a week and clean them regularly. Early infection might then be recognized and treated soon. Chronic ear problems often require surgical intervention to open up the dog's ear canals. If your dog is in top physical condition, this may be your best solution. If not, keep up the medication your vet prescribes and put some perfume behind your dog's ears—for your own sake.

DEAR DR. FOX—When we saw that our dog's ears were smelly and infected, we took her to the hospital, where they anesthetized her and cleaned them. That didn't help, and a vet later operated on her ears to open them up. Poor Tiny is still having trouble; her ears fill up with wax and I have to clean them every day. We thought the operation would cure this. Tiny is very nervous and hides when I have to clean her ears. Please help!—N.H.

DEAR N.H.—Your veterinarian did the right thing to operate on your dog's ears and open up the ear canal. It is unfortunate that you did not notice the problem until it had reached such a serious and chronic state. Pet owners take note: A general veterinary checkup every six months is advisable for all pets so that such conditions can be spotted early and nipped in the bud. Pets, more so than humans, need such regular health checks because they can't tell you when they have a problem. Be patient with your pooch and try rewarding her with food or a walk outdoors after you have treated her ears. This way she will learn to associate some pleasure with having her ears cleaned.

epilepsy (dogs)

DEAR DR. FOX—Our very lovable dog (of uncertain ancestry) is in good health according to the last checkup. Only we forgot to tell the vet about the times when she's very dizzy or fearful—she trembles violently, tries to back away from something in front of her, such as a hole or a cliff; also, she usually vomits. She runs to me on these occasions, which last only about ten minutes. Any thoughts?—K.L.E.

DEAR K.L.E.—From your description it sounds as though your dog may well be having a mild seizure. Epileptic seizures can be triggered by a variety of factors, some of which cannot always be diagnosed or treated. You should return to your veterinarian for a thorough neurological workup.

DEAR DR. FOX—My four-year-old German shepherd recently had an unusual attack. I first noticed that he was rolling on his back. When I called him he came toward me walking sideways, as if he were drunk. His legs then started to give out, and he collapsed onto the ground, saliva pouring out of his mouth and all his muscles contracting. His eyes rolled up into his head and he stopped breathing for about fifteen seconds. Suddenly he began to breathe again, his muscles relaxed, and he got up and walked away. What happened?—C.B.

DEAR C.B.—You have accurately described an epileptic seizure. Dogs will develop such seizures out of the blue, with no prior history of illness or head injury. In older dogs, a tumor should be suspected. In younger dogs such as yours, the cause may never be accurately diagnosed. You should be alert to the possibility that your dog may have subsequent attacks. However, the attacks can be controlled with certain drugs such as primidone, allowing your dog to live a good life.

DEAR DR. FOX—My dog Samantha has fits about once a month. I don't want to give her up, as she is a fine watchdog and also serves as my doorbell (I can't hear). Besides, she gave birth to eight beautiful puppies recently. Can the humane society help her? I'm on social security and must be careful with money.—F.R.M.

DEAR F.R.M.—Samantha may be suffering from the long-term consequences of an earlier bout of distemper. Low blood-calcium could trigger epilepticlike seizures, especially when she is producing a lot of milk for her pups. These fits can also be triggered by some other brain abnormality, which might have been inherited. Certain drugs will help control forms of canine epilepsy, so your dog needs a thorough checkup. Call your local humane society; they may have a resident vet or know of someone inexpensive in the area to help you. Samantha probably should be spayed, too—one litter of pups is surely enough for this pet-overpopulated world.

DEAR DR. FOX—My six-year-old poodle has epilepsy. One vet gave him primidone for approximately two years; the side effects nearly killed him. The next vet gave him phenobarbital—also not good. The next vet gave him phenobarbital and dilantin. I'm worried, because he doesn't seem to be getting better.—C.R.

DEAR C.R.—Epilepsy seems to be inherited in poodles and can be difficult to control. One should avoid overexciting the dog and also avoid switching from one medication to another. This is because it takes time to find out which drug is best to stabilize the dog's problem.

Some dogs do well on primidone after an initial course of phenobarbital. Other dogs do better on dilantin. It is unlikely that you will get complete inhibition of seizures. The important thing is to find the most effective treatment, which will reduce the seizures to once a month or so.

exercise when ill (dogs)

DEAR DR. FOX—We have a toy poodle that has always been a fanatical ball-chaser. Several weeks ago she was diagnosed as having a cervical disc problem, and the vet told us no more ball-chasing ever, because turning her head to get the ball causes pain and limping. We understand this, but the dog doesn't. She keeps bringing us balls, barking and wagging her tail, and we feel terrible. If we hide the balls, she runs and runs and runs looking for them. It's really pathetic. Do you have any suggestions?—D.S.

DEAR D.S.—Many dogs are like children—they need to be protected from themselves when they are sick. They simply can't rest and take it easy. Keep your dog as quiet and unstimulated as possible for four to six weeks, then build her up slowly with a little ball play to start off. Cut it out if she later shows signs of pain. Chances are her neck will improve with time, but it must first be given time to heal. If not, you might wish to explore the possibility of disc surgery for your active pooch. One complication, however, is that there may be subsequent disc prolapses and more surgery needed.

eye infections (cats)

DEAR DR. FOX—What can I do for kittens when their eyes are pasty? My husband washes them so they open up, but that condition only lasts a few hours. We also notice that the kittens' mother is a little listless.—*H.H.C.*

DEAR H.H.C.—Your cat family is ailing, no doubt about it. The first sign of a viral disease in cats is a severe inflammation of the eyes. You should take both the litter and their mother to a veterinarian, because there is a stong likelihood that all are infected with a viral disease. All cat owners, take note: The eyes are very important clues in diagnosing diseases in cats, and signs of redness, tearing, sneezing, and (later) discharge of pus are key indicators of upper respiratory infections or more general viral infections that can be fatal.

DEAR DR. FOX—My cat developed some sort of infection in both eyes. It looked like a flap of skin growing up toward the center of the eye from the bottom lid. The skin was clear but white. After giving her drops in both eyes four times a day, she began to clear up. Then my *other* cat developed the same problem. How do cats get this infection?—*K.V.*

DEAR K.V.—The "skin" that you saw in your cat's eyes is quite natural. It is called the third eyelid or nictitating membrane, and it moves over the eye to protect it when there is an eye infection, or when a cat gets an upper respiratory or other virus infection. Your first cat passed the infection on to the second—probably cat influenza, and your drops were of no use. The eye problem was just a sign of a more serious general problem affecting your cat's entire system. Next time, instead of home doctoring, take your cat to the vet. It could have been a more serious virus disease, and your cats could have died.

eye infections (dogs)

DEAR DR. FOX—My nine-year-old toy poodle has dry eyes (no tears). Nothing seems to help. Scum keeps forming, and she has also developed an ulcer in one eye. Antibiotics were prescribed, but they are slow in bringing about any healing. Please help.—*D.R.*

DEAR D.R.—Poodles are prone to eye problems, and dry eyes can have serious consequences. Chronic infection and irritation, sometimes aggravated by inturned eyelids or eyelashes (which should be surgically corrected), require constant attention.

Some owners apply their own remedies, using the wrong eyedrops or cortisone ointment, which can increase the chances of corneal ulcer formation. The best treatment, under veterinary supervision, is with appropriate antibiotics and frequent daily irrigation of the eyes with drops of normal saline, *not* with human eyedrop medications, since excessive use of these can damage the eyes.

DEAR DR. FOX—Recently my German shepherd's eyes started turning white. My dog and my brother were playing in the snow, and she ran into the fence. That's when it first started. Then she got a cold in the other eye. The vet gave us eyedrops, but her eye is still half white. Can you tell me what it is?—R.M.

DEAR R.M.—Dogs sometimes develop a temporary cloudiness of the cornea after being vaccinated, but this usually clears up quickly. Your shepherd is probably losing her sight and should be examined again without further delay by your vet or one who specializes in ophthalmology. When the eye turns white it can mean the dog may have a corneal disease, very difficult to cure.

eye infections (hamsters)

DEAR DR. FOX—My teddy-bear hamster seems to have a cold or something in his eye; it closes up and gets stuck together by a light scab or dried mucus. I generally pry it open and wipe away the crust. He always gets this in the same eye, but sometimes the other one closes up, too. He's had it for years.—D.B.

DEAR D.B.—All hamster owners should know that pinkeye, or inflammation of one or both eyes, can be a symptom of any number of diseases. Sometimes the infection is limited to the eyes themselves, but other infections can involve the hamster's upper respiratory system. For this reason, the current eye infections should receive veterinary attention. Your animal doctor can prescribe some drops or ointment to apply. Do not get something from the pet store to treat the problem, because your hamster could have more than a simple eye infection, and only a vet will be able to tell.

eye infections (rabbits)

DEAR DR. FOX—My three-year-old pet rabbit has pus coming out of her eye. What should I do? Does she need to see a vet? I also have a Siberian hamster who keeps biting me. What should I do to prevent that?—R.A.W.

DEAR R.A.W.—Yes, your rabbit should see a veterinarian, because any discharge from the eye or nose could mean your rabbit has a chronic infection such as snuffles or pasteurella, or an inflammation of the conjunctiva, which will cause considerable discomfort.

Some hamsters are rather truculent characters and will bite, especially if they are not handled regularly from an early age. I suggest you wear gloves to protect yourself as well as your hamster, since you could accidentally drop it if it bites too hard.

feline acne

DEAR DR. FOX—My six-month-old cat, Norton, has developed a scablike rash all around his mouth. The veterinarian diagnosed it as feline acne. I have never heard of this before—can you tell me the cause of this condition? Also, can we expect Norton to outgrow it, just as teenagers do?—J.M.P.

DEAR J.M.P.—Cats have scent glands around the lips, and when they become blocked, an inflammation, or feline acne, develops. This can be alleviated by applying a mild steroid ointment, but I would first advise you to follow your vet's instructions and medication. If your cat has not yet been neutered, this too may help, since feline acne is linked, as it is with human teenagers, to circulating sex hormones.

feline infectious peritonitis

DEAR DR. FOX—We have just had our second cat put to sleep from feline infectious peritonitis and are now worried sick about our remaining three. Our doctor tells us that no vaccine is currently available. Is it possible to pressure the pharmaceutical houses into intensifying their research?—G.C.S.

DEAR G.C.S.—Rabies causes more concern than feline infectious peritonitis

(FIP), because it can affect humans and other animal species such as dogs, cattle, and wildlife. FIP applies directly to cats and has only recently been recognized as a specific disease. Write to the veterinary school in your state and ask them what you, as a cat lover, can do to help raise funds to support research into this and other feline diseases for which no treatment or protective vaccines have yet been developed.

feline leukemia

DEAR DR. FOX—My cat has just died from leukemia, and I an very anxious to get another. How long should I wait before bringing another cat in? I have rid the house of everything that belonged to the cat, because I hear this disease is very contagious. What else should I do?—*B.E.M.*

DEAR B.E.M.—There is still the possibility that the virus could remain alive on your own body (in your throat or nasal passages), and for this reason alone it would be a good idea to wait for three months before getting a new cat. You might also have the cat you're considering checked for the presence of the virus.

Unfortunately, we do not have all the facts about the transmission of this particular feline disease, but it is well known that some cats are carriers. For this reason, cat lovers, it is always a risk to introduce a new cat into a home where there are other healthy cats. The social stress in a home where there are several cats that aren't getting along smoothly can also trigger an outbreak of this disease.

DEAR DR. FOX—One of my two cats recently died from leukemia. This sickness just hit overnight. There is an 80 percent chance that my other cat will also have it. She will be checked within three months. But she is lonely now—the two cats were together for four years. My question is: If my cat checks out negative, will it be OK to get another cat in three months? I don't want to go through this heartbreak again.—*WORRIED*

DEAR WORRIED—Feline leukemia blood tests are not too reliable. If I were you, I would take the risk after three to four months of adopting a kitten from the animal shelter and give it a chance at a loving family life even if there is a risk of contacting leukemia. This virus is extremely common in cats. Many are born with it anyway and remain healthy. Other succumb because of dietary, social, or other stress.

DEAR DR. FOX—I heard recently on TV that cats transmit leukemia to other cats, and that no research has been done to show if cats can transmit this disease to humans. With more and more people coming down with cancer of all kinds, do you think that the day will come when we realize that cancer is being spread by our domesticated animals?—*A.L.*

DEAR A.L.—Wrong! Considerable research has been done to see if there is any connection between humans and feline leukemia. To date, no connection has been found. This means there are no grounds for concern and no need to avoid cats, since the two diseases are quite distinct. People are naturally immune to feline cancer. Meanwhile, research on feline leukemia continues. Your vet can give your cat a blood test to see if it is clear or not. In the not-too-distant future a vaccine will, I hope, be developed to protect cats from this all-too-prevalent and untreatable viral disease.

fungus infections (fish)

DEAR DR. FOX—Three of my goldfish have died, and they all had some kind of black stuff on them. What was it?—*L.E.*

DEAR L.E.—All fish can suffer from a variety of diseases that appear as discolorations or growths on the scales or as rot on the fins. The diseases are caused by microscopic parasites, bacteria or fungi, such as furunculosis, fin rot, and "ich." Because these diseases are so common, it is advisable to purchase your fish only from a reputable pet store that will offer some kind of guarantee. Also, quarantine new fish for ten to fourteen days to avoid the risk of introducing disease into the tank of healthy fish you already have.

DEAR DR. FOX—We've had two goldfish in a ten-gallon tank for almost five years. One fish has now grown some kind of whitish opaque bubble over its eye and part of its face around the eye. My vet is strictly a dog-and-cat doctor and can't help. Two pet shops suggested we treat it with something called Maracyn and Maracyn 2, but we don't know if we should. Any advice?—M.O.

DEAR M.O.—Follow the pet store's advice. Better stores are familiar with common fish diseases that many veterinarians don't treat, and they have appropriate medication to treat such problems. White lumps on fish are either fungal or parasitic growths and generally respond well to treatment.

If the growth is not too large, cut it off with a sharp knife and apply the medication as directed. Infections develop under the scales, and need to be removed surgically. Change the water every few days and put the healthy fish in a separate container to prevent cross-infection.

DEAR DR. FOX—My fish, Tumbleweed (I'm not sure what kind of fish he is), has had a type of fungus growing on his face. Tonight, when I cleaned out his tank, it looked as if his eye was coming out of his head. What's wrong with my fish? Is he going to die?—C.F.

DEAR C.F.—Poor Tumbleweed probably has lost the sight in one eye. External parasites and fungus infections are common in pet fish, and the sooner the problem is recognized, the better, because many of these infections grow into the fish's body, just like a fungus will grow deeply into the soil.

Others are less invasive at the onset and can simply be wiped off or painted with a medication you buy at a pet-supply store. Also, the water in the tank can be medicated, after changing the water, disinfecting the tank and all ornaments in it, and throwing out any vegetation, which may harbor infective agents. Often having the water too cold or having too many fish in one tank can trigger such diseases.

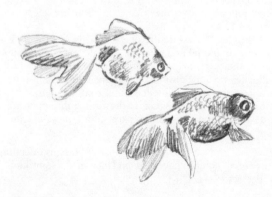

head-twisting (rats)

DEAR DR. FOX—I have three pet rats. I love them as pets and raise their babies to sell. But I am worried about two of them. My champagne rat keeps tilting its head from one side to the other. And my other rat seems to have an insatiable craving and stuffs everything into her mouth—even plastic. Any advice?—*J.M.*

DEAR J.M.—Rats are great pets, aren't they—intelligent, gentle, and very responsive. Head-twisting can mean an infection or disorder of the nervous system. If the condition worsens, get an antibiotic from your veterinarian and put it in the rat's drinking water. That may help. As for your other rat, who craves to get things into her mouth, give her a hunk of wood or a piece of beef bone (sparerib) to gnaw on. It will keep her teeth trim. Rats are curious and dexterous, so plenty of toys are in order, such as an activity wheel, cardboard tubes, paper to shred, etc. The more "enriched" their living space is, the happier they will be.

heart attack and stroke (dogs)

DEAR DR. FOX—Our dog will be fourteen years old in July. Within the past three months she's had what I think are heart attacks. She staggers for a minute, then collapses and lies quietly with her eyes open. She also urinates where she lies. After we pet her for a few minutes, she gets up and seems to be fine. I hate the thought of putting her to sleep.—*MRS. J.C.*

DEAR MRS. J.C.—Your dog could well be having mild heart attacks or strokes. A time comes when death mercifully intervenes. But sometimes the will to live, or supportive medication, keeps death at bay. If there is no suffering, then I say OK, let things be. But to be sure that your dog is not suffering physically or psychologically, have her examined by your veterinarian. Euthanasia—a humane death induced with dignity—is the ultimate act of love and responsible compassion.

hernia (cats)

DEAR DR. FOX—Is it true that when my cat's nose is warm he is sick? Also, my rather heavy one-and-a-half-year-old cat has a hernia about the size of a walnut, which doesn't seem to be giving him any trouble. But can we still play with him and pick him up like we did before?—*D.M.*

DEAR D.M.—In answering your first question, no—healthy cats often have warm noses, as do sick cats, but the latter have other signs to look out for as well, such as a hunched-up, ruffled appearance, lethargy, and disinterest in play and food. If the hernia is in your cat's middle (the navel or umbilical area) it may well require surgery. At any time, a segment of intestine could become trapped and twisted, and this could kill your cat. So if you want to be able to play with your cat and handle him normally, and also eliminate the risk of hernia complications, make an appointment to see your local veterinarian, who will advise you if surgery is needed.

hiccups (dogs)

DEAR DR. FOX—Our three-and-a-half-month-old mastiff suffers from hiccups frequently. As soon as she wakes up, she gets them. They don't last long, but she has many seizures. She has three excellent meals a day (instead of four) as advised by our trainer and vet. Any advice as to cause and prevention?—*J.D.*

DEAR J.D.—Hiccups go along with puppyhood—especially for a fast-growing pup like yours whose digestive system has to work overtime. Things will ease up when your pup's growth rate starts to slow down, when she eats less food and less often. But to be absolutely certain that it's nothing more than mild indigestion, your vet should check the dog's stool for worms, which do cause digestive— and worse—problems in pups.

hip problems (dogs)

DEAR DR. FOX—Our darling five-year-old shepherd-collie stays about ten pounds overweight all the time. As shepherds get older, we've heard they "get down in the hips." Naturally, we don't want to do anything that would make her more susceptible to this affliction. One of the tricks we've taught her is to sit on her hips with her front paws up in the air. Could this "sitting up pretty" bring on hip trouble?—B.G.

DEAR B.G.—Shepherds don't simply "get down in the hips" as they get older, they suffer from hip dysplasia, an inherited disease that gets worse as they get older. Most shepherds have it, thanks to ill-planned breeding for low, racy-looking hips.

You and your dog may be saved from such suffering, however, since she's a mongrel and therefore has a lower probability of having defective hips. Sitting up on her hips won't hurt. Give her regular exercise—warm her up before chasing a ball or stick—and do try to keep her weight under control. This is good preventive medicine for all dogs.

DEAR DR. FOX—Recently I noticed my German shepherd is tender around the hip area when I pet or touch him there. He will sometimes yelp and grab my arm in his mouth, but he's immediately sorry afterward, and I know it's from pain. My vet says *every* German shepherd has hip dysplasia to a certain degree: Is this true?—D.C.

DEAR D.C.—It is rare to find a German shepherd with "clean hips." This is one of the tragedies of the purebred dog hobby. Until recently people bred dogs for looks and not for performance, stamina, and intelligence. Consequently, almost all popular purebred dogs today have physical and often psychological defects. The "clean-up" operation is going to be difficult, and the American Kennel Club (AKC)—the national registry for purebred dogs—should take the initiative and *only* register veterinary-certified sound animals for breeding purposes. Until the AKC and breed clubs get together to clean up this mess, I will continue to advise people not to purchase purebred pups. (I happen to know of a hemophilic purebred Doberman who is being bred and spreading that inherited disease all over the United States.)

DEAR DR. FOX—I have an eighteen-month-old Great Dane whose parents are certified clear of hip dysplasia. His littermates have been x-rayed recently and are also in the clear. I understand that hip dysplasia is hereditary, but I'm still concerned because when my dog was about six months old he seemed to have pain that lasted a few days, coming and going. Also, he's slightly cow-hocked. Are these signs of hip dysplasia?—MRS. G.C.

DEAR MRS. G.C.—Giant breeds such as the Great Dane do actually seem to experience "growing pains." Their rapidly growing body structure requires a variety of essential minerals, especially calcium and phosphorus in the right ratio. Temporary imbalances can cause problems, but with such rapid growth, basic incoordination is the major trouble. Get a mineral supplement from your vet and give your dog vitamin D and A supplements as well (though don't overdo these). With poor coordination the pup is more likely to bruise or sprain one or more extremities. Growing up for dogs like Great Danes is just difficult. As for his being "cow-hocked," you should be glad. Too many Danes are too straight at the hock or ankle (thanks to bad breeding) and are permanently impaired and disfigured as a result.

itching (cats)

DEAR DR. FOX—My ten-year-old cat has a skin condition that causes intense itching with encrustation all over her body. She has had this for almost a year, and we've tried medicated baths and different types of pills, and now she is taking 5 mg of Prednisone. (We also removed her flea collar.) Please advise.— G.L.S.

DEAR G.L.S.—Dermatological problems can be extremely difficult to diagnose and treat. I would be cautious in the use of cortisone over any extended period. I would first suspect a hormonal imbalance and explore the possibility of sex-hormone replacement therapy if your cat has been spayed.

Next, try a different diet; your vet can help you determine if the problem is due to a food allergy. (Allergy to fish often causes skin trouble in cats.) These steps are worth exploring, provided, of course, your cat's skin has been checked for external (mange) parasites and flea-bite sensitivity.

itching (dogs)

DEAR DR. FOX—My two-year-old Yorkshire terrier has severe itching attacks in which he bites and scratches at his hind legs and buttocks. This generally occurs when he awakens in the mornings. The local vet suggests cortisone shots, but I'm reluctant to start them. Any suggestions?—S.J.

DEAR S.J.—Your instincts are on the beam. Cortisone will probably make things worse. Some "hyper" cats and dogs engage in very intense or frantic grooming when they wake up. But it might also be a case of infected or blocked anal glands. Have these checked out. If all's clear, extra attention or exercise may help take the dog's mind away from his obsessive compulsion and break the habit.

DEAR DR. FOX—My Chihuahua growls and chases her tail. The vet says it's her glands, and he has squeezed them a few times. She's still miserable and itching, and I'm at my wits end. What can I do? Would spaying help her? She'll soon be twenty months old. I'm alone and she's a lot of protection—I love her.— J.M.W.

DEAR J.M.W.—Anal glands that are causing constant irritation need more thorough treatment than the occasional squeeze-out to empty them. If they are infected, treatment with drugs is indicated. They can also be surgically removed. Discuss these options with your veterinarian, and feel free to seek a second opinion. Plenty of exercise and some roughage in the diet in the form of dog biscuits, bran, or cooked whole-grain rice will help—especially if you're feeding a moist high-meat diet.

Some dogs do growl and chase their tails as a form of self-play. I trust you and your veterinarian have eliminated this possibility. Your dog could also be acting up to get your attention. All she may want is for you to have a tug-of-war with an old sock. Either way, such games would help distract her and give her beneficial exercise.

lethargy (puppies)

DEAR DR. FOX—Our puppy, not quite a year old, doesn't do anything but eat and sleep. He doesn't want to play, but just wants to be left alone. The problem is that we got him with the idea of making him into a watchdog. How do we go about this? We can't afford a training school.—MRS. D.M.

DEAR MRS. D.M.—Your description worries me, because most puppies are extremely active and playful. From your picture, your puppy could be sick or brain-damaged. Or the puppy could have what veterinarians call the "purebred dog syndrome": the dog is an unresponsive dullard, existing on an eating-sleeping level and returning none of its owner's attentions. I advise you to consult your veterinarian. Good luck!

TRUE OR FALSE? A CAT HAS NINE LIVES

No, a cat has one life, like you and me. But it knows very well how to take care of that one life, and when it's sick, it will not stir for days, giving itself time to recover. This inactivity is a cardinal sign of illness in a cat. The important thing is to know when that inertia has lasted past the normal point and is so serious that you should consult a vet. But every owner should know his or her cat's peculiarities.

---

limping and stiff legs (dogs)

DEAR DR. FOX—My fourteen-month-old long-haried dachshund has a very definite limp, although it's sometimes in the front leg and other times in a rear leg. When playing with other dogs, she has no obvious limp, and jumps up on furniture with no strain. Any comment?—G.C.D.

DEAR G.C.D.—Don't let your dog jump on furniture. Dachshunds should stay low on the ground at all times. With their abnormal structure and keen spirit, they only injure their backs leaping on and off furniture. The problem is that their minds are normal, but their bodies are abnormal. Dachshunds often have grossly deformed legs and are thus more prone to sprains, which result in temporary lameness.

Shifting lameness and pain can also be signs of vertebral disc problems. Arthritis in older dogs is another disorder with comparable signs. Your pooch could also fake being lame occasionally, in order to get your attention.

DEAR DR. FOX—My nine-year-old Labrador has developed a stiff leg. Would aspirin at four-hour intervals help him? He is quite sedentary, so I take him on long hikes every day. Should I cut down on these? I hesitate to take him to our regular vet, except for necessary shots. He absolutely hates that man and has a fear even of the building!—P.D.

DEAR P.D.—Try going to a woman veterinarian. Many animals find women doctors less threatening. Or get a tranquilizer from your present vet and give this to your dog before you go in for the appointment. But get your pet in for an examination. A stiff leg doesn't sound very good to me. Your dog could have a painful

hip disease called hip dysplasia or some other orthopedic problem, which, if unattended, could get worse. Long hikes could be just what he needs—or they could
make things worse. Only the examination can tell you that. Good luck!

moles (dogs)

DEAR DR. FOX—My dog has at least ten moles all over her body. Could you
tell me where they come from and how they are treated? She is in good health and
eats well.—S.C.

DEAR S.C.—Moles and warts are quite common on the skin of dogs, and are
prevalent in certain breeds such as boxers and schnauzers. Moles are also found
more often in older dogs. They are generally best not touched, surgery being indicated only when they become large, pendulous, injured, or infected.

Some of these growths are caused by viruses; others are tumor proliferations of
certain cells, which can sometimes become malignant. This is one of many reasons why older dogs should see their animal doctor every six months. Signs of
malignancy might then be detected early.

motor-control problems (cats)

DEAR DR. FOX—I just got a cat for a present, and there's something funny
about him. He has a march for a walk. Also he can't jump up or climb stairs
without falling. Maybe he was hit when he was young, but the people who gave
him to me don't know. Could it be mental?—D.D.

DEAR D.D.—Cats that seem to "march" when they walk, fall easily, and
can't manage to walk at all when they're blindfolded have a neurological problem. This could have resulted from a blow to the head or, more likely, from an
infection during early life. Some cats are born with a defective or hypoplastic
cerebellum, but these cats learn to compensate for this disorder. Hypermetria
(high-stepping gait) and abnormal righting reflexes are symptomatic. Chances are
your cat is compensating fine, and that its I.Q. is OK. But to be safe and sure,
have your vet check him out.

DEAR DR. FOX—I have taken in the neighborhood tramp tomcat. We don't
know his age, but judging from the condition of his teeth, he is no spring chicken.
In the past four months we have observed about five occasions when he seemed to
lose motor control and staggered considerably. Yesterday he flopped across the
floor and went out flat for a few moments. What is your opinion?—J.J.

DEAR J.J.—Your old Tom could well be having the feline equivalent of a
stroke or heart attack. Have your vet examine him. Medication, if his problem is
treatable, could give him a new lease on life. Pet owners often forget that older
pets need geriatric care and can benefit from appropriate treatment and health-
care maintenance. You sound like a Good Samaritan. I wish there were more.

DEAR DR. FOX—Our eighteen-year-old Siamese seems to be in good health
for his age. The only problem is his equilibrium. Occasionally, if he shakes his
head hard, he will stagger or fall over. Can this be treated, or is it to be expected in
an old cat?—L.U.

DEAR L.U.—You describe signs of progressive neurological deterioration,
which are not unexpected in a cat as old as yours. Congratulations for keeping
him in good health for so long. Have him examined by a veterinarian to determine how incapacitated he is and what signs to look out for that indicate the time

has come for him to be put to sleep (such as crying, loss of appetite, loss of bladder control, etc.). Don't be talked into any extensive medical treatment with pills, injections, and so forth that may well cause more distress and not increase his life expectancy one jot.

mouth ulcers (dogs)

DEAR DR. FOX—I have two scotties. The female has developed ulcers in her mouth, and no method of treatment has helped. The vet said that she is going to have these sores for the rest of her life. I am terriby worried, especially since the male drinks the water out of her bowl. Can you help?—MRS. L.C.

DEAR MRS. L.C.—Since conventional medicine has failed, you should next try unconventional medicine. A number of animal doctors are finding that mega-vitamin therapy (high doses of vitamin C, especially) and putting the dog on a diet of fresh (unprocessed), homemade food will result in dramatic improvement for a wide variety of chronic disorders. (But not if these ulcers are cancerous, which they could be.) Talk this over with your vet, and if you get a totally negative reaction, seek a second opinion; such negativity reflects rigid thinking, which is not an attribute for any healer.

parvovirus (dogs)

DEAR DR. FOX—My German shepherd died from parvovirus. I have heard contradictory information about this disease. Our vet told us that our other dogs could not catch it; another vet said they could. One vet said yes to shots, another said they wouldn't help. What are the facts?—H.M.B.

DEAR H.M.B.—Parvovirus is a highly contagious disease that is rapidly transmitted from dog to dog. The veterinarian who said that your other dogs could not catch it is quite wrong. Because the vaccine to protect dogs from this serious viral disease has been difficult to obtain, many vets have been using a feline panleuko-penia vaccine, which supposedly provides some protection. It is advisable to repeat this vaccination every six months, although experts differ as to the number of shots needed.

The disease is a problem, but no cause for hysteria. Epidemics have been occurring only in certain locales. One theory is that this virus may be a mutant form of a feline virus that has now become infective to dogs. Whatever the origin, it is advisable to consult with your veterinarian and to have your dogs protected against this disease, especially if they are going to a boarding kennel or a dog show, where they're likely to be under stress or exposed to dogs infected with this virus.

pyorrhea (cats)

DEAR DR. FOX—The vet says my cat has pyorrhea, and warns that it may be necessary to remove all her teeth. I can't believe this! How would she get along without any teeth!—B.R.

DEAR B.R.—Pyorrhea is as serious in cats as it is in humans, but probably much more painful. Your vet knows that if the infection has spread to the roots of your cat's teeth (aside from inflaming her gums) there may be no alternative but to remove them via surgery. The vet will also give her treatment with antibiotics and steroids.

A toothless cat can adapt very well for its whole life on a diet of soft food, never fear. At least, she won't be in pain.

radiation from TV (cats)

DEAR DR. FOX—My cat just loves to stretch out on top of my TV set while it's on because it feels nice and warm. I recall reading that radiation coming from TV x-rays is unsafe. Is this true?—*D.M.*

DEAR *D.M.*—Several researchers believe that it is bad for any living organism, and that includes cats as well as human beings, to spend any length of time near electrical equipment. Various electrical frequencies may be hazardous to the body, which is, essentially, a delicately balanced bioelectrical field. Pending concrete evidence, which is difficult to come by, why not play it safe? Don't allow your cat to remain for any length of time on top of the television.

radiation therapy (dogs)

DEAR DR. FOX—If humans can be given radiation therapy to kill lingering cancer cells, why can't dogs receive similar treatment? My Marden is nine-years-old and weighs fifty-five pounds. Is there anything I can do other than wait for more tumors to appear in my dog?—*S.J.*

DEAR *S.J.*—There are certain forms of cancer in dogs that can be treated with radiation or cancer chemotherapy, but few veterinarians have such techniques available. Your dog's doctor can advise you if such treatments are available at a state veterinary school. Often, because of time, expense, and the kind of cancer the dog has, little can be done except limited surgery and supportive medication.

seborrhea (dogs)

DEAR DR. FOX—What is the cause of seborrhea? Is there a cure? My poodle has had it on his tummy and chest for years. Now it's also on his feet. They are swollen and sometimes bleed. He is a sweet, playful dog, and I grieve to see him suffer.—*S.&D.Mc.*

DEAR *S. & D. Mc.*—Seborrhea has many underlying causes and can be either dry and flaky or extremely oily and sometimes itchy. Some forms respond well to supplementation with fat-soluble vitamins, A, D, and E, B-complex, and polyunsaturated fat (vegetable oil) in the diet. Discuss these options with your veterinarian and explore making up your dog's daily food from entirely fresh produce.

I have found that zinc and selenium supplements help in some seborrhea-type skin conditions. Shampoos containing selenium can also be effective. For awhile, avoid feeding your dog foods containing wheat. Cereals can interfere with the absorption of essential trace elements such as zinc and, in large breeds, contribute to fatal "bloat."

DEAR DR. FOX—My six-year-old German shepherd has a bad case of seborrhea, resulting in loss of hair, oily, thick skin, and a lot of scratching. My vet prescribed medicines that gave the dog only temporary relief. He said that the only cure would be to have my dog neutered, as he is producing too many hormones. Could neutering be the answer?—*L.E.I.*

DEAR *L.E.I.*—Seborrhea can be difficult to treat. Your dog should have a thorough clinical examination, including allergy tests. I doubt that castration will help, although some forms of seborrhea do sometimes respond to castration or estrogen treatment. Poor thyroid function may be involved instead.

Attention to diet is especially important—too much carbohydrate can aggravate skin problems. Also, have the dog checked for mange and fleas, since flea hypersensitivity can cause severe itching and skin reactions. A bacterial culture and antibiotic sensitivity test should be run to rule out the possibility of a bacterial skin infection.

sensitive back (cats)

DEAR DR. FOX—My eight-year-old cat has recently put on weight. Also, he has become very sensitive from the middle of his back to his tail and keeps trying to reach that area to bite it. The result is that he falls over and bites his paw. My vet is perplexed. The cat is otherwise normal and playful.—MRS. M.C.

DEAR MRS. M.C. —Hypersensitivity along the back in cats can be related to a number of problems, from hormonal imbalance associated with neutering to infected anal glands, kidney trouble, or a partially herniated "slipped" disc in the spine. A very thorough veterinary examination is needed, so perhaps you should seek a second opinion. If he checks out OK, you'll have to face the fact that some cats are hypersensitive for no apparent reason and do fine, living a full and contented life—so long as no one strokes them from the middle of the back on down to the tail. Heads and necks only, please! That's a small price to pay for the company of a pet.

sensitive nose and ears (cats and dogs)

DEAR DR. FOX—Our all-white cat has been diagnosed as having cancer on his ears. They bleed and have crusty sores. The vet says he may need to have his ears cut off. We feel so helpless. Is there any cure? Could a cat live without ears?—A.P.

DEAR A.P.—White cats do sometimes become photosensitive (hypersensitive to light), especially on the tips of their ears. Repeated exposure to sun, just as in sensitive human beings, can eventually lead to skin cancer. Your vet is not talking about taking your cat's ears off, but surgically trimming them, which is necessary surgery for cancer.

After the surgery, keep your cat indoors away from sunny windows until the ears are completely healed, and apply a strong sunscreen every day. This is an example of how domestication can create disease. Breeding white cats increases the chances of genetically linked deafness as well as photosensitivity. In the wild, white cats wouldn't survive, so these problems wouldn't develop.

DEAR DR. FOX—My redbone coonhound has this nose problem—the skin gets dry, cracks, and peels. He licks it continuously, making it more tender. I've had him to three different veterinarians, but their ointments or astringents don't seem to help much.—R.L.B.

DEAR R.L.B.—Your dog may have photosensitivity, which causes him to get sunburned easily. This is quite common in collies, so the ailment has been nicknamed "collie nose." Some dogs, after recovering from a bout of distemper earlier in life, may develop hyperkeratosis of the nose and sometimes also of the foot pads.

If the latter cause is more likely, ask your vet for a mild cortisone and antibiotic cream to apply. Vitamin A and D ointment may also help. If you suspect sunsensitivity, a regular human sunscreen ointment will help. Chronic sore noses rarely heal, and the best you will probably be able to do is to stop things from getting worse.

DEAR DR. FOX—We have two Heinz 57s. One of them, a large brownish-orange dog, is bothered by biting flies all over his muzzle. We have put everything on it, but nothing works. Could you suggest something?—M.T.

DEAR M.T.—Biting flies usually attack a dog's ears and not the muzzle. I suspect that your dog may have a sun-sensitive muzzle and actually gets sunburned. Sore spots and weeping blisters (which may attract flies secondarily) can develop on a sun-sensitive nose. You should see your vet to confirm the diagnosis, and apply a suitable sunscreen as a preventive measure.

shaking (rabbits)

DEAR DR. FOX—When I put my Netherland dwarf rabbit into her cage, sometimes she just lies there and shakes. Do you know what causes this and how it can be treated?—M.S.

DEAR M.S.—Shaking or trembling can be a sign of fear, brain malfunction, or neuromuscular disorder. Have your vet give your rabbit a thorough neurologic checkup; this will help put your mind at rest. Chances are it is a benign disorder and not likely to progress into something more serious, each as convulsions or paralysis.

skin infections (dogs)

DEAR DR. FOX—My boxer has big boils or blood blisters between her toes, and they give her a lot of trouble. She also gets small cracks or sores underneath her feet. The vet gives her shots and medicine for staph infections, but even that clears it up only temporarily. Can you help my poor pooch?—B.B.S.

DEAR B.B.S.—Boxers are prone to skin problems, and some are very resistant to treament. When a particular bacterial infection is involved, sometimes a vaccine made from a culture taken from your dog will help. This is called an autogenous vaccine and is worth investigating. Supportive treatment with multivitamins and local treatment (for short periods only) with a steroid-antibiotic combination may also help, as might a changeover to a homemade diet of rice and lean meat. You should explore these possibilities with your veterinarian.

skin infections (guinea pigs)

DEAR DR. FOX—Our three-year-old guinea pig seems to be healthy, except for a big black spot on a swollen front paw. The black spot is on the bottom of its foot and is about the size of a dime. It bleeds sometimes, and we apply an antiseptic solution from time to time. We keep his cage clean and dry, and his water is in a bottle. Perhaps you could comment.—B.A.B.

DEAR B.A.B.—Guinea pigs, just like humans, all develop skin infections, possibly from an injury or abrasion. If the wound is not properly treated, a chronic inflammation may set in. I advise you to take your pet to a veterinarian, who will clean and dress the afflicted area properly; if it is not cleaned thoroughly and all dead tissue removed, it will never heal.

staph infections (dogs)

DEAR DR. FOX—Can staph infections be successfully treated? My Siberian husky has had open sores on his face, around his mouth, and in his ears for several weeks. I am growing concerned. Three visits and $34 later his skin condition has not improved satisfactorily, even with Panolog for the exterior sore, erythromycin pills, and lidocaine pills. At first, the medications helped, but then their effects wore off and new sores appeared.—R.Z.

DEAR R.Z.—Staphylococcal infections in dogs are extremely difficult to eradicate. They are often a symptom of stress, which could be social or related to a nutritional deficiency or food allergy. Constitutional factors, such as genetic susceptibility and hormonal dysfunction (such as hypothyroidism), can also contribute.

You have the option of following these leads (and I would begin by putting your dog on an all-natural diet of rice, vegetables and lamb, eggs, cottage cheese, or fish for protein) or having an autogenous vaccine made from a culture of your dog's infection.

sudden death (cats)

DEAR DR. FOX—Six months ago we lost three nice cats. One became ill and would not eat or drink the next day; he was dead less than a week later. The other two cats died the same way, showing no pain. They were fed at a pan with four other cats whom we still have, so it couldn't have been the food. What could have caused such quick deaths?—MRS. E.H.

DEAR MRS. E.H.—Without doing an autopsy on your cats, I can only offer an educated guess. Cats that play outdoors can get into rat poison and are more likely to pick up a contagious viral disease from sick stray cats in the neighborhood. Chances are your cats died from feline distemper or panleukopenia, which can kill cats so quickly it looks like they have been poisoned. So follow the basic rules—have your cats protected with vaccinations and avoid letting them roam free outdoors if you value their lives and health.

swim bladder malfunction (goldfish)

DEAR DR. FOX—I have a goldfish, raised from an egg, that has been swimming belly-up for more than five weeks. I keep the fish alive now by placing it in a shallow dish for feeding, after which it is returned to a large tank. What caused this condition? As a last resort, should I puncture the bladder with an insulin needle?—C.F.L.

DEAR C.F.L.—All fish can develop a malfunction of the swim bladder, so that it expands and prevents them from being able to dive. It also disrupts their sense of balance, and as a result they swim upside down. Infection, overfeeding, or sudden temperature change can bring on this condition. For severely distended fish the needle can be a lifesaver, just like relieving a cow of bloat. The process is risky, and the fish might die. You will have to make the final decision.

swollen toes and lip (cats)

DEAR DR. FOX—My kitten is about five months old, and repeatedly her toes swell and a smelly, clear liquid seeps out. Now her lip is swollen. Could the condition be related? I have been to our vet with her, but the problem lingers on. Incidentally, the swellings do not seem to be painful, but please answer. I am worried.—I.F.

DEAR I.F.—Your cat could have a herpes-type virus infection. Cow pox is another possibility if you live on or close to a farm. Recent studies in England have discovered that cats can and do get cow pox, which, fortunately, has a low transmission rate to humans. You might ask your cat's doctor to arrange for a consultation at the state veterinary school and hospital.

tear-duct problem (dogs)

DEAR DR. FOX—My six-year-old poodle's eyes are so wet all the time that even his chest and the side of his face get damp from the secretion. The hair under his eyes sticks together. Also, one of his eyes has a white cloud over the center with a dark spot in the center of it. Any suggestions?—D.L.D.

DEAR D.L.D.—Your poodle probably has defective tear-duct drainage, which leads to tear-staining on the face. Sometimes an inturned eyelid or eyelash can be causing the chronic irritation. If so, it can be corrected surgically. The white spots in the eyes could well be early cataract formation—a common affliction in poodles. I would suggest a trip to the vet for your poodle.

tongue flipping (dogs)

DEAR DR. FOX—Our seven-and-a-half-year-old Yorkshire terrier sits with her tongue flipping in and out at a fast pace. It must come out almost two inches. It makes me nervous to watch her. Have you known other cases?—R.K.M.

DEAR R.K.M.—Dogs will engage in "air licking" or "licking *in vacuo*" for many reasons. Sore gums, tonsillitis, or even an itch on their backs that they can't reach can trigger this behavior. Considering your dog's age, I would suspect a minor neurological malfunction such as low-grade epilepsy. Don't be too anxious about your dog's quirk—unless it becomes more frequent and intense. Medication with an antiepilepsy drug may even rectify the problem.

tumors (cats)

DEAR DR. FOX—When my cat stopped eating, the veterinarian told me he had enlarged kidneys and that there was nothing that could be done. I don't understand—isn't there a medicine for this condition?—MRS. G.O.

DEAR MRS. G.O.—Your veterinarian was trying to be kind; by "enlarged kidneys," he probably means cancer. This is one form that feline viral leukemia can take—tumors invading various internal organs. There is no cure, no magic pill or miracle surgery. Seek a second opinion if you wish, but if you must, put your cat humanely to sleep. Don't feel guilty. It's an indulgence to try to keep a pet alive at all costs regardless of its suffering, as too many pet owners do.

tumors (dogs)

DEAR DR. FOX—My dog has what the animal doctor called a "fatty tumor." He said it's not dangerous—only disfiguring. One of my friends says vitamins can cure this condition. Can you tell me which vitamins?—C.A.

DEAR C.A.—Some people think vitamins are magic! I have never heard of vitamins dissolving away tumors. Lipomas, or fatty growths such as your dog has, are best left alone if they are small, and operated on if they become unsightly, ulcerate, or get in the animal's way. There is no simple home remedy for such growths. Surgery is the solution.

DEAR DR. FOX—Our three-year-old boxer has been getting tumors on her lip and back. We are concerned about her getting them while still so young. We had another boxer who didn't have tumors until she was eight years old. Why do boxers get tumors? Should I give her a special diet to avoid the tumors? Would the tumors cause her to be hyper?—L.G.

DEAR L.G.—Skin tumors are prevalent in certain breeds, especially boxers. Most are benign, but some can turn malignant or get damaged, enlarged, and infected. You should consult your veterinarian. Chances are these will be nonmalignant and easily removed. There's no special diet to control this problem, and I doubt that there's a significant relationship between temperament and this particular affliction.

DEAR DR. FOX—Our darling miniature schnauzer has patches of little red bumps that sometimes break open in little crusty pimples. We give her one cortisone pill every other day, and a cream, Dicort-V, for relief, but she still itches. If there anything else we can do? What causes this problem?—J.&M.D.

DEAR J.&M.D.—You are describing a common schnauzer skin problem. Viruses and sometimes abnormalities in the cellular structure of an animal's skin can lead to the development of pinkish or gray-brown "moles." These are benign tumors, but they should be carefully checked at regular intervals for signs of infection or malignancy. This is the kind of breed-linked disorder that requires further research.

It is quite probable that with careful attention to the frequency and distribution of this schnauzer skin problem, breeders would eventually eliminate it. Meanwhile, all you can do is live with it and follow your veterinarian's advice.

tumors (hamsters)

DEAR DR. FOX—I have a teddy-bear hamster named Ted. Lately, Ted's stomach has swollen. He also has cataracts. I've had four hamsters and never encountered this problem. Is it a tumor? What do you think?—X.

DEAR X.—Since your hamster has cataracts, he's probably quite old. He would have expired in the wild long ago. Little wonder that he has developed a chronic abdominal problem, which is most likely a tumor. When he begins to lose weight rapidly or is no longer active and interested in food or life, it will be time have him put to sleep.

tumors (parakeets)

DEAR DR. FOX—My pet parakeet has developed a growth at the lower part of his mouth near his beak. The growth looks like a swelling, but during the last three months, it hasn't grown any bigger. Do you know what it could be?—D.T.

DEAR D.T.—Parakeets often suffer from growths or tumorous outgrowths on various parts of the body. Some can be operated on by a veterinarian. However, an anesthetic must be given, and this is a risky procedure since birds don't withstand surgery well. Your vet will determine if the growth is operable or not. If it is, good luck. If not, you and your bird can still live happily with this minor problem, I'm sure.

urinary infections (cats)

DEAR DR. FOX—Help! For two years our black Burmese cat has behaved wonderfully and has been affectionate. Recently we had him declawed to save our living-room furniture. Our vet also found a urinary infection, but ten days of medication has not cured him. Coincidentally, we have been feeding an abandoned stray cat. Since then, our cat has been obsessed—running from window to window and now urinating anywhere in the house.—M.R.M.

DEAR M.R.M.—What a lot of coincidences. And all could be stressful to your cat: claw surgery and the presence of an intruder in his territory are enough to bring on an acute cystitis, combined coincidentally with a need to mark his territory with urine. I would suggest another urine test to see if the bladder infection is still present. Then buy a leash and harness and walk your cat outdoors as often as possible. Confine him to one room in the house (with litter tray and plenty of attention) for a couple of weeks. If he is unchanged, light tranquilization with Valium may do the trick.

ANNOUNCEMENT FOR CAT OWNERS

As all cat owners know or should know, feline urolithiasis, also known as the feline urological syndrome, is a common cat killer and a cause of much suffering. Fine stones or "sand" form in the urine and block the urinary tract so the cat is unable to urinate.

Research funded by the Morris Animal Foundation at Colorado State University says high levels of magnesium and phosphorus in catfoods can cause these stones to form. Acidifying the urine by mixing ammonium chloride (obtainable from your veterinarian) in the cat's food helps prevent and dissolve urinary stones.

---

warts (dogs)

DEAR DR. FOX—Our scottie has been troubled by warts for years. They are pink and grow quite large. The vet removes them, but they grow back. We hesitate to anesthetize him again. Can you help us?—E.G.

DEAR E.G.—Dogs do suffer from classical warts—a transmissible virus infection of the skin that results in benign, tumorlike growths. There are also other benign skin growths that look like warts but don't seem to have any virus origin. Such tumors can become malignant, however, so I advise that you always have your vet check. If the vet is suspicious, he or she will take a biopsy sample to find out exactly what you are dealing with. Minor warts can be treated with silver nitrate stick (ask your vet), but regular tumors cannot; these should be removed, but only when they get in the way. The less cosmetic removal, the better for the animal.

DEAR DR. FOX—My dog, Sam, has a growth on his right eyelid that looks like a wart. How can we dissolve it?—M.R.D.

DEAR M.R.D.—If you apply wart remover to your dog's eyelid, chances are it will get into his eyes, and that could lead to serious complications. Please, don't try home doctoring. A small wart can be easily and safely removed by a veterinarian. The cost should be minimal and well worth it, since your dog will not only look better, but have vision that is not occluded all the time. Warts are caused by viruses, and home doctoring could cause them to spread.

wet-tail (hamsters)

DEAR DR. FOX—My hamster got wet-tail two weeks after I purchased her. How can I treat this?—P.T.

DEAR P.T.—I get this question repeatedly in my mail because wet-tail is the most common problem affecting hamsters. Wet-tail can mean one of two things: you are feeding her too much greens and moist food, which is causing loose stools, or it could be an intestinal infection that will require putting veterinary medication into her drinking water for a few days. If treated soon, wet-tail can be quickly corrected.

DEAR DR. FOX—I bought a teddy-bear hamster about a month ago and it soon died of wet-tail. I know wet-tail is a common disease; before I buy my next hamster, could you tell me what to do to prevent it?—P.F.

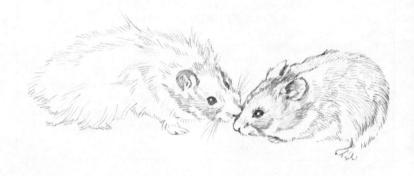

DEAR P.F.—Wet-tail isn't a specific disease, it's a symptom—a sign that the hamster has a serious intestinal infection. Hamsters with wet-tail and runny droppings require veterinary attention. Before you get a new hamster, be sure to clean the cage and utensils thoroughly with hot water and a strong disinfectant and detergent. Then let the cage and other gear and utensils stand in the direct sun for a few hours. Ultraviolent light (which is in the sun's rays) is a super antibacterial sterilizer.

ALLERGIES

asthma (cats)

DEAR DR. FOX—My all-black cat, Inky, recently diagnosed as having asthma, gets medication for his spells. Is there anything else I can do to make him comfortable?—H.C.

DEAR H.C.—Asthma is not a disease, but a symptom. I suggest that you ask your vet to try to track down the possible cause. If your vet won't take the trouble, find one who will. Your cat could be suffering from allergic reaction, or his asthmatic attacks may occur when he gets too excited or upset by certain goings-on in the household. Be on the alert from now on to spot what is triggering the attacks. Therein may lie the solution.

bee stings (cats and dogs)

DEAR DR. FOX—I have a dog and two cats, and I was wondering what could happen if they were stung by a bee. Do animals have allergic reactions the way some humans do? If so, what do you do about it?—D.D.

DEAR D.D.—Yes, animals do suffer from bee and other insect stings just as we do, and the sting causes pain and inflammation. These can be alleviated somewhat with baking soda or antihistamine cream. Sometimes the insect's stinger may need to be removed. If your pet has difficulty breathing or its hair stands up in tufts, then it may be having an allergic reaction, and that calls for emergency veterinary treatment.

finding the cause

DEAR DR. FOX—With no set pattern, large lumps appear on the head of my sheltie, sometimes closing his eyes completely. Two different vets comfirmed allergy as the cause. One suggested shots, the other Benadryl. The season seems to make no difference. The dog stays in the house and is also allergic to fleas. Any suggestions? The lumps disappear as quickly as they appear.—*P.F.*

DEAR *P.F.*—Allergies seem to be on the increase in pets and people alike. Since there is no seasonal difference, you must check on such things as certain table scraps, floor polish, and hand cream you put on yourself.

We live in chemically complex and often hazardous environments. It will be up to you to pinpoint the triggering cause. Vacuum the house thoroughly every other day (to remove dust and pollens), and fumigate the house if needed to get rid of any fleas that spend part of their life cycle off the dog in cracks, crevices, and carpets. Good luck. Allergies are a plague.

pollen and grass (cats and dogs)

DEAR DR. FOX—Our calico cat is constantly coughing and has a hard time breathing. We take her to the vet every year, and he gives her a shot plus pills. He says it's pneumonia. But I think it's something else, because it occurs every spring and lasts all summer. My other question is, how can you tell how old a cat is?— *G.S.L.*

DEAR *G.S.L.*—It is extremely difficult to tell how old a cat is. Since a cat's front teeth are so small and don't wear down like a dog's teeth, there's no wear-index to assess age.

Your cat's spring and summer respiratory problem could be an allergic reaction. Cats, like people, do become allergic to pollen, grass, etc., and a course of treatment with suitable allergy-relieving medication is indicated. Keeping your cat indoors may also help.

DEAR DR. FOX—Our Norwegian elkhound has developed a blueness first in his right and now in his left eye. The vet gave him medication, and although the eye sometimes clears, the condition returns the following day. Any advice?— *MRS. J.S.*

DEAR MRS. *J.S.*—Your dog is probably suffering from an allergic reaction to grass and other pollens. Don't allow him to rub his face in the grass, which he'll tend to do to alleviate the eye irritation, and which will only make things worse. Alternatively, he may be having an eye reaction to a viral infection such as canine hepatitis, or chronic eye irritation from inturned eyelids or lashes.

If an allergy is likely, keep him out of long grass, and continue with the medication your vet has prescribed. Many forms of allergy in dogs have an inherited basis and could be cleared up by owners not breeding dogs with such problems that might be transmitted to the pups.

DEAR DR. FOX—I have a Welsh Highland white who spends July until the first frost with a constant itch. The vet suggested four Allerests a day. This accomplished nothing. What shall I do?—*MRS. G.J.*

DEAR MRS. *G.J.*—Popping pills into a pooch may help alleviate the symptoms, but symptom-oriented medicine isn't usually the best. When medicine doesn't work, more extensive tests and alternative medications are needed to get to the root of the problem.

Your dog may well have an allergy. A veterinarian can run tests and provide some medication to make your pet's summer easier. Meanwhile, a regular mild shampoo and a light jacket to keep pollen and grass off his coat (especially on the undercarriage) will also help.

synthetic materials (cats and dogs)

DEAR DR. FOX—In your column I read about a cat who had a skin problem involving encrustation. My cat had the same problem, and I cured him by removing all vinyl and nylon from his sleeping places and replacing or covering them with cotton and wool. I understand a lot of cats have this same allergy—and a dozen cotton diapers is a lot cheaper than medicine.—J.N.

DEAR J.N.—Thanks for sharing your experience. Yes, both cats and dogs (and people) can suffer from contact allergies, and do better if contact with vinyl, plastic, nylon, and other synthetic materials is lessened. Handling such problems is an integral part of what is now called ecological medicine, so you are right on target with your alternative of natural cotton.

INJURIES AND EMERGENCY CARE

accidental imprisonment (cats)

DEAR DR. FOX—Our three-year-old cat was accidentally shut in a large bureau drawer filled with sheets. When we found her two weeks later, she was in amazingly good condition and quite calm—there was no trauma, no incredible appetite—and now she is her normal self. Can you explain how this could be possible?—M.R.

DEAR M.R.—It's amazing that you cat didn't howl the house down. Some cats will claw and try to escape before giving up. What obviously kept your cat alive is her good physical condition and the fat stored in her body together with her natively minimal water requirement. Since cats were originally desert animals, they have a metabolism that actually helps conserve water.

Your letter should serve as a reminder to all cat owners who think their lost cat has slipped outdoors to check all rooms, closets, and drawers. Pet owners who are deaf or hard-of-hearing should be especially careful, because they won't be able to hear their cat calling.

EMERGENCY AID: ACCIDENTAL BREEDING

A common emergency for owners of both female dogs and female cats is accidental breeding. To avert pregnancy, get the animal to a vet, who will give her an injection of a hormone. But you have only twenty-four hours leeway from the time of mating. There are side effects—cats may die—so it's a risk-filled decision (and another reason for spaying in advance).

---

bloody noses (gerbils)

DEAR DR. FOX—My pet gerbils get bloody noses every once in a while. Then the blood dries up on their fur and looks pretty messy. Any clues as to why this is happening?—K.F.

DEAR K.F.—The trouble can be caused if gerbils are allowed to chew sharp materials, or have a cage with sharp edges between which they can push their noses. So check your cage out very carefully. Also, make sure it's not really a discharge from the animals' noses, which might need veterinary treatment. And don't worry if you see a red discharge coming from your gerbil's eyes—gerbils secrete a bloody, red-brown material in their tears, called porphyrin.

eye injuries

DEAR DR. FOX—Recently, my cat, Laurel, got into a fight with another cat, who cut Laurel's eyeball. It has pus all over it and is swollen. We don't have money to take him to a vet, but we found out that we should put an eye ointment on it and clean it with warm water. When we didn't have eye ointment, we used boric acid. Is this OK?—*CANDY, AGED NINE*

DEAR CANDY—There are no two ways about it—injured eyes should be treated by a doctor, otherwise certain injuries can lead to blindness. Could you face that? It's a pet's right to be examined by a veterinarian when it's sick—and an owner's responsibility. People who say they can't afford it should think twice about owning a pet. It's a good idea to put spare change into a piggybank for your pet's future needs.

falling (cats)

DEAR DR. FOX—I have a kitten whose leg was broken when she was thrown down. She is now in a cast. I always heard that cats land on their feet when they fall. If this is true, why did her leg break?—*J.D.*

DEAR J.D.—Cats do normally land on their feet when they fall because they have a very fast righting reflex triggered by gravity receptors in their ears. But a cat that is *thrown* down, or one that falls from a considerable height, could fracture a leg. Very often, the jaw is broken or the spleen ruptured from a severe fall. Also, some cats—particularly Siamese—do have a brittle-bone disease and require special treatment and careful handling.

DEAR DR. FOX—Is it possible for my one-year-old cat to have brain damage? Since falling out of a four-story window onto a concrete sidewalk six months ago, she goes to the bathroom on the floor about four feet from the litter box. Also, before the fall, she was very introverted, and now she is very friendly to everyone.—*TIRED*

DEAR TIRED—Your cat's sudden friendliness after the accident is probably less of a sign of brain damage than of a positive response to the tender loving care she received. The erratic use of the litter tray could have many causes, from a sudden insecurity relating to a new home situation to wanting an extra-clean litter tray. Brain damage usually includes some abnormal neurological signs, and long-distance diagnosis of this nature is not possible; if in doubt, have your cat thoroughly evaluated by your veterinarian.

limping (dogs)

DEAR DR. FOX—My two-year-old miniature schnauzer has an odd habit. When he gets up after he has been lying down for a while, he limps. When he walks around, the limp immediately goes away.—*E.D.*

DEAR E.D.—Your dog is too young for arthritis, which causes older dogs to be lame, especially when they first wake up. Possibly your pet has a sprain or even a more serious injury such as a torn knee ligament or cartilage. Avoid strenuous exercise for your dog and have him examined by a vet. The problem could get worse rather than better.

HEALTH REMINDER: HEATSTROKE

Come the "dog days" of summer, and your car can become a hazard to your pet.

Never leave your animal in a parked car when the temperature is over 70 degrees. If you park in the shade, remember the sun moves. Even with windows partly open, the temperature in a car can reach 160 degrees in a very short time. Dogs and cats do not perspire like people; they cool themselves by panting, and with only overheated air to breathe, your pet may die of heatstroke.

Symptoms of heatstroke: increased panting, red to purple coloration of the tongue, glazed eyes, vomiting, and convulsions leading to collapse.

Treatment for heatstroke: Gradually immerse the animal in cool water, or if possible spray it gently with a garden hose; apply ice packs to its head and neck and under its tail. Once you get the temperature down, take your pet to the vet immediately.

---

loss of claw (crabs)

DEAR DR. FOX—I have heard that if a crab loses one of its claws it will grow a new one. Is this true? the other day I found a sand crab, and a guy on the beach broke off two front claws so we could handle it. He said the crab felt no pain and could grow new claws. But about three hours later, it died.—*S.G.*

DEAR S.G.—Crabs can pinch off their own claws, without bleeding, and it is true that they will eventually grow new ones. Crabs need their claws for many purposes, especially for defense. Removing both claws leaves the animal quite helpless, and even if we are not sure that it hurts, it is inhumane to so mutilate any creature. Having two claws torn off could well have killed the crab from shock; they, like all creatures, are not totally insensible. If only crabs and other silent creatures could scream—then humans might have empathy and respect them more!

poisoning

DEAR DR. FOX—What are the chances of a complete recovery for a kitten who got into some phosphate-type poison in the form of Shell Ant and Roach Spray for only ten minutes or so? He apparently got it on his fur and then licked it off for nearly a week until we discovered what had happened. He was given the antidote at the hospital and sent home presumably well, but he doesn't eat or play much. At times he wants to bite, lets out little whines, and is not obedient.—*J.F.*

DEAR J.F.—It really is tragic the number of pets (and children) who get into harmful chemicals that are in the house—especially when it is so easy to stow such hazards out of pets' reach. Your kitten will take many weeks to recover, and there may well be residual internal damage that will require careful vigilance. Be careful, however, not to overindulge and fuss over him excessively, since this could set up other problems, such as finicky eating. Exercise moderation—even in tender loving care.

porcupine quill removal (dogs)

DEAR DR. FOX—I recently heard that if a dog encounters a porcupine the hard way, vinegar may lessen the pain and soften the quills. I was wondering if this same method can be used if a dog runs into a cactus.—*D.H.*

DEAR D.H.—Vinegar is an acid, and acids sting. It certainly will not help reduce pain, but vinegar could have some slight antiseptic affect. For cactus thorns and procupine quills, the only answer very often is a general anesthetic or knock-out dose with a tranquilizer. An easygoing dog may not need to be sedated, and with a dog who trusts you and has a high pain tolerance, you may be able to remove the offending "points" yourself. Wash the wounds well with mild soap and water and apply a first-aid cream. Keep a lookout for any warm lump that may develop later. This would mean an abscess is forming, and veterinary treatment should be sought. Cut the quills in half before you tweeze them out so they can "breathe" and will be easier to remove.

SUMMER HAZARD—SKUNKS!

If your inquisitive pooch gets itself sprayed by a skunk, come vacation time:
1. Wash its eyes with a solution of boric acid.
2. Give it a soap-and-water bath.
3. Give it a second dousing with a few cans of tomato juice.

SNAKEBITE

Animals , like people, can be bitten by a snake when on vacation. What to do?
- Apply a tourniquet above the bite.
- Keep the animal quiet and warm to combat shock.
- If you're caught without a snakebite kit, make a single incision between the fang holes and then suck and squeeze out the venom.
- Get your pet to a ranger station or to the nearest human hospital if veterinary help is not available, so that antivenin can be administered to the animal.

---

tail protection (dogs)

DEAR DR. FOX—When excited, my sister's Gordon setter bats his tail on furniture and doors. This splits the end of his tail so that blood spatters everywhere. Is there any salve or medicine you could recommend that might heal the tail?—*K.E.B.*

DEAR K.E.B.—So many dogs suffer from what I call the Peter Pan-Perpetual-Puppy Problem. They never seem to grow up, remaining hyper, solicitous, playful, tail-wagging creatures who exhaust nearly everyone.

Chances are that by now the tail has some minor infection associated with the traumatic lesions, so you should have it thoroughly cleaned and medicated by a veterinarian. A lightweight tail protector of plastic tubing slit down the side may help if you can't keep a bandage on. Ask the vet for an adhesive-type bandage and keep the tail covered and protected for at least a couple of weeks. Once it has a chance to heal, it may cease to be a problem. If not, part of the tail may eventually have to be amputated.

INTERNAL AND EXTERNAL PARASITES

feather lice (parakeets)

DEAR DR. FOX—My parakeet has lost almost all his feathers. This has happened before, but never this badly. He talks, eats everything, and doesn't appear sick. He just looks dreadful. Help!—J.D.

DEAR J.D.—You're describing a perennial problem of parakeets. Some of them preen excessively and self-mutilate to the point of looking like plucked chicks. Others shed because of a sudden stress, or lose their feathers because of hormonal imbalance. Feather lice—which literally cut off the feathers at the base—can ultimately create a bald bird. The best hope for your bird is a veterinary examination. Just as in people, there are many reasons for baldness, and your vet might be able to cure your bird. In the interim, keep him warm.

flea repellants (ultrasonic)

DEAR DR. FOX—Do ultrasonic flea repellants really work? They are for sale, either to attach to your pet's collar or in large units to use in the house.—D.L.

DEAR D.L.—This is the latest consumer ripoff. I wish the Food and Drug Administration would intervene. These devices, which claim not to affect pets, have no effect on fleas but do drive some pets crazy.

One woman's cat ran away as soon as she switched on her ultrasonic unit in the room. Imagine poor dogs wearing these devices all day and night. Dogs and cats are sensitive to ultrasound, while fleas are quite resistant to it. So protect your pet and your pocketbook and don't buy these quick gimmicks.

fleas (cats and dogs)

DEAR DR. FOX—Help! What do millions of pet owners do to keep fleas from their homes? We had none until we took our four-year-old white Persian to be declawed; he came back full of fleas. I sprayed him and put a flea collar on him, but I'm finding fleas throughout our home. If I don't get rid of these fleas, my husband will make me get rid of the cat—so please help.—F.C.

DEAR F.C.—Fleas have part of their life cycle developing off the animal in cracks, crevices, and thick carpeting around the house. So, vacuum everywhere. Then put your cats in a safe place after dipping or powdering them. (Ask your vet to recommend a dip or powder.) Call in a pest-control company to fumigate the house. Repeat this after approximately three weeks to get any fleas that may have been in a resistent phase in their life cycle. After that, don't let your pet roam free—he can pick up fleas outdoors. And forget about that flea collar—it's not a good preventive, especially on long-haired cats and dogs. Stick to dips and powders.

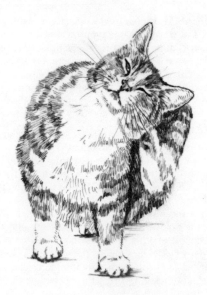

SUMMER FLEAS

Fleas are a late-summer problem in most areas, and a year-round one in warmer states. Fleas may be present if there are red, itchy bites on you or your children and if your pet scratches often. One or more itchy, moist spots may mean an animal has flea hypersensitivity. Examine the "pile" of your pet's fur; you may see pinhead-sized, brownish fleas moving quickly, or black "dust" that looks like coal flecks. Brush or pick it out and place on wet white paper. If the paper turns a reddish-brown, it means there are fleas (the coal flecks are flea feces). To fight fleas, use a veterinary-approved dip or powder, and consider having your house fumigated.

DEAR DR. FOX—My cat has fleas. Can fleas get on people and still live? Do they sometimes live in the ears of the cat?—*L.A.D.*

DEAR L.A.D.—Yes, fleas can get on people and live and bite (or more correctly pierce your skin and suck your blood). The bites cause much itching and at first glance look like chicken pox. But dog and cat fleas don't live long on the human body; they prefer their natural hosts.

If your cat is scratching its ears, it may have earmites, which are invisible to the naked eye. These can cause irritation and a brown, tarry buildup in the ear canal. If you suspect this, take your cat to your animal doctor.

DEAR DR. FOX—The flea season is coming, and I don't want my cat to suffer as she did last year. What do you think of flea collars for cats?—*M.M.*

DEAR M.M.—If used with extreme caution, flea collars on cats can be effective. But if you use one, you must be on the alert constantly, because they can produce rather serious toxic reactions. Examine your cat every day under the collar to see if an allergic skin reaction is developing. Never let the collar get wet. Some cats do get quite ill from the chemical in the collar, showing symptoms of uncoordination, refusal to eat food, increasing weakness, anemia, and other complications. Unless you know you can be fully alert to these possibilities, stay away from these cat collars.

DEAR DR. FOX—You recently wrote about flea collars. My Persian cat became paralyzed in the hindquarters and then nearly died before it was realized that her condition was due to wearing a flea collar. Isn't it true that Persians or any longish-hair cat should *never* wear a flea collar?—MRS. H.W.A.

DEAR MRS. H.W.A.—Now is the season for pet owners to be especially alert to the problems that flea collars can cause in both cats and dogs. Not all brands of collars and not all pets will react as acutely or as severely as your Persian, but chronic exposure can have a cumulative effect or stress the pet so that it is more susceptible to other problems too.

Many pesticides suppress the immune system. So please take the flea collar off your pets and use them only in emergency, and only for a few days. Fleas get resistant quickly. On very furry pets, like Persians and large dogs, collars aren't effective. The more potent the collars are, the more likely your pet is to get sick.

DEAR DR. FOX—Our dog suffers terribly from fleas, so last summer our vet gave us Proban for him. This medication apparently "poisons" the dog's blood, and when fleas feed on the dog, they die. Proban has worked well for us, but we wonder what the drug's long-term effects are.—P. AND A.B.

DEAR P. AND A.B.—I would not use this drug on dogs that are hypersensitive to fleas and who develop allergic dermatitis and "hot spots" from their irritation, because the drug goes into the dog's blood and kills fleas only after they have bitten. Systemic poisons are always risky.

Some holistic veterinarians suggest making a strong tea of one lemon rind chopped up into one pint of boiling water. Let it steep overnight, then on the next day anoint your dog's body with it. Repeat every three or four days through the summer with an occasional regular shampoo and flea dip.

DEAR DR. FOX—Do you approve of Proban as well as the prolonged use of flea collars? Does the flea get resistant to Proban?—M.D.

DEAR M.D.—So many people ask about Proban. I do *not* approve of Proban. It is an oral insecticide which, in higher doses, would kill your dog as well as the fleas. Lower doses, though not poisonous, could still cause problems. With repeated use, this insecticide may lower the animal's overall resistance to disease.

There are safer ways to get rid of fleas. One of the first steps, of course, is to train your pet cat or dog to stay indoors and not roam free, since the more it roams, the more likely it is to come home with fleas. Regular dipping or powdering plus fumigating your house are safer remedies. Also never mix pesticides by using more than one flea treatment at once, since your pet may well become poisoned.

DEAR DR. FOX—Is it safe to use the new "deflea" treatment on a pregnant cat? I refer to the treatment where the medication is rubbed on the back of the cat's neck, or the cat is injected. I understand the treatment works on the nervous system, and all the fleas drop off.—P.D.H.

DEAR P.D.H.—I would not use any injectable, systemic insecticide on any pet, and least of all on a pregnant one. The possibility of causing damage to the developing fetuses, especially during early development, is very real. The fewer chemicals in our lives and in our pet's lives the better, not simply because one particular chemical may be hazardous, but because there are so many contaminating our air, food, and water that the potency of one can be enhanced by others. This is called chemical synergy, which means that it is silly to talk about "safe" levels of PCBs, pesticides, and other industrial and agricultural chemicals in the environment, as our government does today—especially when there are at least 60,000 to be concerned about.

DEAR DR. FOX—I have heard from numerous people that sprinkling yeast on cat or dog food once a week will keep fleas away. It supposedly makes the fleas dislike the odor of the animal's coat. Is this so?—V.N.

DEAR V.N.—Some people do make this claim about fleas—and mosquitoes, too. Some even say that eating yeast or taking vitamin B tablets repels mosquitoes from attacking people! I would like to think so, but to my knowledge it has not been researched or documented. However, it's certainly worth a try, since yeast is a good source of essential B vitamins. Because of the taste, some animals will refuse to eat food that has yeast sprinkled on it, so only give a pinch to begin with and no more than a teaspoonful every three or four days once your pet accepts it.

flies (dogs)

DEAR DR. FOX—We have a fine Siberian husky who is the constant victim of biting flies during summer. Her ears are a heartrending sight, and we are desperate and anxious to bring her misery to an end. Can you help?—S.C.

DEAR S.C.—I have found that Cutter insect repellent is extremely effective in keeping biting flies off dogs. It is a sad fact that these flies can eat the ends of a dog's ears off in one summer, and they do drive some dogs crazy! Cutter insect repellent can be bought in stick or cream form from any outdoor sporting goods store. An alternative is lemon oil and oil of citronella. But don't buy any repellent in spray-can form; sprays scare dogs and get in their eyes.

heartworm (dogs)

DEAR DR. FOX—My beautiful nine-year-old Irish setter developed heartworm last summer. A couple of months later, I took him to the vet, who said there was nothing he could do because the dog is too old. Now the dog is beginning to show the effects of heartworm, and I wanted to know if you could tell me more about the subject.—MRS. A.

DEAR MRS. A.—Heartworm is a canine disease transmitted by mosquitos, which enter the dog's bloodstream when the insect feeds off the dog. These young worms eventually mature inside the dog's heart and disrupt its functioning, causing very serious problems. Treatment can be worse than the disease, because when the worms die, they break up and can block circulation. The drugs used have side effects, so that a highly infested old dog would probably not survive the treatment. All dog owners should give their animal preventive medicine during the summer, but not carcide, which contains stirid. Stirid has caused a variety of problems in dogs, including severe and chronic diarrhea and infertility.

DEAR DR. FOX—I have just gone through the process of having my two dogs treated for heartworm, followed by two rounds of treatment with pills before they were declared "clean." They are now on preventive pills. When I was in the East about ten years ago, I had never heard of the problem. Is it more prevalent in the Midwest?—*B.M.*

DEAR *B.M.*—Canine heartworm, once most prevalent in the South, is now a widespread problem in most states. Unfortunately, no vaccine has yet been developed, and the only prevention is daily medication—a pill or liquid in the food.

Dogs must first have their blood checked and receive treatment if they are afflicted. Fortunately, this parasite only rarely affects cats, and very occcasional cases in human beings have been reported.

hookworm (dogs)

DEAR DR. FOX—My puppy has hookworms and roundworms. I've taken her to a vet, but the medicine doesn't seem to help. Is there anything else I can give her?—*M.X.*

DEAR *M.X.*—Pups often need two or more treatments to get rid of worm infestations. Your vet should examine her stools about two weeks after treatment to be sure she's OK. However, if you put your pup out in the yard, chances are she will be reinfested from contaminated soil, hence her recurrent infections. Ploughing up your garden or building her a concrete run, and cleaning up all droppings thoroughly, may help break her of this cycle.

DEAR DR. FOX—Could you tell us how a dog gets hookworms and how soon a litter of puppies should be checked for this problem?—*C.D.L.*

DEAR *C.D.L.*—Pups can be born with hookworms, so their stools should be checked at six, ten, twelve, and sixteen weeks of age and the animals treated as needed. The eggs passed in the feces develop in the ground; in this way the dog becomes reinfested, especially if he frequents a heavily contaminated yard. Regular checkups are better than giving the animals preventive medication in case they do pick up an infection. Prolonged treatment can be harmful, so checkups pay off.

DEAR DR. FOX—One of our friends claims that papaya seeds—dried and ground and sprinkled on pets' food—will kill hookworm parasites. Is there any truth to this?—*F.J.B.*

DEAR *F.J.B.*—Papaya seeds are supposed to have some beneficial effects in ridding a pet of certain internal parasites. But I would not prescribe such treatment without good evidence and objective test trials. To my knowledge, there are none.

mange (dogs)

DEAR DR. FOX—My three purebred adult boxers are my "kids," and I love them very much. They were all diagnosed as having demodectic mange, and I am puzzled as to how they got it. I read that it is hereditary, but none of my three dogs are related. I am most anxious to get by dogs back to normal.—*M.R.*

DEAR *M.R.*—Demodectic mange is an all-too-prevalent, distressing, and disfiguring canine skin disease. Strictly speaking, it is not inherited, but pups do become infested from their mothers. They may show no symptoms until much later in life—during stressful growth phase, heat, pregnancy, or disease such as hookworms or distemper. A "good" parasite lives quietly and peacefully on its host, but when its relationship with the host (your dog) is disrupted by some new condition, then trouble starts. It's not in the best interests of the parasite to kill its host.

DEAR DR. FOX—When our dog developed a severe case of mange, none of the prescribed treatment benefited her, and the vet finally recommended that she be put to sleep. Dixie was nearly covered by raw areas and scratched constantly. One day in my absence, a neighbor made a mixture of burned motor oil and flower of sulfur and dipped Dixie in it. The itching stopped. After two weeks and several dips, Dixie began to heal and recover her beautiful coat. My neighbor is a hunter and saw this done on hunting dogs with good results.—M.G..

DEAR M.G.—The mixture your neighbor used was a "kill-or-cure" treatment. Dogs are more often killed than cured, especially when kerosene or turpentine is used instead of motor oil or axle grease (which supposedly smothers the mites). It's a matter of luck. Many veterinary pharmacologists are now taking a fresh look at some of these old remedies because of the cost and frequent bad side effects of many modern drugs. Exercise caution, though, and please check with your vet before trying Grandpa's elixir!

DEAR DR. FOX—When we lived in Guatemala, our Welsh terrier suffered severely from mange. The gardener suggested flower of sulfur mixed with petroleum jelly, which worked well. I'm writing this because I was horrified recently to hear that some people use burned motor oil and, worse, kerosene and turpentine to mix with the flower of sulfur. It's not necessary to inflict such pain to get the healing effect.—J.M.D.

DEAR J.M.D.—Thank you for your confirmation of the benefit of sulfur and petroleum jelly, which supposedly smothers the mange mites. However, it is not a panacea. Dogs in poor condition, run down, with a heavy worm infestation, or with a defective immune system often succumb to mange. Without treating these auxiliary stressors, mange treatments often fail. Good diet is an essential part of treatment too.

Folk remedies often get confused, so little wonder people apply petroleum or turpentine instead of petroleum jelly mixed with powdered sulphur. This should not be fed to the dog, but applied daily to the mangy areas on the skin.

DEAR DR. FOX—Our purebred puppy developed a little spot about the size of a pea on top of her head. The vet said she had the red mange and prescribed an insecticide in tablet form to be taken orally and a liquid to be put on the bare spot. Now she has developed a larger spot on her hip. Is this the usual treatment for red mange? Can we expect a complete recovery?—G.R.

DEAR G.R.—The kind of mange your dog has is difficult to treat. It is very important for your vet to make sure she has no other problems, such as worms, which could delay her recovery and response to treatment. Your dog should be on a top-quality, high-protein diet that includes one teaspoon of vegetable oil, a pinch of brewer's yeast, kelp, wheat germ, and multivitamin capsules (one adult dose per day). You should also tell the breeder about the problem. You may be doing another buyer a favor, as the breeder may have some other sick animals around.

DEAR DR. FOX—We love our dog as dearly as we do our own son. The problem is the dog has mange and the vet's treatment—pills and shampoos every day—have not helped yet. He is still itching terribly and losing hair. Now, is it possible that my husband got mange from the dog? He has itchy pimples over his body and hands and red spots on his feet that hurt and burn. The doctor says he's allergic to something, but doesn't know what. What should we do—put the dog to sleep? What should my husband do?—*MRS. W.D.*

DEAR MRS. W.D.—Yes, it is possible for humans to get mange—one or another kind of skin parasitic mite that causes itching and dermatitis. But it is usually easily cured in people, once a doctor recognizes it.

Mange treatment takes time in dogs. Very often there is some other factor that is lowering the dog's resistance, and so the treatment of mange alone doesn't always help. Your dog could have a concurrent worm infestation, for example, which needs treatment as well as a rich diet to build up his resistance. Some dogs seem to have an impaired immune system, so other supportive medication is needed. It's best to buy a pup from a local breeder who will guarantee that your pet is healthy.

mites (cats)

DEAR DR. FOX—One of my Siamese cats picked up earmites somewhere, and now they both have them. I've had them to a vet, but when they started taking medicine, they got into big fights, so I gave up. What can I do to get rid of the pesky mites?—*J.U.*

DEAR J.U.—Your cats fought because the ear medication changed their familiar smell and they took each other to be strangers. This is an example of instinct-control, when animals cease to be rational. My suggestion is that you keep the two cats separated for a few days while they are being medicated. That way they should get used to the new odor on their bodies. Return them to the vet first, since their ears will probably need another good cleaning out before you start treatment. Earmites are very common on cats and can cause much distress. I suggest all cat owners check their pets today; any black tarry secretion in the ears could mean your cat has earmites and requires treatment before the problem gets worse and almost incurable.

DEAR DR. FOX—I recently got a cat, and since then I've broken out with little pimplelike sores that itch. I'm not allergic to cats, as I've had them in the past with no reaction. Do you think it's a parasite or fleas? What medication should I use?—*L.M.R.*

DEAR L.M.R.—Your cat might well have infested you with a rare mite, called *Cheyletiella parasitivorax*, which causes pimplelike, itchy sores. This mite is a microscopic creature, and you should have your vet examine your cat. Rabbits are often infested with this parasite. Treatment with rotenone or pyrethrum is effective. There's no need to panic or get rid of your pet. If the vet finds that your cat is not infested, perhaps you infested yourself outdoors with chiggers.

mites (mice)

DEAR DR. FOX—My pet mouse's ears keep bleeding. Once they start to heal, Patches scratches them and squeaks as if someone were murdering her. What can I do?—*A.O.*

DEAR A.O.—Mice do suffer from various skin diseases, and a common one is caused by irritating mites. In order to help the healing process and to stop the animal from scratching, it is advisable to put tape on the hind and front paws or to fix a little cardboard collar around the animal's neck. However, one of the best cures for many mouse skin problems is to have another mouse in the same cage. It will groom its companion, and its saliva will have a powerful healing effect. Mice that are kept alone have more skin problems in areas like the back and ears, which they can't easily reach to groom. Your vet should also make sure that Patches doesn't have a serious contagious disease such as mouse pox.

mites (parakeets)

DEAR DR. FOX—My parakeet's beak itches and is very dry-looking around the nostrils. His dry feet also itch. I've been noticing small feathers all over the cage. What could be the problem?—*J.G.*

DEAR *J.G.*—I get dozens of letters like yours. Your bird is suffering from a very common and widespread affliction of birds—an infestation of small parasitic mites that borrow into the bird's beak. This results in a dry, scaly crust, and the beak can become deformed, softened, and much larger. It is extremely irritating to birds. Mites can also burrow under the scales on birds' feet and legs. Your veterinarian can prescribe a relatively nontoxic insecticide for you to paint on your bird's beak and legs. But you must disinfect the cage with hot water and strong detergent and get a new perch once your start treatment. This is one of the most common and easily recognized cage-bird diseases. The parasite can be destroyed if caught early.

ringworm (dogs)

DEAR DR. FOX—My dog has ringworm. It started on her back and spread to her stomach. Patches appear in the dog's coat and hair falls out. The veterinarian prescribed Conofite to her coat once a day, and a half tablet daily of Griseofulvin 250 M.H. Do you know of any additional medication I may use?—*J.K.*

DEAR *J.K.*—Ringworm is not actually a worm, as some people think, but a fungus that grows on the animal's skin. Under ultraviolet light you can see it glowing on the shafts of the animal's hair. What your veterinarian prescribed sounds like adequate treatment. You must be careful to avoid getting this disease yourself, since it is transmissible to humans. Fortunately it is easily diagnosed and cured.

Your dog will be helped further by being on a well-balanced diet supplemented with a tablespoon of vegetable oil and a teaspoon or less of brewer's yeast plus vitamins E and A. Sunlight is sometimes helpful for certain skin conditions.

tapeworm (cats)

DEAR DR. FOX—Every day my cat goes out, eats mice, and comes home with worms. We have had her dewormed, but then she goes out and starts all over again. Dr. Fox, it is too expensive to have her dewormed every week. What do I do?—*WORRIED*

DEAR *WORRIED*—You certainly do have a dilemma. The obvious solution is to break the cycle and stop your cat from going out and picking up the tapeworm infestation from the mice that she kills and eats. It is also important to check that she does not have fleas, because there is another species of tapeworm that has its life cycle in fleas that cats, but not humans, will pick up. Do *not* deworm your cat every week. It is surprising how well cats adapt to having tapeworm in their systems. Even if you cannot prevent your cat from going out and hunting, stop the worming unless she becomes very run down and seems unable to tolerate a high parasitic infestation. Generally, these parasites live quite well in their hosts and do not cause undue suffering or sickness, except when the animal is stressed.

tapeworm (dogs)

DEAR DR. FOX—Our German shepherd has tapeworms constantly. We de-worm him every other month, and the veterinarian bills are piling up. Pooch is kept tied most of the time, but his friends come to visit him. When, why, and how does he get tapeworm?—J.A.

DEAR J.A.—Your vet is not doing a thorough job. What he has to do is find out what kind of tapeworm is infesting your dog and take steps to eliminate the source. It could, for instance, be from dead rabbits. More likely, since he's tied up, your dog is getting reinfested because he also has fleas, and fleas are the inter-mediate hosts for a very common dog tapeworm. Vets who give pills for the worms and don't do anything about the fleas need a refresher course in parasitolo-gy—or ethics.

tapeworms (parakeets)

DEAR DR. FOX—I have an eleven-year-old parakeet. She has two long tape-worms, which come into her throat and choke her. I've called every vet I know, but they only treat dogs and cats. Do you know of a remedy for this problem?—WORRIED.

DEAR WORRIED—If you really believe your bird is in danger of choking, you need a veterinarian immediately. Ask friends of yours who have birds to rec-ommend a "bird doctor," or call your humane society for a name. Ask the vet to prescribe tapeworm medication, calculating the dose in proportion to your bird's weight. But it is possible that you are imagining that the bird is choking. Many wild animals have such parasites and live in harmony with them, if they have adequate food and are not stressed. You should not treat the bird unless it is losing weight and not eating well, because treating cage birds for intestinal parasites is risky since the drugs used to kill the worms can kill the bird, too.

tapeworms (transmitting them to people)

DEAR DR. FOX—My veterinarian says our three-month-old puppy has tape-worms. Can my small children catch it from the pup?—D.W.

DEAR D.W.—Most of the tapeworms that infest dogs cannot infest people, partly because we are immune and partly because the worm don't use humans as hosts in their life cycle. Dogs get tapeworms from eating their own fleas, mice, and squirrels in which the tapeworm is in a cyst or larval stage. Considering all the diseases that can affect pets, it is fortunate that so few affect us and vice-versa. Be sure that if your pup's tapeworm is the kind that develops via the dog's flea, that you get rid of fleas, otherwise your dog will get reinfested with worms.

tick identification

DEAR DR. FOX—My malamute has a tick under her skin. It is lodged on top of her head, right near her ear. I've tried to squeeze it out, which is not easy when holding a ninety-pound dog. My dog shakes her head quite a bit and holds that ear at "half-mast" sometimes, so I'm sure this tick is still there. What can I do to get it out? Her hair is quite thick.—A.C.

DEAR A.C.—I knew a psychology professor who thought he had a blood blis-ter on his arm that was getting bigger and bigger; my then six-year-old daughter looked at him incredulously and said, "Don't you know that's a tick?" It's not always easy to tell, but you should know that ticks suck blood, get fat, and drop off. They don't stay on a dog more than a few days. Your dog has either a sebaceous cyst or a skin tumor. Have a veterinarian treat it.

DEAR DR. FOX—My light-colored cat picks up ticks (even in the winter) when he goes out. I keep him in most of them time, but is there any medicine I can give him? We have lots of squirrels around our neighborhood. Any connection?—*C.D.*

DEAR C.D.—Sorry, you can't blame this one on squirrels (though they will harbor ticks), and no, there's no medicine that will keep ticks away from your cat. This is one reason why I encourage cat owners to raise their kittens to be indoor cats. Free-roaming cats bring home ticks, fleas, and a host of other problems. It is possible that by now your house is infested with ticks. Fumigation may help that. Try to make your cat stay indoors and take him for short walks on a leash if he will accept it. Keep him away from underbrush and thick vegetation: ticks don't like exposed sunny areas.

SUMMER HAZARD: TICKS AND THEIR REMOVAL

Examine your animal regularly for ticks in summer months. Ticks are brownish-black. They will usually cling to your pet's ears or between its toes.

To remove a tick, paralyze it first by soaking it with nail polish remover, linseed oil, or petroleum jelly; then pull it out firmly with a pair of tweezers. Flush ticks down the toilet; otherwise they seem to have nine lives.

---

worms (transmitting them to people)

DEAR DR. FOX—Our Siamese cat likes to sleep in our bathtub all the time, and I was wondering if it is possible for us to get worms from him when taking a bath, since he has been infested with them a few times.—*L.C.*

DEAR L.C.—No. There is no cat worm that you could pick up from the bath where your cat chooses to nap. But what an odd place to sleep—cold, smooth comfort indeed, surrounded by white walls like some isolation tank for a deep meditator.

Cats are such wonderful individualists. If your cat is an indoor cat, check for fleas, since these are one source of worms. Another source might be mice or other creatures your cat may eat outdoors. So keep him inside, but not confined to the bath.

worms—treatment (cats and dogs)

DEAR DR. FOX—Is it always necessary to worm a new puppy? I really don't find any worms in his stool and have a large enclosed yard in which he frisks about happily.—*E.M.*

DEAR E.M.—It is usually necessary to worm pups and kittens because they are often born already infested with worms. These parasites aren't always present in the stools, but their eggs are and can seen only under a microscope. Take a stool sample to your animal doctor for analysis and in the meantime, get your puppy his protective vaccination shots.

It's a good idea to have your pet checked over each year and a stool sample analyzed every spring and fall, especially if your animal spends time outdoors where it's likely to pick up hookworms. And don't forget: blood tests are needed if heartworm, a common canine killer, is present in your area.

DEAR DR. FOX—Even though my kitten was eating well, he stayed thin. The doctor confirmed he had roundworms and gave him a blue pill. At the same time, he gave him a distemper shot. Two days later the kitten had diarrhea and was so weak he couldn't stand, much less eat. When he died, the doctor said it was from the worms. Was it? Or was the pill too strong? Is this a common reaction?— MRS. R.M.

DEAR MRS. R.M.—Medicine given to a sick animal can sometimes make it sicker; this is called iatrogenesis, or treatment-induced illness. It wasn't a good idea to stress the cat with a vaccination while it was ill. However, a more likely explanation is that your kitten got to the vet too late. The diarrhea was related to the fact that it was seriously ill. A severe worm infestation can indeed kill kittens, or reduce their ability to withstand other diseases that eventually cause them to die. That is not uncommon. This is one reason I urge all pet owners to give their kittens a routine veterinary checkup.

SURGERY

anesthesia (dogs)

DEAR DR. FOX—Five months ago our dog suddenly developed a bad limp. We thought it was merely a pulled muscle, but x-rays showed that she had ruptured the ligaments in her knee. The vet recommends surgery to replace the ruptured ligaments. She is eight years old, and I am worried about her having anesthesia. Also, what will her future be like?—C.B.

DEAR C.B.—Surgery on your dog is to be recommended, since the longer it is put off the more likely it is that more crippling arthritic changes will take place. There are risks with anesthesia, but if your dog is healthy and not overweight, the risks are greatly reduced. I would urge you to have her operated on. She will then have a new lease on life. The injury is common in dogs and is best avoided by keeping a dog trim and well exercised.

DEAR DR. FOX—Our fourteen-year-old overweight dachshund needs dental work because her breath is terrible. Our vet wants to clean and scale her teeth, which requires putting her under anesthesia. She was anesthetized before, but she was younger. Needless to say, our concern is that she's old and might not survive. I've asked two other vets for opinions—one said yes and the other no. Your answer will be the deciding one.—MRS. G.J.

DEAR G.J.—There is always a risk in giving an anesthetic to an animal or human being. The older the patient, the greater the risk. However, if your dog is otherwise in good condition, except for the obesity, it would be advisable to have her teeth attended to, since infected gums and teeth can cause chronic ill health and suffering.

With modern tranquilizers and short-acting anesthetics, the risks have been greatly reduced. A veterinarian who is a competent anesthetist and aware of the risk involved will know whether or not your dog should be operated on. Trust.

bone fractures (cats)

DEAR DR. FOX—When our cat was struck on the left top part of his leg, the vet operated on him for a fracture and installed a pin in that area. About ten days after the operation he moved around fairly well on his three good legs, but since then he won't move at all. Sometimes he goes into a spasm or fit for two or three seconds and utters a heart-rending scream. Our vet says it's normal and gave us some medication for him. He goes back soon to the vet to remove the pin.—J.H.R.

DEAR J.H.R.—There are many complications that can arise after orthopedic surgery. I hope your veterinarian gave your cat an analgesic. Animals don't always clearly show how much pain they are in, and it is advisable, especially after painful bone surgery, to give a painkiller. Readers anticipating bone surgery for their animals should bear this in mind.

When your cat is fully healed, I trust you will train him to live indoors and to walk on a leash. Free-roaming cats are too often killed or injured by automobiles.

cherry eye (dogs)

DEAR DR. FOX—The vet has suggested that our five-month-old puppy might be a candidate for "cherry eye" surgery soon. Is this step serious, dangerous, and/or really necessary? What exactly is cherry eye?—C.P.

DEAR C.P.—Cherry eye—or a red, inflamed conjunctiva—is developed by dogs for many reasons. The fact that your veterinarian recommended surgery leads me to believe that your pet is suffering from entropion. This is an inward curling of the eyelids that results in the eyelashes irritating the surface of the eye, causing a chronic inflammation. It is extremely unpleasant for the afflicted animal, and I would therefore recommend that if this is the case you should have your dog operated on as soon as possible.

postsurgical trauma (cats)

DEAR DR. FOX—I recently had my cat spayed. For two days she hid under the furniture then she started crying and hasn't stopped. Since she never cried before, it's getting to me. Is this a stage—or do you think she'll be sad from now on?—O.R.

DEAR O.R.—There's always a chance that your cat is crying because she's sick. However, my guess is that she is suffering from a transient traumatic reaction to surgery, and the best way to deal with that is to get mild tranquilizer from your vet after he or she has examined your cat thoroughly. Give it to her for a few days along with lots of tender loving care, and watch your crybaby quiet down.

DEAR DR. FOX—My cat always loved to be petted and would sit on my lap for hours while I studied. Then he was declawed and neutered. Since the operation, Patches will not let anyone pet him; sometimes he will even bite me or kick me with his back claws. He also avoids visitors by hiding under a bed. What is the reason for such behavior, and what can be done about it?—W.J.N.

DEAR W.J.N.—Fortunately, it is most unusual for a cat to develop such a postsurgical or posttraumatic phobia, which is what your cat is suffering from. Forced contact to resocialize your pet won't help, but mild tranquilization for several days may be of benefit. Your vet can prescribe such a medication to reduce your pet's fear reactions, and then you should be able to get close and start "contact therapy." Reduce the dosage gradually and keep up the contact, petting, grooming, playing, etc.

slipped-disc surgery (dogs)

DEAR DR. FOX—Our schnauzer-poodle was operated on two years ago for a slipped disc, and he is now walking and running. His hindquarters are still weaker than the front, but he sure has it mastered. It's a miracle after seeing him in a walker at the hospital.—*M.P.*

DEAR *M.P.*—Thanks for your letter and personal success story. Yes, surgery has helped many dogs with herniated intervertebral disks. But a word of caution: Such dogs should never be bred, since there is a strong hereditary factor in this disorder. Regular exercise and a sensible diet to keep your dog lean rather than overweight is one of the best preventives. An enzyme injection (to dissolve ruptured disks) has recently been developed in Canada for humans. This may also soon be available for dogs.

tumors (dogs)

DEAR DR. FOX—Our thirteen-year-old dog is partially paralyzed in one leg and hip and has cataracts, but despite these he gets along quite well. Our real problem is that the vet found a tumor on his testicle and recommends surgery "before it metastasizes, as it is malignant." One, how could he know it was cancer without a biopsy? And two, do you recommend surgery of this kind on an old dog?—*R.B.*

DEAR *R.B.*—Certain tumorous growths in particular parts of the body, such as the testicle, are more likely than not to be malignant and to spread (metastasize) throughout the body. Not doing a biopsy saves you money and also saves the dog the trauma of anesthesia. Anyway, at his age, he doesn't really need his testicle. And if he's well enough for surgery, you should waste no time and have the enlarged one removed. The old boy has plenty of life left in him.

undescended testicles (dogs)

DEAR DR. FOX—My Pomeranian (six-and-a-half-years-old) has one testicle on the outside and one on the inside. The vet said an operation is needed to correct this condition. We lost one dog after an operation that may not have been needed. Please tell me if this operation is essential. If he doesn't have to have it, how harmful would the symptoms be for him?—*P.M.*

DEAR *P.M.*—Undescended testicles are quite common in dogs, especially in some of the smaller toy purebreds such as the Pomeranian. The testicle that is still inside the dog could change and start producing female sex hormones, which could feminize your dog. Removing the testicle would certainly be a preventive measure. However, a more conservative approach would be to wait and see. There is a chance that your dog will not have any problems whatsoever; he *is* already on in years. Meanwhile, do not use your pet for breeding, because the problem is inherited.

AGING AND EUTHANASIA

behavior changes (dogs)

DEAR DR. FOX—We have a beagle, who is a pretty old girl. She has this habit of patrolling the kitchen, lingering at our feet and following us. If we're not careful where we step, we fall over her. In the evening, she'll start to whine, whimper, or howl, even though she's not hungry. Does she want attention in her old age? Is she getting senile?—*P.Y.*

DEAR *P.Y.*—Dogs do begin to act in odd ways when they get older, some becoming more irritable, others more dependent. I wonder if they have any concept of growing old and of death. Wanting to be close to you in the kitchen simply shows that she doesn't want to be alone or left out of things. Whining at night may also be a sign of her needing more attention. And when she gets it, she learns to whine or howl even more to maintain your attention. This way, through manipulation and reinforcement of their owners, older dogs' behavior begins to change. I would advise a veterinary checkup every four months or so, since older dogs do need extra attention and geriatric care, about which your veterinarian can advise you.

bladder problems (dogs)

DEAR DR. FOX—Can anything be done for our sixteen-year-old, terrier-mix, spayed female's leaky bladder? She spends most of her days in the house sleeping and often wakes up in a puddle. Except for this problem and being practically deaf, she is in good shape.—*B.F.*

DEAR B.F.—Poor thing—she's not alone. Treatment with estrogen may be helpful since "leaky bladders"sometimes are linked with spaying. Older dogs do sometimes urinate in their sleep. A diaper would certainly help. Tuck the diaper under her when she goes to sleep and restrict her sleeping area to a disposable cardboard box into which she can easily crawl and feel safe and comfortable. Some aging dogs become distressed when they have such accidents.

For those, I feel that being put to sleep is a humane answer. A time comes when the body functions begin to fail, and it is selfish and inhumane to keep an animal alive when it is suffering emotionally or becoming a vegetable. Of course, only you can judge how your dog is taking her problem.

gray hair (dogs)

DEAR DR. FOX—Can you please tell me why dogs, and I am speaking of golden retrievers in particular, get gray around the mouth and nose area at such an early age? My golden is only four years old and is already turning gray.—*MRS. M.DeR.*

DEAR MRS. M.DeR.—The loss of pigmentation of the hair is part of the aging process in pooches and people alike. Some breeds, like the golden retriever, age faster than others—many an eight-year-old golden retriever looks like a fifteen-year-old mutt. Why certain breeds age faster is a mystery. I'm surprised that medical researchers aren't looking more into this dog problem, since it would seem that the medical industry could profit well from helping those people who want to remain young forever. I like gray hairs myself, but in the age of narcissism, it's *passé!*

methods of euthanasia

DEAR DR. FOX—In a recent article, you advised that one should make sure that local animal shelters use a humane way of putting animals to death—a shot of sodium pentobarbital, not the decompression chamber. At our local shelter, where I volunteer, we use the decompression chamber.

We were told that it's like going up in a airplane—the pressure goes up, and the animal just goes to sleep from lack of oxygen to its brain. It seems simple and painless, and it takes about sixty seconds.—*VOLUNTEER*

DEAR VOLUNTEER—Decompression is not a humane way of killing animals. The jet-plane analogy is exceedingly misleading; the cabin of a passenger plane is pressurized, so the change in altitude is not experienced at all. A decompression chamber, in contrast, produces a very rapid drop in pressure, which can be extremely painful for the animals. For more documentation and to help get this cruel system banned, write to The Humane Society of the United States, 2100 L Street N.W. Washington, D.C. 20037.

DEAR DR. FOX—I am concerned about the use of live animals for experiments, but I also wonder what might befall a pet when it has to be put to sleep. My apprehension is so strong that if for some reason my cat would have to be put to sleep, I would want to stay with her until she is cold. Am I overly worried?—L.H.

DEAR L.H.—You are right to be concerned. In some animal shelters, pets are sent to research laboratories instead of being humanely destroyed. It is most unlikely, however, for this kind of thing to occur in a private veterinary hospital. It is possible that a vet may not wish you to see your cat being injected, for various reasons that I can understand. You should, therefore, request to see your cat's body after it has been put to sleep if the vet will not allow you to be present when the injection is given.

proper care for older pets

DEAR DR. FOX—My dog is elderly, but he's been a great friend. I'd like to know if there's a form of senior-citizen care for older dogs. How can I make his life easier—and possibly longer?—MRS. F.R. JR.

DEAR MRS. F.R. JR.—Your concern is touching and your question intelligent. There are many things that can be done to make life easier for an aging pet. First, take him to a veterinarian every four to six months. Second, give him regular exercise, play sessions, and grooming.

Older dogs need a special diet high in good-quality protein, such as cottage cheese, lean meat, and cooked eggs. I also recommend some vegetables and well-cooked whole-grain rice. Older dogs also need a constant supply of fresh water, because they often develop kidney problems. Your dog is lucky to have you as a friend.

HEALTH REMINDER

As animals grow older, their bones tend to become brittle. To offset problems, add some calcium lactate or sterilized bone meal to your senior pets' diets. Also, sprinkle in sme wheat germ, which provides vitamin E, and brewer's yeast for vitamin B. And don't forget a few drops of vitamin A and D at each feeding. Caution: Don't overdo it.

DEAR DR. FOX—My husband and I are in complete disagreement as to the proper way to handle a problem with our nine-year-old dachshund. Annie has a difficult time negotiating stairs and jumping down from the couch and such. My husband insists she is just lazy and in no pain and should be forced to go up and down stairs. He says I spoil her by picking her up to help her. Could you settle this problem for us?—G.F.

DEAR G.F.—Your husband is wrong—very, very wrong, and if he gets his way, he could turn your dog into a cripple. Jumping off a sofa or being forced to negotiate stairs can lead to slipped-disc problems, acute pain, and paralysis. Perhaps your husband is jealous of the attention you give to your pooch.

No older dachshund, especially if overweight, should be allowed to jump up and down from furniture, but should live on the floor and be carried up and down stairs. A stair gate to prevent an overeager spirit from injuring itself will help too.

CHECKUP FOR SENIOR CITIZEN PETS

Old animals, like old people, begin to lose hearing and vision. You'll know your senior citizen pet is going deaf if it does not respond as usual when called or when another dog barks. When it starts colliding with objects and doesn't recognize you from a distance, it's probably losing its eyesight; you may also see a clouding over the lens. Deaf or blind cats and dogs fare well and remain happy, but they should never be allowed outdoors, unless on a leash.

---

respect for aging pets

DEAR DR. FOX—My dog, Rebel, is fourteen years old, and our vet said he's in really good condition for his age. He has gray hair around his muzzle and his back legs shake a little, but does that give people the right to say, "He's useless—he can't do anything"? It's not true, and it makes me feel very bad to hear things like that. I hope this is a reminder to people that if they don't have anything nice to say—don't say anything at all.—*P.K.E.*

DEAR P.K.E.—Sounds like you have taken good care of Rebel if the vet says he's in top condition and he's fourteen years old. Be proud of your dog. So he can't frisk around like a puppy—so what? Think of all the good times you've shared, and he's still a good and faithful companion. When your friends put your dog down, saying "He can't do anything," tell them that he's already done everything—and that they'll be lucky to keep their dog in such good shape as yours for fourteen years. It makes me sick how people despise and demean (and even destroy) their old dogs. Who wants a perpetual puppy?

when euthanasia is best

DEAR DR. FOX—It seems that you frequently advise someone to put their pet to sleep. You suggested recently a crate for a peke a poo with bad chewing habits. If that didn't work "put him to sleep." Recently, you suggested a chain collar for a biting poodle, or putting him to sleep. How cruel! Who knows what that dog has been through? All my children were biters. Would you have told me to destroy them, or to take the time and patience to teach them right from wrong? Sometimes a dying or critically injured animal is better off being put to sleep. But they deserve every possible chance at living, and, surely, because an animal has a bad habit isn't reason to kill it.—*K.R.B.*

DEAR K.R.B.—We really agree, although you don't think so. I also feel that animals should be put to sleep when they are suffering and cannot be helped in any way. But what of a very old dog or cat that is not obviously suffering but is urinating everywhere, or an animal with a very unstable temperament that cannot be corrected and is a danger to children? In such cases, euthanasia is generally best. Even so, I often suggest some alternative (such as keeping a house-wrecking dog in a crate for short periods) because it's better than putting it to sleep. I am only too aware of how ready people are to have their pets destroyed. I'm totally opposed to killing healthy pets that are "too much trouble" for uninformed owners, but limits must be set for destructive and/or suffering animals.

DEALING WITH YOUR PET'S DEATH

incurable illness (cats)

DEAR DR. FOX—Boris, our beautiful four-year-old cat, had to be put to sleep last week. It was terrible. He was always a picky eater, so when his appetite dropped off I blamed it on the onset of summer. But when he kept getting thinner and thinner I took him to the vet, and in a few minutes be diagnosed it as cancer. Now I'm filled with self-recriminations. Could I have saved him if I had taken him to the vet sooner?—D.S.

DEAR D.S.—Please don't—as so many pet-owners often do—put yourself on trial following the death of your pet. Your animal's doctor should have reassured you that cancer in cats is incurable, and the kind your cat had, which was probably related to feline leukemia virus, is lethal. There's simply no cure, and no one's to blame. Some people place the blame on the vet—which doesn't help either. I know it's hard to accept death and defeat, but don't make it harder by filling yourself with reproaches. You loved your cat, and he did have a good life with you—didn't he?

BURIAL SERVICES

Do you know that burial services, gravestones, and/or cremation for pets are all available at a modest fee? City dwellers who cannot simply bury their beloved deceased birds, puppies, etc., welcome these alternatives. Some ceremony is meaningful in making death real and dignified for a child, whether in the backyard or in a graveyard.

6

Breeding
and Pregnancy

aiding the birth (cats)

DEAR DR. FOX—My cat is expecting kittens, and I would like to know how to make a place for her that she will accept as the "delivery room."—*P.S.*

DEAR P.S.—Let your cat choose the place, but help her in the process. Put four or five cardboard boxes in various parts of the house—in dark corners, open closets, or wherever you would like her to have the kittens. Also put newspaper and a piece of old blanket or towel in each box. As your cat's hormonal system triggers her nest- or den-seeking behavior, she will choose where she wants to have her litter. She may not want to be too far away from you, especially if she sleeps with you. A nest box under or beside the bed could be ideal.

DEAR DR. FOX—Alas, I realized too late that my twelve-year-old silver-tip Persian was in heat. Now that she is pregnant, my problem is that she recently lost both her front lower teeth—the two that are sharp and pointed. Her uppers are intact, as well as all the other teeth. My immediate concern is how she will sever the umbilical cords. I hesitate to interfere with Mother Nature, but when, how, and should I?—*P.D.H.*

DEAR P.D.H.—Your Persian cat must be in good health to have a litter. She will cut the umbilical cord with her back molar teeth—the carnassials—not with her "fangs" or canine teeth that have fallen out. Have your vet check her teeth—they may be infected and need cleaning. Also, since this breed has such large-headed kittens, she may need a cesarean. You should consider having her spayed later.

143

artificial breeding (dogs)

DEAR DR. FOX—I have a beautiful Labrador, which I have tried four times to breed. First we tried to breed her with our own male; although she is pals with him throughout the year, she won't go near him when she is in season. Then we took her to a professional breeder, but she tightened up so badly he had to take her to a vet for artificial breeding. She still has not produced a litter, and the vet said he would start her on hormones next time she comes in season. Is there anything else that would be helpful?—J.M.

DEAR J.M.—I have mixed feelings about using artificial methods to get a dog pregnant. She may have a hormonal or behavioral anomaly that might be passed on to the offspring. Some bitches will actually come out of heat when taken to a strange place to be bred. Others seem to have an incest taboo and refuse to mate with the dog they live with. Give her one more try and possibly bring an experienced and confident male to her. Some bitches are just very picky.

birth defects (cats)

DEAR DR. FOX—Our cat, Bubbles, gave birth to a kitten with no hair, and to another that had his intestines hanging out. How could this happen? She also has had miscarriages.—D.T.

DEAR D.T.—There are many reasons why cats have miscarriages and deformed kittens. A virus infection is often involved. Sometimes the development of the fetus is disrupted so that parts of its body do not form properly, so you get harelips, cleft palates, hydrocephalus, and hernias.

Some umbilical hernias need to be repaired surgically. Have your cat spayed, since next time she may not have a normal litter. Even if she does, a visit to the local humane society will convince you that there are too many kittens being born as it is.

birth defects (dogs)

DEAR DR. FOX—My dog had a puppy before she was even one year old. This pup has problems with her hips. We think her body isn't shaped right, and that she might even be slightly retarded. But she is very lovable. My problem is that every time we separate the two dogs, the daughter panics. If the mother were to die, would the daughter survive?—G.R.

DEAR G.R.—It is quite possible that your new pup has multiple congenital abnormalities. I have seen cases of dogs with deformed limbs and jaws associated with mental retardation. Others suffer from a low-grade hydrocephalus (water on the brain) together with other physical abnormalities. You should have the pup examined by your vet.

Otherwise, you have a case where the mother is extremely protective of her offspring—or at least the pup is dependent on its mother. If you plan to keep this pup, you should spend as much time as possible getting her attached to you, because she could, being kept with her mother, become too "dog-oriented." The dog would then be less responsive to you, possibly never becoming sufficiently attached to you to appreciate you as a supportive "parent" or guardian.

cannibalism (rabbits)

DEAR DR. FOX—Whenever my female rabbit has babies, she eats them. We would really like to have some baby rabbits. What can we do?—K.R.

DEAR K.R.—Some female rabbits have a vice of eating their babies, which is virtually impossible to prevent. Once the habit seems to be developed, the mother will devour litter after litter. It is important to separate your male and female rabbits as soon as the mother shows signs of nest building. Provide her with a nest box, and then *do not disturb the nest*, since disturbances can trigger cannibalism in rabbits and other caged pets, especially hamsters. The less interference, the better. I wish you good luck next time around. You can also check my book *Understanding Your Pet* for more details on rabbit care and psychology.

change in behavior toward newborns (cats)

DEAR DR. FOX—Our cat, Lady Gray, is hostile toward her son. She hisses, growls, and sometimes strikes him. Has she gone mad? We really think she hates her kitten, who is now six months old.—H.A.

DEAR H.A.—Your cat has had a temperament reversal, related, I believe, to her need to dominate and control her offspring. While some cats mature and remain closely attached to their offspring, others really wean them for good and have no enduring attachment. This is probably how the domestic cat's wild ancestor reacts toward its offspring. Your solution, other than living with the tension, is to find a home for the young cat, who may well be under considerable stress and would be better off in another home.

egg-laying cycle (cockatiels)

DEAR DR. FOX—Four months ago, our eighteen-month-old cockatiel began to lay eggs. This was a big surprise—we thought it was a *he!* In four months she had laid five batches, or whatever you call them. Isn't this too much? We provide fresh water daily and a balanced diet with calcium and mineral cakes. Is there anything else we should be doing?—C.W.

DEAR C.W.—Yes. Perhaps it's time for you to be providing a mate and a nest box. Many people think that hens need a rooster around before they can lay eggs. The truth is that hens, parakeets, canaries, cockatiels, and others will lay eggs by the dozen once they mature. The main thing to look out for is egg-binding or constipation and also gradual loss of condition. A strict diet of a little water and salt-free toasted bread crusts for three or four days may switch the trigger and break the egg-laying cycle.

egg-laying cycle (parakeets)

DEAR DR. FOX—We recently bought what we thought was a male parakeet. But then Tweety started to act funny. He had large droppings and sat on one of his toys at the bottom of the cage. Then, to our surprise, we found an egg there and realized that Tweety is a female. How often does a female bird lay an egg? We have no intention of raising young parakeets.—MRS. J.R.

DEAR MRS. J.R.—Many parakeets produce eggs in this way, but without a male in her cage, Tweety won't have any babies because her eggs will be infertile. Give Tweety a nest box and let her enjoy sitting on her eggs for a week or so. It is part of the bird's natural rhythm to lay eggs, and all you need look out for is an egg becoming "stuck"—impacted or egg-bound. A little warm olive oil in the right place should help. You may wish to inhibit her totally by removing her toy "friend," but I personally wouldn't frustrate her unduly by depriving her of such stimulation.

encouraging mating (mice)

DEAR DR. FOX—I have three mice, two females and one male, and all are healthy. The females are about eighteen months old, and I bought the male about four months ago. They live together in one cage and get along like one happy family, but why haven't they produced any babies?—M.R.

DEAR M.R.—At the rate mice multiply, many people in your place would be thankful. Are you sure your new male *is* a male? If he's subordinate to the females, then little wonder he's impotent. It's also possible the females are now too old to breed and probably quite content without producing litter after litter of mice. It looks to me like you may just have to accept zero population growth.

encouraging mating (parakeets)

DEAR DR. FOX—I purchased two parakeets a year ago. They kiss each other, dance, and are a fine pair. I've been trying to get them to mate, and I have bought all the necessary equipment for mating, but no luck. Each pet dealer tells me a different story about when the female is ready to mate. Could you please explain the problem?—V.H.D.

DEAR V.H.D.—A nest box and a large cage often do the trick. However, many animal species that are raised together seem to have some sexual inhibition, analogous to an incest taboo. This could possibly be the problem, so why don't you separate the birds?

Then put them together for a couple of hours once every four or five days over a period of a couple of months during late spring and early summer. If they don't become more amorous, then forget it. They just may need a long, long time to get their act together—if ever.

frequency of pregnancies (cats)

DEAR DR. FOX—How many times a year can a cat get pregnant? Our calico stray has had four litters this past year. If it happens again we shall go mad.—E.W.

DEAR E.W.—Four litters of kittens in one year must certainly be a record. Most cats average two. You are in a dilemma—you are a Good Samaritan in caring for a calico stray, but you are contributing to the pet overpopulation problem by keeping her healthy and thus in fine shape to keep having litter after litter.

Your most logical choice is to have the cat spayed as soon as possible. That is better than putting all her kittens to sleep. The truth is there's nothing natural about so many litters in the first place, and it only results in more homeless cats and more destruction of wildlife in rural areas.

handling newborns (cats)

DEAR DR. FOX—My one-year-old Katie should be delivering her first litter any day. I plan to keep one male—we live on a farm and I want him to be a mouser. I'll find homes for the others. How long should I wait after the kittens are born to have Katie spayed? How old should the male be before I have him neutered? Also, is it necessary to have him neutered at all?—G.B.

DEAR G.B.—Don't take the kittens away from the mother until they are about eight weeks old. You can have the male kitten you choose neutered any time after five months and have the mother fixed about two months after the kittens are weaned. She and the male kitten should have shots around the time all are weaned. Tomcats roam a lot, so if you want a stay-at-home, have the male of your choice neutered. If his mother is a good mouser, chances are he will be too.

handling newborns (hamsters)

DEAR DR. FOX—I have a pregnant female hamster. When she has her babies, will it be OK to leave one of them with her, or will they fight? Also, is it better to keep a female baby or a male baby?—J.A.

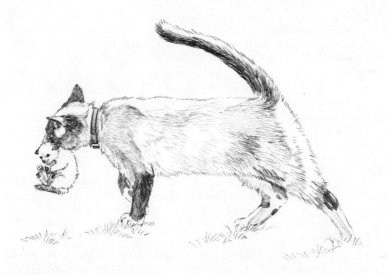

DEAR J.A.—I strongly advise you to separate the litter from the mother as soon as they are well weaned and eating solid food by themselves. Be sure that the father is separated before the mother gives birth. Do not disturb the nest. This may sound like a lot of precaution, but alarmed mother hamsters will sometimes kill and even eat their offspring. Hamsters prefer to live alone once they reach maturity, so it's not a question of male or female—I don't advise keeping any of the litter with the mother, because they may fight and one or both may get injured.

handling newborns (rabbits)

DEAR DR. FOX—I know that you're supposed to separate the parent rabbits when they have babies or the male might kill them. But how long must I wait to handle the babies and take them away from their mother?—A.P.

DEAR A.P.—You have the first rule right: Separate the male from the female partner. Rule No. 2: Do not disturb the mother for at least four days after the litter's birth, or she too might kill the babies. Bunnies can be weaned at four weeks, but it is best to keep them with the mother until they're about eight weeks old and let the mother wean them naturally. You'll enjoy noting how the mother pulls out her belly fur to line the bunnies' nest and seeing how rarely she nurses them—just one or two feeds a day! Segregate the sexes by the time they are three months old to prevent early breeding. Rabbits are precocious and prolific creatures.

heat cycles (cats)

DEAR DR. FOX—How many times in a year is a cat in season? Also, are they in pain during this time? If so, what can you do for them?—D.C.

DEAR D.C.—Cats come into heat differently, some twice a year, some many times over several weeks. They become more active, sometimes more irritable or affectionate, and may call or yowl—a mating call that is often misinterpreted as a sign of pain.

Some cats, especially Siamese, become almost hysterical, acting restless, rolling, rubbing, and licking repeatedly. Neutering is probably a kind solution and certainly a responsible decision, since there are too many kittens born every day. Thousands are put to sleep every twenty-four hours by animal shelters across the country.

DEAR DR. FOX—Does it take the presence of a tomcat to trigger the onset of heat in a female cat? Does an older female cat go through a menopause? If so, will she stop conceiving?—J.H.

DEAR J.H.—No, a tomcat won't trigger a female cat to come into heat. Queens come into heat cyclically. But during intercourse, the male does stimulate the female to ovulate. Some cats come into heat soon after one heat has finished, if they aren't pregnant.

Yes, aging cats and dogs do go through a form of menopause. But since older cats can still have kittens, I advise that they be neutered early in life, because there are too many unwanted kittens in the world. A visit to your local animal shelter will convince you of this. Depriving your cat of breeding has no adverse psychological effect.

DEAR DR. FOX—We have three male Siamese cats and one female. Is there anything to give the female to keep her out of heat so she doesn't get bred?—D.M.

DEAR D.M.—There is no hormone that is safe to give a cat to keep her out of heat. Side effects of various hormones can be harmful; you must seek a safer alternative. As I suggest in my book *Understanding Your Cat*, if you stimulate the female with a cottontipped swab she may reflexively ovulate, have a false pregnancy, and thus go out of heat. The other obvious alternative is to isolate your cat from males. She will cry and holler and may then have repeated short-heat cycles. A mild "shock" of four or five days in a dark room, with plenty of human contact but restricted food, may break the cycle.

heat cycles (dogs)

DEAR DR. FOX—Is there anything to the rumor that the new parvovirus shot would cause a dog not to come in heat? Our beautiful Rhodesian ridgeback, a champion, will soon be four years old. She came in heat when she was eight months old, then again a year later. We had anticipated another heat a year later, but it didn't happen. We have a beautiful mate picked out for her. Any advice?—M.G.

DEAR M.G.—I m glad your vet is reluctant to give your dog hormones to bring her into heat. No—I haven't heard that the parvo vaccine stops dogs from coming into heat. Young dogs are sometimes irregular. The presence of other female dogs can help bring on a heat cycle.

The stress of social isolation may disrupt things, as on a visit to a dog show or to a veterinarian for shots. I have known of dogs so stressed that they either missed a heat or had it abruptly terminated just as they were entering their heat cycle. Heartworm medication called stirid caricide could also be the cause. You'll have to do some detective work.

importance of mates (birds)

DEAR DR. FOX—I have been given a conure. Should these birds have a mate for a better environment? I know they are not too easy to get to talk, but I almost have him saying hello. He is really loud and noisy. Will he be able to talk?—C.F.

DEAR C.F.—Your bird would definitely be better off if it had a cage mate of the opposite sex for company. And remember, the larger the cage the better. But your bird is more likely to "talk" if he's more dependent on you and doesn't have a cage mate. I personally wouldn't deprive him of the company of his own kind just so I could have a pet that would parrot a few words.

Of course, I wouldn't have a bird that wasn't bred, hatched, and raised in captivity. Many exotic birds like yours are imported from foreign countries, and statistics from the Humane Society of the United States indicate that some 80 percent of all birds caught in the wild for sale in pet stores die before they ever reach someone's home. Imported birds are also a threat to poultry farmers, since exotic birds carry Newcastle disease, which could ruin the poultry industry.

interbreeding (cats with dogs)

DEAR DR. FOX—Can a cat and dog mate and produce offspring? Some people seem to think so. What are the facts?—G.R.

DEAR G.R.—There are rumors of cats producing doglike or rabbity-looking kittens after they have been seen with a dog or chasing rabbits, but it's all nonsense. Such kittens are all cat, but they have some kind of birth defect.

Cats and dogs cannot interbreed because they are genetically so different. Even after artificial insemination (with dog sperm), cats won't have any offspring. But close friends do engage in and seem to enjoy sex play. It's quite natural for house pets of the same or different species and sex to sometimes behave sexually toward each other. So don't think such practices are weird. It comes naturally as a result of their being raised together and developing a close affection.

mismating (dogs)

DEAR DR. FOX—I have a quite small Labrador retriever–water spaniel mix who is less than a year old. She is already four weeks pregnant by our much larger dog—a mix between a German shepherd and a wolfhound. Will her young age and small size make delivery unsafe? If so, what could be done about it?—J.G.

DEAR J.G.—Mismating such as you describe, particularly in an immature female dog, can indeed mean problems when the pups are due. Have her checked over by a veterinarian and keep the hospital emergency number on hand. She may need a cesarean operation. Sometimes nature protects in that a small mother creates a small placenta, which means the offspring will be small—even when the father was very large. Let's hope this will be the case with your dog, but be prepared, just in case.

nursing (cats)

DEAR DR. FOX—My cat had a litter of five kittens several months ago, which she weaned. Now she has another litter, and she is letting the older offspring nurse the kittens. I'm afraid they will starve if she continues to do this. The young ones are under the house where I cannot even get to them.—B.M.D.

DEAR B.M.D.—Try to keep the older kittens away from the newborns, and they will turn to the mother again. Actually, I would be more worried about the poor mother cat being sucked raw and dry by two successive litters. I suggest you clean up your cat colony. It could reach epidemic proportions once the others start to breed. Have the mother spayed and the others neutered and adopted. That's the best thing to do for the cats under your house.

sexual maturity (horses)

DEAR DR. FOX—How old does a stallion have to be before he's fertile? My friend owns a stallion that is ten months old, and he has been left out in a paddock with a pony mare for a few weeks. Is it possible for her to become pregnant?—M.B.

DEAR M.B.—Young colts reach sexual maturity, physically, by the end of their first springtime—at around a year of age. But psychologically they mature more slowly. They are not assertive and dominant enough to mate, because older mares psychologically "castrate" them. Still, they may engage in some courtship and sex play from a very early age. If the pony mare comes into heat, she will probably refuse him. It's best just to keep an eye on things. It is unlikely that he will be amorously inclined until he is more psychologically mature.

show-quality animals (dogs)

DEAR DR. FOX—My daughter has a blue Labrador that she bought as a show dog only to find out after a year that it had a hip problem. My daughter is still determined to get a show dog—how does one go about it?—MRS. D.W.S.

DEAR MRS. D.W.S.—The best way your daughter can find a show-quality pup is to go to a dog show and talk to the handlers and owners. An alternative is to buy one of the many purebred dog magazines that carry breeding kennel advertisements, and then go visit the kennels.

Does your daughter really plan to show her dog? I'd sooner have a sturdy field-trial black Labrador, but I would think twice about keeping it confined alone all day. A companion cat would help. Your daughter should get the pup at six to eight weeks old when the kitten has matured and is about six months old. They should get along fine then.

DEAR DR. FOX—My Irish setter is a year old now, and his hair is still not very long. I'd like to breed him, but if his hair never gets long, what's the point? I paid quite a lot for him, so I feel it's a shame not to breed him.—L.G.

DEAR L.G.—Some Irish setters do not develop their full "feathers" until

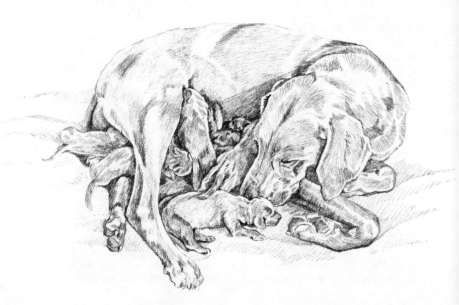

they're fully mature—between two and three years of age. And some never develop a long, silky coat. You can't expect a guarantee. But I certainly do not regard your dog as being worthless, no matter how inferior his coat is—nor should you. You may end up with a loving, intelligent companion, even if he isn't a star in the show ring.

CAT SHOWS

Your cat doesn't have to have a pedigree to win a cat-show award. Domestic cats are judged on their beauty and condition. The first step is to register your pet with one of the cat clubs that exist everywhere in the United States. Joining the club will automatically make you a member of the Cat Fanciers' Association. Ask your local cat club for details.

---

signs of pregnancy (cats)

DEAR DR. FOX—How can I tell if my cat is going to have kittens without taking her to a vet? If she is going to have kittens, how many will she have? Will I have to do anything to help her?—B.O.

DEAR B.O.—Your cat will begin to swell, and if your run your fingers very gently on her sides, you will feel some little "lumps" that sometimes move after the sixth week or so of pregnancy. Your cat could have anywhere from a couple of kittens to six or seven. You can provide her with a nest box in a warm, quiet, dark corner of a closet in which to have her kittens.

Get a book on cat care from the library. Once the kittens are weaned and you have found them good homes, have mama cat spayed—there are too many kittens and not enough homes for them in the world.

signs of pregnancy (hamsters)

DEAR DR. FOX—I put my hamster with a male several times, and now I think she might have babies soon, because she feels heavier than usual. She also is making a very large nest. Are there any other symptoms?—D.M.

DEAR D.M.—Yes, there are other signs when a hamster is "expecting." First, of course, she won't show her usual heat cycles and will have no interest in a male hamster. Next, if you look at her tummy every few days, you will see her nipples enlarging. Her abdomen will also swell, and you should be able to see the babies moving inside when your hamster is sitting still or quietly restrained on her back. Nest-making is, of course a good sign of an impending birth. Don't touch the nest—because if you disturb the mother she could reject her pups or even kill them. Have a quick look in the nest, using a pencil to open it up, when the mother is out of it eating. The babies are pink and hairless when born. Don't handle them at all until they crawl out of the nest by themselves. Remember, hamsters like to live alone when they grow up—not with other hamsters.

sterility (cats)

DEAR DR. FOX—We have a black hybrid Himalayan kitten. I remember reading somewhere that females can have kittens, but the males are sterile. Is this true?—J.T.

DEAR J.T.—The Himalayan variety of cat doesn't normally have sterile males. The only variety that does is the calico-colored cat. Fertile males are extremely rare, because the genes for this coat color are sex-linked with a sterility factor that is transmitted via the fertile mother to most male offspring.

vaccinations during pregnancy (dogs)

DEAR DR. FOX—My eleven-month-old Chinese pug is coming into heat the second time, and we plan to breed her. Is she too young? Do you think she could handle the puppies? Also, all her shots are coming due soon—will these shots affect the puppies? How much of a chance does she have of getting rabies or parvovirus if she doesn't get these shots?—*B.W.*

DEAR B.W.—It's illegal not to give your dog a rabies shot. And it is advisable to have her vaccinated against the common canine virus diseases as well. I would not advise vaccinating her while she is pregnant. You should wait until her third heat before breeding.

Being a small breed with a large head, she may have difficulties giving birth, so find a veterinarian who can help you and your dog cope with possible complications. Unless she's a show-winner, I suggest not breeding her. If you do, please avoid mating her with a close relative—because this could lead to genetic defects that are all too common in highly inbred breeds.

when not to breed (dogs)

DEAR DR. FOX—I have been trying to mate my teacup poodles. But when the female accepts the male's advances, it frightens him and he backs off into a corner to escape her. When he finally gets up the courage to mate with her, he loses interest and soon walks away. Can you explain his behavior?—*M.F.*

DEAR M.F.—Teacup poodles are adorable, but they have low viability and are often very sickly, leading short lives punctuated by frequent illness and trips to the vet. I think the inability of the two dogs to procreate is perhaps a reflection of the old saying, nature knows best. Under natural conditions, these little creatures would never survive. Is it right, therefore, to endeavor to propagate them under artificial conditions (many have to be delivered by cesarean section) when the chances are they will never live normal, healthy lives? I think not.

7

Neutering

DEAR DR. FOX—I intend to neuter my English springer spaniel soon. I never intend to use him for stud purposes and don't want him taking off after females in heat. But I've been getting a lot of criticism by self-styled experts who say that I'm crazy, that neutering will make my dog fat, lazy, and good for nothing. For other readers who are truly responsible and caring animal owners, would you please enlighten us on the pros and cons of neutering?—B.F.

DEAR B.F.—The advantages to owners and pets of having pets neutered far outweigh the disadvantages, which incidentally crop up very rarely. These include obesity, which can be easily corrected with diet and exercise, and other hormonal-imbalance syndromes, which can be rectified with hormone replacement therapy. Most pets, like humans, adjust well. After neutering, male cats and dogs roam and fight less, and both sexes "stay at home." Prostate problems are reduced in males, and breast cancer and uterine and ovarian diseases are reduced in females. Reasons enough? Most men don't object to neutering cats or female dogs but get very defensive when it comes to castrating a male dog. Little wonder why.

DEAR DR. FOX—I am writing for your opinion on whether to neuter my one-year-old male cat. I am going away to college. My cat is independent and free-spirited, although he stays inside with me in the evenings. I don't want to change his personality, but I don't want him running away from his new home. Advise me, please.—D.S.

153

DEAR D.S.—Neutering your tomcat will help him become more of a stay-at-home, less motivated to go out and roam, court, and fight. And he will be much less likely to spray indoors and stink up your rooms. The sooner it's done the better, because the more he gets a taste of the outdoors, the more difficult it will be for him to readjust.

In the new house, keep him indoors for at least the first week. Why not try to adapt him to living indoors all the time and get a harness and leash so he can go out safely for a regular stroll with you? A female kitten companion may make home life better while you're away during the day.

DEAR DR. FOX—I have read that neutering will make a cat less hostile, less prone to spray the walls, and less likely to roam. But since my cat does not spray and is not hostile and I neither let him out nor ever intend to, why should I have my cat neutered?—MRS. R.C.

DEAR MRS. R.C.—Your cat is still young, but as he matures his sex hormones will make him more aggressive—not to you but to rival males. He will probably want to go out, court, and fight and may well spray and smell up the house if he's frustrated or can't go outdoors. If he gets out, he may well come home repeatedly beaten up and develop bite abcesses from fights with other toms. Castration at around eight to ten months will eliminate these problems pretty well *before* they develop. Castrating an older cat, once he's got a taste for the outdoors, is often too late, so have him neutered as soon as possible.

best age to neuter (cats)

DEAR DR. FOX—How old does my kitten have to be before she can be spayed? And about how much does it cost? Also, will spaying change the way she behaves?—L.W.

DEAR L.W.—Spaying per se has no known adverse effects on a cat's psyche. She may be prone to put on weight and to develop skin problems, but these can be rectified by dietary control and hormone replacement therapy. The advantages far outweigh the minor and not-so-common complications.

Your vet will tell you at what age spaying is best done—vets do vary in their preferences, but most choose around five or six months. The price will vary, but it tends to be fairly uniform in a given area. It can range from $40 to $80 or so.

Spaying (or castrating) a cat is a responsible decision and one of the best contributions a pet owner can make to help reduce the pet overpopulation problem.

effects on hunting dogs

DEAR DR. FOX—My husband and I do volunteer work for the local humane society. It is the society policy (as with most humane societies) to require the neutering of any dog or cat adopted. We often find that a prospective owner who wants the dog as both a companion pet and a hunting dog will refuse to agree to have the dog neutered, believing that this will destroy its hunting instinct and ruin it for hunting. Because of this widespread belief, a dog may be deprived of the chance to be adopted into an otherwise potentially good home. Could you comment on the truth of this idea?—E.J.

DEAR E.J.—From what is known about the effects of castration on hunting behavior per se, it is unlikely that castration will have any significant direct effect on hunting dogs' performance in the field. Female hunting dogs do well without testicles and male sex hormones. My feeling is that it is a myth. However, since so many hunters, for reasons of their own ego-involvement with their dogs, find castration unthinkable, I suggest vasectomy; the dog will still be entirely male, but his sperm will not be able to reach a female dog.

miniature dogs (problems with)

DEAR DR. FOX—I have a miniature crossbreed—the mother is a Yorkshire terrier and the father is a miniature poodle. I took her to be spayed at seven months, but the vet could not sedate her because of her small veins and suggested I forget it. What is your opinion? The dog now is eight months old.—*R.B.*

DEAR R.B.—You have a Yorkshire pudding by the sound of it—a great crossbreed indeed. Sure, she has small veins and is probably a little hyper, too. So a vet could give her a pill or a shot into the muscle to calm her down before anesthetizing her. Any vet who can't spay your dog because her veins are too small shouldn't be doing surgery on dogs. More likely, the vet is apprehensive about operating on a small dog—toy breeds are a surgical risk. Find a vet who has more confidence and go ahead with the spaying—and soon.

8

Travels With and Without Your Pet

airline travel (cats and dogs)

DEAR DR. FOX—I am moving to another state and want to know if I should sedate my cat, place her in her carrier box, and drive by car (six hours), or take her with me by plane in her carrier box next to me. Please, help me decide.—*H.L.D.*

DEAR H.L.D.—Some airlines will allow you to take your pet into the passenger compartment, provided you use a regulation-type carrier. You should call the airline you're flying to make sure. It they give you the OK, arrange to pick up the carrier a week or so ahead of departure, so that your cat can sit, sleep, and play in it. Then she won't be afraid of it when the time comes.

If the airline says your cat must go in the baggage compartment, then by all means take her by road instead, inside a large wire cage with a litter box on hand under the seat.

I do not recommend tranquilizers for animals being transported unless they are extremely fearful creatures. If your cats only protest vocally and don't scream or claw at the bars, I wouldn't drug them.

DEAR DR. FOX—We live in New York, and for family reasons are planning a trip West this summer. The only way such a lengthy trip is feasible with a child is by airplane, but we are in a quandary as to what constitutes the best (most humane) provision concerning our dog. Should we take her with us on the airline, in cargo, or leave her for the two weeks at the home of a trusted neighbor, who owns a female golden retriever?—*J.R.*

DEAR J.R.—Because there's no way of predicting or controlling human behavior, I would not entrust your pooch to the airline baggage compartment. No matter what protective rules and regulations we have, there is always an element of risk in sending a dog by air freight.

If she gets on well with the neighbor's dog, I would take that option. It's only for two weeks, after all. Be sure she's had her booster shots and wears a tag on her collar in case she gets lost.

car seat (dogs)

DEAR DR. FOX—My small Boston terrier loves to ride in the car so he can look out the window. Because he's small, the only way he can see is if someone holds him, so I tried to buy him a car seat. Due to the design of most car seats and the fact that I have bucket seats, nothing worked out. Finally, I bought him a beanbag chair and shaped it to the desired height. I set the dog in with his harness and leash attached to the seat-belt bracket, and it's terrific!—*MRS. K.K.*

DEAR MRS. K.K.—You are most ingenious to think of using a beanbag chair so your dog can enjoy sightseeing. I commend you on securing your dog; small dogs, like children, can get thrown and injured when the brakes have to be put on quickly. Keep the window closed to protect your dog's eyes. However, I do not advise cat owners to use your trick. I have come across a number of cases where cats kneaded the filler (it feels like kitty litter to them) and used the living-room beanbag as a toilet.

car travel (fish)

DEAR DR. FOX—I'm going to be moving in about three weeks and I'm going to be taking my large tropical fish. It will be a two-hour trip. How do I move him without spilling water or depriving him of air?—*WORRIED*

DEAR WORRIED—For short trips, a large, tough plastic bag two-thirds full of water taken directly from the fish tank and one-third full of air, with fish inside and the top well tied, is the best way to transport your fishy friend. Put the bag inside another one for safety and keep it out of direct sunlight so you don't cook your fish in transit.

car travel—overcoming problems with (cats and dogs)

DEAR DR. FOX—We are planning on moving from Atlanta to New Jersey in a few months. Our cat is mild-mannered, except when she's in her travel carrier. Do you think we should send her home by plane or let her travel in the car? She hates the car even for a short ride to the vet.—*J.E.*

DEAR J.E.—Considering your cat's fear of the car and carrying case, I suggest you have your vet prescribe a tranquilizer. Give it to the cat just before you put her in the container. Then have her flown to your destination. She will be traumatized either way, but the journey will be shorter by air. That would be my preference, if I were her.

DEAR DR. FOX—We have a Doberman/German shepherd puppy approximately three months old. When we take her for a ride in our car, she drools by the bucketfull. We have had numerous dogs and never had this problem.—*J.N.*

DEAR J.N.—Your dog could simply be experiencing motion sickness, so you might try giving her Dramamine before you set out on a car ride. Also, drooling is a very common sign of nervousness or anxiety in a dog. If that's the case, simply sit in the car beside your puppy as often as you can, with someone else in the driver's

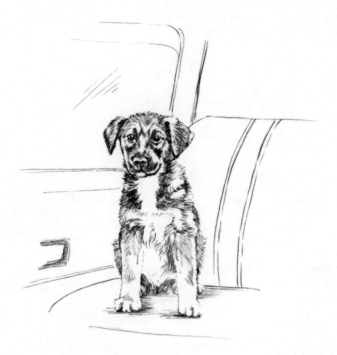

seat. Talk to her, pet her, and give her a food reward, and she will become desensitized to being in the car.

Next, switch on the engine and let the animal get used to it. After several days, drive slowly around the block at various times. Such gradual building-up of the pet's sense of comfort in a car works extremely well for both animals with anxiety and those suffering motion sickness, which may be in part psychosomatic. A nervous or erratic driver can also contribute to the problem.

DEAR DR. FOX—Why does our golden retriever act so strangely in the car? She's always anxious to get in, but the second my husband is behind the wheel, Samantha jumps at him, nipping and growling. (You can almost see a mischievous look on her face!) Then when we get going, instead of sitting down, she paces back and forth.—M.C.H.

DEAR M.C.H.—Dogs do develop a wide range of quite bizarre behavior patterns related to riding in automobiles, from chasing their tails to panting and yelping continually. Try playing with Samantha before she gets into the car—strenuous games such as tug-of-war with a towel, catch-the-ball, or retrieve-the-stick. This may help discharge some of her excitement and playfulness. As for her pacing back and forth, she may well be an anxious backseat driver. Better go easy on the brakes and accelerator.

DEAR DR. FOX—Our golden retriever has developed a sudden, strange habit. She always loved to ride in the car and went along happily. Now she goes wild whenever anyone else is in the car or even near it. She jumps and sometimes growls and snarls. I am afraid she may hurt someone—even our child.—*L.J.G.*

DEAR L.J.G.—Such triggered aggression is extremely difficult to inhibit. You should begin by putting your dog through obedience school so that she learns to sit, stay, etc., and comes to regard you as the leader. Then she should be easier to control.

Severe discipline will be needed in the car. Certainly, riding with such a dog is not advisable. The dog might even redirect its aggression and bite you or the child. So take no further risks. The prescription is obedience school, and no driving with the dog until her behavior is corrected.

DEAR DR. FOX—Do you have a remedy for dogs who bark in cars at all moving objects and become hysterical when they see other animals and trucks? I have tried squirting my dog with a water pistol and even gone through the desensitization steps suggested by a psychologist (sit in the car, turn on the engine, etc.), but as soon as the engine is turned on she starts barking, so she's never gone beyond the second step! I live alone and want her to travel with me, but so far she's had to go to the kennel.—*FOILED-BY-A-DOG*

DEAR FOILED—Provided you have a full tank, your car can run far longer than your dog is likely to bark. You gave up too soon. MANY repetitions of putting the dog in the car and leaving the engine switched on (in an OPEN garage or driveway) are needed until she settles down and you move on to step three: a slow drive around the block. A mild sedative from your vet may help speed up the desensitization program. But, above all else, you need patience and perserverance.

car travel (variety of animals)

DEAR DR. FOX—I will be moving soon and will be taking three cats, eight hermit crabs, and two large, expensive goldfish. All the animals are dear to me, and I can't part with any. Please suggest how I might pack and transfer these friends from one coast to another.—*A.P.*

DEAR A.P.—Assuming you plan to travel by road, I suggest separate cat carriers for your felines, with a leash and collar for each cat so they can be let out and allowed to walk around and use a litter tray at intervals of every three to four hours.

The hermit crabs will do fine packed in moist seaweed or moss. The goldfish can be left in their tank half-filled with water. Place the tank inside a large plastic bag and open the bag every three or four hours to let fresh air in. Both the goldfish and the crabs will manage without food for a few days, but offer them some, since they may feel like eating.

Feed the cats in the evening when you are all settled into a motel. Call up ahead of time to confirm that they will accept your cats; most motels will. Have identity tags on your cats' collars just in case you do lose one on the way.

hotel and motel stays

DEAR DR. FOX—Is it true that you can't register at a hotel if you have a pet with you?—*M.T.*

DEAR M.T.—In some cases yes, and in some cases no. There are approximately 4,000 hotels and motels that welcome pets. Some even have kennels on their premises. However, you will only know by phoning in advance and can reserve accordingly. Some hotel-listing guides indicate each hotel's pet policy.

TRAVELING TIPS

To avoid trouble when traveling with your pet, keep these hints in mind:
- Have it wear a collar and identity tag.
- When traveling by car, keep your cat in a traveling case and your dog restrained.
- Never travel with the car windows all the way down.
- Take a supply of your pet's regular food along, since it may not be available where you're going.
- More than 4,000 hotels and motels across the country welcome pets and their owners. To make vacationing simpler, some even have kennels. Check out pet reservations when making your own to avoid disappointment.
- Be aware that bus lines prohibit pets from accompanying passengers, although some independent lines will allow it if the pet is an approved species. Animals may ride in the baggage cars of rail lines, and you may visit them at any stop that exceeds ten minutes.

---

pet sitters (cats and dogs)

DEAR DR. FOX—I would like your advice on this problem. We are going away for three weeks, and I can't decide what to do about my twenty-two-year-old cat. I could possibly get someone to come in once a day to feed her, or I could put her in a local kennel. Which alternative do you suggest?—J.C.

DEAR J.C.—People write to me often with your dilemma. My advice is that keeping an aged cat at home rather than at a local boarding kennel is usually less stressful, if it can be managed. Adding the strain of unfamiliar surroundings to the stress of separation could cause your vintage cat to pick up an infection at a kennel. When you keep her at home, leave a radio on for company. Have a cat-sitter—a neighbor or student—come in twice a day. Have the phone number of your veterinarian on hand. Take it with you too—in case of emergencies or simple questions you might need to ask.

DEAR DR. FOX—What do you do with a cat if you have to leave town for four days? Is it harmful to leave the cat alone in the house with plenty of food and water?—C.A.

DEAR C.A.—I think that four days is too long a time to leave a cat at home unsupervised. There's always the risk of the cat getting sick, which happens to some cats as a result of the stress of solitude. (A relapse of cystitis—bladder trouble—is quite common.) I suggest you find a high-school student close by, or make friends with neighbors who would be more than happy to keep an eye on your house and come in to feed and check up on the cat while you're away. Leave your own phone number where you can be reached in case of an emergency and your veterinarian's name and telephone number. Then you can enjoy your four days without worrying about your pet.

DEAR DR. FOX—My three-year-old Lhaso apso is very close to me, as I am to him. In the two times that I left him to go on vacation, he moped around at my sister's house and ate very little. As she said, it was very evident he missed me and his home. My problem is that my whole family and I are dispersing on vacation for two weeks, and I am afraid my dog will get very sick from loneliness at my sister's again. Can a dog die from a broken heart?—A.B.

DEAR A.B.—Have you thought of finding a house-sitter? A good neighbor or student could stay at your home and take care of your pooch. He will be depressed without you, but he will have the comfort and security of familiar surroundings plus a sympathetic dog-sitter. That will help your dog weather the separation. The chances of your dog dying of a broken heart are slim, although animals have passed away from loneliness. It is a fact that pets can become very depressed, like homesick children off at camp for the first time. Trouble is, pets can't understand, so they can suffer more. What a responsibility, indeed, for those of us who care!

pickup trucks (dogs)

DEAR DR. FOX—Having dogs ride in the back of pickup trucks seems to be quite a fad. I can't believe that intelligent owners don't realize the danger posed to both their pets and other motorists. Could you say something about this? Maybe owners who see it in print will realize their negligence.—J.S.B.

DEAR J.S.B.—Good point, indeed. It is surprising how a dog who's used to it can travel safely in a pickup. But untrained dogs can jump in traffic to play with or challenge a dog on the street. I've seen that happen, with dogs getting run over and worse. One driver took a corner so fast that his dog flew right off the back of the truck. I was behind him and gave him a piece of my mind.

public transportation (dogs)

DEAR DR. FOX—Some time ago, you mentioned in your column several countries that do not allow animals on public transportation. It brought back a memory I'm sure you and your readers will enjoy. I boarded a bus in Ireland and found myself amid three canine commuters. If you pay for your animal's seat, they go right along with you, all the way. I felt like a part of a cartoon—a refreshing atmosphere, compared to our rigid rule-conscious society.—E.C.

DEAR E.C.—Thanks for your anecdote. I remember tearooms in England and restaurants in other European countries where one could often see a well-trained, polite dog sitting by someone's table.

America has many virtues, but the phobia about disease, the irrational fear of dogs, and rigid rules that only permit blind persons to be with their dogs in various public places are sources of exasperation. One of my friends pretends to be blind; that way she can travel on airplanes, trains, and buses and go into restaurants with her dog, whom she has rigged with a guide-dog's harness.

quarantine (international travel)

DEAR DR. FOX—Our family will be transferred to London, England, soon. The quarantine laws are rather stiff—six months—and we are asking ourselves if it would be harmful to subject our dog to such a confinement. She loves to run (she's our daily running companion) and is a super "people's dog."—E. & M.E.

DEAR E. & M.E.—If your dog is young and adaptable by nature, it might not be too much of an ordeal for her to be in quarantine for six months. Many quarantine kennels allow owners to visit, and you could do so. However, if you are going to be transferred from country to country—which could mean more sojourns in quarantine for your dog—then find her a good home, since your lifestyle might not be really compatible with quarantine laws and traveling with a dog.

sailing (cats)

DEAR DR. FOX—My dad just bought a sailboat, and I would like to know if I could risk taking my Siamese cat on it for a weekend. He loves to ride in a car.—*M.L.M.*

DEAR M.L.M.—Judging from those cats I have been to sea with, cats make darned good sailors. They seem especially to enjoy watching the waves. But be sure to keep your cat on a harness and leash for the first couple of sails, just in case he panics or accidentally falls overboard. Cats are good swimmers, and your animal is unlikely to drown if he does fall in, provided you can get to him within a reasonable period of time. If yours is a squinty-eyed Siamese, as so many are, think twice about taking him aboard. Such cats have difficulty perceiving depth and could well finish up in the briny deep.

DEAR DR. FOX—We take our cat sailing with us every weekend, and every weekend she gets seasick. She loves to go to the boat but dislikes sailing. We have tried several seasick pills and tranquilizers with no success.—*B.L.Mc.*

DEAR B.L.Mc.—It is unusual, from what I have heard, for cats to get seasick. You just don't have a sailor—there are always exceptions. Having been afflicted once myself with seasickness, I would say that your cat must be suffering considerably each weekend.

Since medication hasn't helped, I would put her comfort ahead of your need for her company on board. Buy her a leash and harness and take her for walks on terra firma.

sailing (dogs)

DEAR DR. FOX—We are happy owners of a Lhasa apso and keeshond. Both dogs love to play in lakes and rivers. This summer we would like to take them for rides in our canoe. Does anybody have floatation devices, life jackets, for dogs?—*B.F.*

DEAR B.F.—Dogs come in so many different shapes and sizes and the market demand is so meager that I doubt any entrepreneur has entered the doggie life jacket market! Dogs are excellent swimmers, and I personally would worry that a flotation device would interfere with their natural balance and buoyancy. An inflated rubber collar around their necks would probably be best—experiment with the inner tube of a bicycle tire. Or try to design your own life jacket out of Styrofoam and waterproof canvas and see if it works in some safe situation.

9

Dealing with Strays and Unwanted Visitors

animal shelters

DEAR DR. FOX—My apartment is filled to the brim with stray cats and dogs. When I see a skinny, dirty, matted stray, my heart breaks. Now I don't know if I should take the strays to the shelter or turn them loose on the streets again. Why do I feel so skeptical about bringing animals to the shelter?—L.L.

DEAR L.L.—Unfortunately, there is no single simple solution to the problem of strays. Local and national humane societies need public donations to help them educate pet owners to keep their pets from roaming free and to have them neutered. And municipal authorities need stricter laws and stricter enforcement. As for collecting strays and giving them to the local animal shelter, you're skeptical because you know that most will be destroyed, since not all strays are adoptable. Be sure your shelter uses a humane method of destruction such as an injection of sodium pentobarbital—not the decompression chamber or T61, a compound that can cause respiratory paralysis before death, like the curare-type drugs that some vets still use. A humane death for a sick, homeless, and starving animal that can't fend for itself outdoors may be a greater kindness than throwing it into a survival struggle. Some 15 to 20 million unwanted cats and dogs are killed each year, and no local authority could afford to keep a fraction of this astronomical population. The ultimate solution lies with the owner.

discouraging pigeons

DEAR DR. FOX—I hope you can help me get rid of the dirty pigeons on my patio—the smell is terrible. I must clean the mess every day, and it's getting me down, especially as I've just gotten out of the hospital and would like to sit on my patio—*MRS. B.L.S.*

DEAR MRS. B.L.S.—Some people would be happy to have the pigeons so close, regardless of the mess or smell. There's no catering to all tastes, I guess. One of the best pigeon deterrents is a cat, so I hope you like cats. If not, you can hang on strings around the patio some mobiles to clash and bang. This will scare off the pigeons and make it hard for them to perch. A third alternative is to put food out for them—but near someone else's patio so they can perch there instead—and, I hope, be tolerated.

discouraging skunks

DEAR DR. FOX—Part of the basement floor of my old home is composed of dirt. Skunks have dug underneath the steps and are living in the basement. Please tell me what I can do to get rid of them.—*M.L.B.*

DEAR M.L.B.—I think you would probably cause more of a stink getting rid of the skunks than trying to live quietly with them. Actually, skunks are very useful in eliminating all kinds of insects, slugs, and snails that might otherwise ruin your vegetable garden. If you really want the skunks to go, call the local animal-control or humane society, and try to specify that humane box-traps be used, rather than cruel steel-jaw traps or poison bait.

discouraging sparrows

DEAR DR. FOX—Please tell me a humane way to discourage sparrows from nesting inside my garage every year.—*R.K.G.*

DEAR R.K.G.—Birds have to nest somewhere, and with so many trees being cut down in urban and suburban areas, plus the hazards of free-roaming house-cats, birds are in trouble. So why not offer your garage as a haven? I would.

However, if you really must discourage the birds, get a cat. Or better still, simply keep the garage doors shut. But isn't it more fun and satisfactory to live with, rather than against, Mother Nature?

finding homes for strays

DEAR DR. FOX—We have five cats—two of our own and three strays. I am going broke with catfood bills. I can't find anyone who will take the strays. Why doesn't someone start a pet adoption column? I would be willing to pay a fee to advertise.—*MRS. E.P.*

DEAR MRS. E. P.—What a great idea! The trouble is that papers won't want to mention a pet adoption that isn't in their area. Since you are willing to pay, why not put a suitable ad in the "pets" section of your local paper or, if the paper carries my column, give the editor a call—they might run your ad at the end of my column in a special box.

While it's often easier to take stray and unwanted pets to the local animal shelter for adoption, few people realize that most will never be adopted. The majority never find homes and are either put to sleep or sent to an animal dealer who supplies research labs and universities with animals for experimental purposes. This is called "pound seizure" and many animal welfare organizations are pushing for legislation to prohibit the practice. The state of Massachusetts has been the first to ban pound seizure.

taking care of strays (cats)

DEAR DR. FOX—When I found my cat, he already had a taste for the outdoors and couldn't be made into a house-only cat. Two weeks ago he brought home a buddy—an old tomcat that looks pretty beat-up and skinny. I've put food outside so he won't starve, but now he's bringing friends around. I don't mind feeding strays, but it breaks my heart to see so many starved cats. Am I doing the right thing by feeding them, or should I take them to the ASPCA?—*K.D.*

DEAR *K.D.*—That's a touching story—your cat bringing home the hobos and bums of the cat world. Be sure your cats are well vaccinated against infectious diseases that they might pick up from these strays. I would take obviously sick ones to the local humane society for treatment. If you can afford it, take all the strays to be neutered. Otherwise, you can't really legitimize feeding homeless cats, since they will be more likely then to reproduce and you will help aggravate the pet overpopulation problem.

taking care of strays (dogs)

DEAR DR. FOX—I recently took in a stray dog who followed me for some time while jogging. I took him in only briefly—he had a collar but no tags, smelled terrible, and would not eat. But I was fearful of handling him since he was so dirty. What are the risks, if any, from cleaning up and caring for a stray?— *M.R.*

DEAR *M.R.*—A dog such as the one you describe (with collar) is most probably lost, and though dirty, he's not likely to have any disease transmissible to you. Rather than feed a stray and then turn him out, it would be advisable to call the humane society, for the city is no place for a free-roaming dog. Nevertheless, I commend you for being a Good Samaritan.

taking care of strays (rabbits)

DEAR DR. FOX—A tame black-nosed white rabbit has been visiting us daily for two months and now allows us to pet and feed him. We're fearful that he can't defend himself against dogs. Could he survive in the wilds through the winter? Could he be an abandoned Easter bunny?—*RABBIT SAMARITAN*

DEAR *RABBIT SAMARITAN*—If I were you I would build this rabbit a nice hutch and run and put him inside it to give him protection from the elements and from predator cats and dogs. Yes—it is possible he's some child's pet who accidentally escaped, so why not put up a few notices around your neighborhood and in the local schools? I doubt if he's been free for long, since he's still so tame.

10

Cruelty to Animals and What You Can Do About It

animal welfare groups

DEAR DR. FOX—I frequently make small contributions to animal organizations. How can I find out which ones are legitimate and if the money really goes to help animals?—H.G.G.

DEAR H.G.G.—You're to be commended for supporting animal-welfare groups. Unfortunately, some organizations are in it for the money and are quite unethical, doing very little, in fact, for animals. Others are idealists who raise funds with sensationalist propaganda and then do little to educate the public or to get humane laws enforced or new protective legislation passed. One of the most ethical and effective organizations is The Humane Society of the United States, 2100 L Street N.W., Washington, D.C. 20037. Support this organization—and your local society, too—if you care for animals and their welfare. All contributions are tax deductible, since these are nonprofit organizations.

animals in classrooms

DEAR DR. FOX—My daughter came home from grade school last week in tears. One of the pet gerbils they had in the classroom had died. Don't you think keeping such animals in schools is cruel and should be stopped?—S.R.

DEAR S.R.—Animals in the classroom for younger children can be incredible learning catalysts, especially if the pets are well cared for and serve a valuable purpose in the curriculum. Even the death of one can, with the right teacher, be an important lesson for children. But I am opposed to keeping wild creatures in classrooms and to any kind of experimentation (other than direct observation), such as giving the animals drugs or deficient diets for science fair competitions.

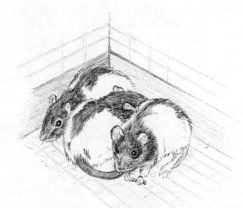

catching fish

DEAR DR. FOX—In all the books and articles about animals that I've read in the past few years, I've seen no reference to fish suffering when caught on a hook. Can you cite any material on this issue?—*MR. H. McG.*

DEAR MR. H. McG.—It has been proven that fish caught on a hook and removed from the water do experience pain, because natural opiates that dampen the painful effects on the entire organism have been found in the hooked fishes' brains. Most fish also probably experience anxiety, since they have a similar biochemical system in their brains to one we have—the so-called benzodiazepine receptor system, which Valium blocks. Swedish researchers have also found that earthworms produce these substances when they are injured, so we should also question the humaneness of putting a worm on a hook. Probably the most humane way to catch fish is in a net, provided, of course, that the net is not left in the water; fish that are caught by their gills would suffer considerably. Hooking fish and immediately killing them would be more humane. All fishermen should be informed and encouraged not to leave live fish tied to their boat on a stringer.

circus animals

DEAR DR. FOX—I recently attended the large Ringling Brothers Circus, and as an animal lover I am curious as to the care the animals receive. Are the animals ever given tranquilizers or drugs?—*D.P.*

DEAR D.P.—If circus animals were drugged for their performances, they would really goof up and could be dangerous. Generally, the bigger circuses take reasonable care of their animals. You will be happy to hear that The Humane Society of the United States has a full-time investigator for zoos and circuses, because they recognize the fact that abuses are still common in some instances when animals are used for "entertainment" purposes. Abuses by animal trainers, especially in the film industry, are a continuing problem, along with neglect of animals that aren't hired out and live in small cages. Crass exploitation indeed.

eating animals

DEAR DR. FOX—I love horses. Do you think it's right for people to eat horse-meat?—A.D.

DEAR A.D.—Hindus respect all creatures and eat none, especially cattle. Americans eat cattle but wouldn't touch dog, which is an Oriental delicacy. Japanese slaughter and eat whales and see nothing wrong with that since, as they point out, their European and American critics eat cattle, sheep, and pigs. Personally, I think we eat too much meat. Nutrition studies show we would be healthier if we ate less meat and animal fat. Horses should be ridden and loved, not eaten, unless we're starving. We're not.

importance of animal rights

DEAR DR. FOX—My wife often reads your column to me, and I wonder why you waste your time and talent on animal problems when there are so many human problems. Child abuse, wife-beating, crime, and drugs are surely far more important and better warrant the time and newspaper space given to the issues you raise.—R.T.

DEAR R.T.—It's not so much a question in my mind as to the relative importance of animal vs. human abuse and suffering. Both stem, I believe, from the same causes, notably ignorance, indifference, lack of respect for others' rights, and a pathological lack of empathy in society.

Children who learn to be humane toward animals are likely to be better citizens. Studies have shown that criminals often have a history in childhood of abusing animals. I wish the courts would recognize not only animals' rights but also that animal cruelty and neglect are signs of serious emotional disturbance in people. And I interpret the wholesale exploitation of laboratory animals in research and the stressful incarceration of farm animals on "factory" farms as a form of collective insanity. A humane society is a sane society.

mousetraps

DEAR DR. FOX—I recently saw an article about the cruelty of Stick-em mousetraps. Apparently, our local supermarket did too, because they withdrew them from the shelves. Are you aware of this product, and what are your thoughts?—A.G.S.

DEAR A.G.S.—I agree that these mousetraps are unbelievably cruel. The poor animal becomes slowly entangled in thick glue and eventually dies of exhaustion or suffocation. It's a sad reflection on society that such inhumane products are manufactured and purchased, and I am gratified that your supermarket—and others, I understand—are removing them from their shelves.

neighbors' treatment of their pets

DEAR DR. FOX—I live in a small apartment building, and every night when my neighbor comes home, I hear her yelling at her dog for chewing something, followed by numerous hard swats. Every morning the dog cries when the owner leaves. She says the dog is "spiteful," but I believe it's cruel to punish a dog like this every day. I will leave your reply in her mailbox if you explain the reason for her dog's behavior.—D.D.E.

DEAR D.D.E.—Your neighbor, like many people who hit and abuse their pets (and children), never ask themselves why the animal is acting "spitefully." Many dogs will destroy things in the home out of boredom and frustration when their owner is away. Calling a dog spiteful is judgmental and achieves nothing.

Perhaps if you explain in your note that the dog misses her all day, your neighbor will feel flattered. Explain that a dog's destructive behavior is neither natural nor spiteful, but a means of communicating loneliness and boredom. You are a Good Samaritan. There should be more humane citizens like you!

DEAR DR. FOX—Will you please say a word to your readers with regard to the countless people who keep dogs chained outside year round, day in and day out, and neither walk nor pay attention to them? The statistics of these incidences would floor you, and yet the humane society will do nothing to intervene if the dog is being fed.—E.V.S.

DEAR E.V.S.—Unfortunately, humane societies cannot do much to bring charges against a person who keeps a dog more or less permanently chained up in the yard, provided it is given adequate food, water, shelter, and veterinary care. The law of the land still regards animals as objects of property, and their rights are not recognized by the law, even though we feel differently in our hearts.

Hence the need for humane education in schools to teach children about animals' needs and rights. Educators who are interested in this should enquire about the new Humane Education Curriculum Guide published by The Humane Society of the United States (2100 L Street N.W., Washington, D.C. 20037). If more people showed your concern, the world would be a better place.

pet shop cleanup

DEAR DR. FOX—I am totally disgusted. How can people be so inconsiderate? The pet shop at my shopping mall stinks. The water is yellow; there are dead or suffering fish scraping at the rocks; the filter needs to be cleaned; algae is all over the glass; and the fish have to swim in all that muck. What can I do to stop them from doing this? (I have my own clean aquarium and a cat.) I would like to be a cat psychiatrist when I grow up—or a cat-book writer or maybe a veterinarian.—S.L.

DEAR S.L.—I advise you to discuss your concerns with one or both of your parents. Take them to the store for a look-see at the fish and then have them with you when you ask to see the manager. Of course, store managers are busy and can't supervise everything. But the person responsible for caring for the fish should be duly reprimanded by the manager or told what to do. It is possible that no one ever informed the assistant how to take care of the fish properly.

Even if you want to be a cat psychologist or a cat-book writer, it's best to become a veterinarian. This means you'll have to get good grades at school so that you'll be admitted to a veterinary school. Good luck!

poisoning of your pet by neighbors

DEAR DR. FOX—My husband and I would like to purchase a standard shepherd. The problem: One of the families living near us poisoned and killed two valuable German shepherds belonging to our neighbors. We're afraid the same thing will happen to us.

Is there a federal, county, or city agency that our neighbors can contact to take action against these people? One of the dogs had a prolonged and painful death.—A.F.

DEAR A.F.—Poisoning is difficult to prove and when proven, courts are usually too lenient with offenders of animals' rights. Courts often miss the significance of much animal abuse; such cases usually indicate a psychopathic personality and emotional problem within the family.

Free-roaming and barking dogs can make neighbors irate and cause them to resort to poisoning. So if you do get a dog, train it to be quiet, have it secured in a well-fenced yard, and when venturing into alien territory, keep it on a leash.

racehorse treatment

DEAR DR. FOX—I can't believe what I saw on TV recently—that nearly all racehorses are doped. What's the country coming to, and why don't veterinarians take a stand to protect these abused animals?—*A.G.*

DEAR A.G.—Unfortunately, some veterinarians are no different from any other professionals, and will get involved in illegal or unethical practices for financial profit.

On some race tracks an estimated 80 percent of horses are on "medication," especially painkilling drugs that make the detection of "dope" during the urine tests more difficult. It is a sad story—crippled horses are doped and overraced, so that competitors often are obliged to dope their horses, too, if they are ever to win.

So what to do? Write to your congressperson and local representatives. State and federal laws are needed, together with more effective enforcement. Anyone or any syndicate group caught racing a doped horse should be barred from going near a race track.

ANIMAL CARE NEWS

Two bills have recently been passed by the Florida state legislature by overwhelming votes.

One is mandatory sterilization of all cats and dogs adopted from animal shelters and animal-control agencies. This is the first of its kind in the nation, and will go a long way to help reduce pet overpopulation.

The other first is a prohibition on "doping" horses—many racehorses are treated with various drugs before they race. Good work, humane societies of Florida.

---

research animals (monkeys)

DEAR DR. FOX—I heard that there are some nationwide demonstrations being organized to protest the use of monkeys in research. What's the scoop? Was this just another antivivisection campaign, or was it legitimate?—*E.S.*

DEAR E.S.—What you're hearing about were mass public demonstrations that were organized nationwide for April 24, 1983, at the major government primate research centers—Atlanta, Wisconsin, New England (Boston), and Davis, California. The demonstrations were aimed not at abolishing legitimate use of animals in research but at the poor conditions under which monkeys are often housed (rhesus monkeys are often kept alone in tiny cages for years on end) and at the lack of scientific accountability and credibility of many animal research studies, which contribute little to human health. Demonstrations of this type are occurring more frequently, reflecting growing public concern over such issues as trapping, factory farming, and vivisection. For more information, contact: The Humane Society of the United States, 2100 L St. N.W., Washington, D.C. 20037.

NEWS BULLETIN

Congratulations to New York State, which now has a law prohibiting the use of the decompression chamber for putting animals to death. It's a very inhumane method that all states should outlaw.
Do you know if it is used in your state?

---

seal hunting

DEAR DR. FOX—In a recent article you criticized hunters who club seals of subjecting animals to unnecessary suffering. Isn't a blow on the head more humane than to grow old and die of illness or starvation? All animals must die sometime. I thought this was the approved method for slaughtering all animals. Also, the people who slaughter seals do it for a living, not for fun.. I would like to have you explain your position.—*S.R.*

DEAR S.R.—You raise important questions. But first, let me ask you one—is it right to kill wild animals for nonessential purposes? Food is essential, but we don't really need to wear seal skins. If sealers need the money, I say let them find another job. Slavetraders found new jobs when slavery was abolished thanks to recognition of human rights. Now the animal-rights movement is underway. You might want to read about it in my new book, *Returning to Eden: Animal Rights and Human Responsibilities*. If it is humane, as the Canadian government claims, why is there a Canadian welfare group studying shooting of seals as a more humane method? And why did the Canadian government refuse to allow any foreign humane societies to observe this year's seal hunt? (I, too, was denied permission.) Sealing is essentially an unethical exploitation of wildlife and should be abolished.

PART TWO

PSYCHOLOGY
AND
BEHAVIOR

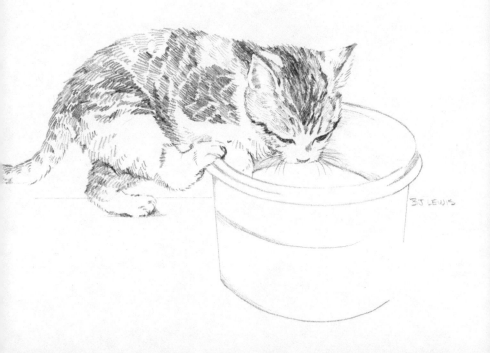

I n this second part of the book, we will look at the psychology and behavior of
our companion animals. Like us, they have a variety of needs, and they
communicate their wants and intentions in distinct ways. You will also learn how
to help animals make the emotional adjustments they need to adapt better to our
homes, and you will find out about training procedures as well. Animals can also
suffer from a variety of emotional problems, often expressed as disobedient or
troublesome behavior; an understanding of these will heighten your ability to
empathize with animals and help prevent behavior problems and emotional
distress.

I must clarify one of my interpretations of animals' behavior that may be
misjudged and dismissed as being too anthropomorphic. Animals *can* experience
a feeling such as jealousy (see Chapter 15). My dog Benji barks furiously
whenever I give loving attention to our other canine companion, Tiny. And if I
continue to ignore Benji, he will "neurotically" go to his food bowl and eat
whatever food is left. Benji is showing jealousy, not of Tiny, but of my *attention*
to Tiny.

This is a subtle distinction that I made through the following simple
experiment. Tiny was out of the large outdoor cage in which the two spend their
time when I am at work. I left the gate open and went in pretending to pet Tiny in
the usual place where she sleeps—on top of her kennel. Benji immediately
barked furiously, then went to his food bowl and started eating. It wasn't the
presence of Tiny that made him jealous, but rather my displaying any affection to
any creature other than him when he is present. He wants all of me—not when
I'm simply reading a book, but always when I embrace my wife in front of him!

If Benji were jealous of Tiny or my wife, he would show animosity, or at least bear them a grudge. Some dogs do bear grudges, just like humans—but this reflects a higher level of reasoning, objectification, and identification. Benji, like most dogs, doesn't do this. Like a very small child, he operates at a level psychotherapists refer to as "primary process thinking." It is simple and straightforward: he doesn't blame Tiny for his neediness. He is not jealous of her; he expresses his neediness when I pet her, and this can be interpreted as a display of jealousy over not receiving my undivided attention.

Furthermore, his jealous behavior is an expression of frustration, deprivation, and desire, which we can all empathize with once we accept that many animals, and especially cats and dogs, are emotionally very similar to preverbal children. This is not meant to imply that pets are incapable of reason or insight. Rather, their immature psyches (primary process thinking) prevent most, but not all, from bearing a deep-seated resentment. In their innocence, they are indeed forgiving and do not blame us for our faults, neglectfulness, and even deliberate mistreatment. Yet by the same token, they are more vulnerable to suffering frustration, deprivation, fear (especially of abandonment), and jealousy. They lack the protective powers of rationalization. How much easier it is for us to blame someone else and redirect feelings of jealousy toward him, rather than to bear the pain of our need for another's attention and affection.

This is part of the appeal of ever-trusting, innately forgiving, accepting companion animals, and it is a great responsibility for us to understand their psyches. For example, it is no use punishing a dog for showing jealousy in the form of needy barking for attention, since this will only add to its suffering and confusion. But if the dog directs its jealousy toward another in the form of aggression (as older-child sibling rivals will do), discipline is appropriate; the animal is no longer acting at a primary process level.

Always remember in dealing with animals that they can suffer in ways more similar to little children than to most of us adults, and we must be attuned to this aspect of their psychology and behavior.

11

Why Do They Do That?:
Instincts and Habits

NOCTURNAL BEHAVIOR AND BIORHYTHMS

early risers (cats)

DEAR DR. FOX—Our Persian has gotten into the habit of waking up between four and six each morning and meowing to be put outside. We're exhausted from losing sleep. Whenever our Persian is outside he is on a leash attached to the porch. We can't let him run free. How can we discourage this awful meowing?—*MRS. A. N. S.*

DEAR MRS. A. N. S—You do have a problem. Basically, your cat's bio-rhythm is out of phase with yours. One solution is to construct an outdoor pen or windowsill cage so he can go in and out as he pleases and do his meowing outside. You could also cut a small flap door into the bottom of the back door. Or set up a "tube walkway" or a ladder encircled in wire netting that leads into an outdoor cage or windowsill sun porch. Then your Persian can be outdoors but safely confined.

DEAR DR. FOX—My three-year-old cat (from the humane society) is perfect in every way except one. She gets up between 5:30 and 6:00 every morning to start her day. If I confine her in a small room she cries, scratches, and pesters me until I get up. How can I get her to sleep later?—*K. L. D.*

DEAR K. L. D.—Felines who are early risers are clamoring for attention and breakfast. A little discipline is in order. This will mean a few disturbed mornings where you do not give in. Let your cat onto the bed, but put her at the foot of the bed where she must learn to bide her time until you're ready to get up.

Hiss and say "NO!" and push her away if she solicits you. A quick spray with a plant mister will help. Be sure to put out a little food for her just before you retire at night. Cats learn not to pester each other. Yours can learn not to pester you, too.

UNCANNY CATS

Cats, similar to homing pigeons, have an internal "time clock." A wildcat knows just what time a rival hunter may be out. A domestic cat adjusts its rhythms to the household so that it rises at the same hour as family members, sometimes acting as an alarm clock. A lost cat can navigate several miles and find its way home by using this internal clock, which is set to local time and the position of the sun. Cats (like pigeons and humans) also have iron salts in their brains that act as a geomagnetic compass—another hidden sense.

---

nocturnal activity (cats)

DEAR DR. FOX—I received an adorable kitten as a gift from my neighbor, but every evening this little creature runs and jumps around the house in the craziest way. Is this normal?—A. Z.

DEAR A. Z.—What you're describing is the typical playful activity of a healthy kitten. You should remember that the wild cat had room and need to run, stalk, chase, and hunt; this is inherited behavior and very natural. One of my neighbors got so worried about her cat's wild behavior that she gave it a tranquilizer, but I don't recommend such action. As time goes by and kitty gets older, she'll quiet down. You may eventually miss her show of high spirits!

nocturnal activity (hamsters)

DEAR DR. FOX—My hamster is very lonely and sleeps day and night. She seems unhappy and won't let me pick her up without a fuss. My mom won't let

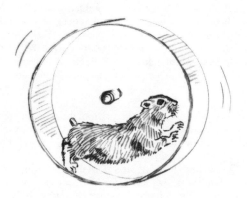

me have another hamster, because she thinks they will fight or have too many babies. Is she right?—*H.E.L.P.*

DEAR H.E.L.P.—Your mother is right (they usually are, you know!). An adult hamster prefers to live alone and will fight when another one is put in its cage. Hamsters sleep all day because, like bats and owls, they are night creatures. Nighttime is playtime for them, and it's the best time to observe and handle your pet. I think I would fuss too, if someone woke me up to play, so try to avoid disturbing her during the day. Keep in mind that hamsters prefer to explore rather than be cuddled when they are awake.

DEAR DR. FOX—I need help fast. I recently got a hamster for a science project, and I am running him in a maze. He sleeps all day, and when I wake him up, he nips me and crawls out of my hands. Once when I was carrying him, he crawled out and fell to the floor, and now he's still scared of me. How can I gain his friendship? Please help me fast—my grade depends on it!—*S. E. J.*

DEAR S. E. J.—Hamsters aren't the best maze-runners. Also, since the hamster is a nocturnal creature, your pet should be studied at night. How would you like to go to school when you're in deep sleep? Your hamster may do better on an activity wheel, and if you can get a revolution counter attached to it, you might design an experiment both you and your hamster partner will like, and get an A + in the bargain.

sleeping habits (cats)

DEAR DR. FOX—I have a darling two-year-old Persian and also a darling tabby who is ten. Tabby sleeps with me all night long, even though I never trained her to. I want my Persian to do this also, and I try to keep him awake during the day so he can sleep at night with me. But I just can't seem to keep him awake. Can you help?—*CAT WAKER*

DEAR CAT WAKER—Please appreciate that cats like to spend much of the day sleeping. This is natural to them. All cats, wild and tame, take frequent "cat-

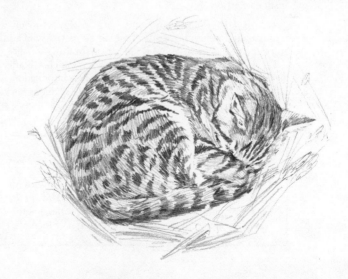

naps." We have one cat who sleeps on our bed, and the other must sleep in the living room because he's subordinate and is driven out of the bedroom by the other cat if he dares to come in. This is probably what's happening with your cat. So let things be, and let your cat sleep where he likes. Many cats, regardless of which is dominant, prefer to sleep and walk alone.

DEAR DR. FOX—Our Siamese cat persists in sleeping in our bed underneath the covers all night long. How can this cat stay under the covers and not smother?—R. J. S.

DEAR R.J.S.—How indeed! It amazes me how little air a cat needs when it crawls between the sheets. Some air will pass through the sheets, and as you turn over in bed you will help circulate some air beneath, so don't worry.

I've never heard of an adult cat suffocating in bed. A cat would wake its owner with its claws and struggle long before it passed out. But I would think twice about allowing a very young kitten way down under the sheets. Also, you don't indicate if your cat goes outdoors. If it does, you never know what it might bring home—fleas, mites, ringworm—not the best to sleep with.

WAYS WITH FOOD

"burying" food (cats)

DEAR DR. FOX—Our Siamese cat, Miss Marple, constantly scratches around her food dish, as if trying to bury it. This can go on for as long as ten minutes before she eats. Can you tell me why she does this?—MRS. H. W.

DEAR MRS. H. W.—In the wild, your cat would be simply hiding its leftover kill from scavengers, with the intent of returning to it later. The odor of the food will also stimulate the cat to keep scraping as though to cover up or mask the odor. Burying is an instinctual behavior, triggered by the odor and presence of food (or feces in the litter box). Your cat's behavior seems odd since there's no earth beside the food to be covered, but it is quite natural for those creatures who are under instinct-control.

DEAR DR. FOX—When my cat, Muffin, is given water, she claws or scratches at the floor before drinking. She's six years old and has been doing this since she was a kitten. What is the reason for this?—C. F.

DEAR C. F.—Cats will paw around their food bowls after they have eaten; it's a common practice, and I often interpret it as burying behavior. A wild cat will hide its kill this way and then return to eat the remains later.

Sometimes natural behavior patterns get out of sequence and occur in a typical

---

HOARDER AROUND THE HOUSE

Hamsters are prudent creatures who hoard any extra food they have. In fact, the German verb *hamstern* means to hoard. Perhaps you've noticed the cheek pouch of the hamster; it can be distended two or more inches if necessary when filled with nesting material or food.

situation or out of context. Being domesticated and kept under conditions that do not allow the full expression of instinctual behaviors probably contributes to such idiosyncrasies. One of my cats carries socks around as though they were her kittens and then proceeds to kill them as though they were rats. Cats are so adaptable, yet still natural in their ways—and that's why we love 'em.

finding worms (birds)

DEAR DR. FOX—I've always wondered how robins always find worms. Do they really hear them?—J. B. J.

DEAR J. B. J.—Birds not only listen with their ears (you can see them tilting their heads from side to side to get an accurate auditory "fix"), they may also feel vibrations in the earth through their feet. They also go out worming when the worms are most active, in the early morning. Worms are also active at night and are favorite food (when in season) for foxes and badgers. Worms are important creatures, keeping the soil aerated and enriched, so never use worm-killer on your lawn or garden.

regurgitation (parakeets)

DEAR DR. FOX—My parakeet has started throwing up whole seeds, followed by heavy saliva drippings. Also, I'm sure she's losing weight. She does not appear to be in any pain and is fairly active and chipper. What could be wrong? —W. L. H.

DEAR W. L. H.—If your bird is regurgitating over a mirror or plastic toy in the cage, it may be "in love" with its reflected image and engaging in misplaced feeding of a would-be mate or fledglings in the nest. The heavy saliva is crop milk, a nutritious fluid.

Remove the mirror or whatever stimulus may be triggering this behavior until your bird regains her strength. (Males see their image in the mirror as a female to court and feed, and females see it as a fledgling to nurture.)

Throwing up of food can also be due to sour crop, or intestinal parasites. A veterinarian experienced with cage birds should examine your parakeet.

salivary reflex (dogs)

DEAR DR. FOX—When my cocker spaniel is around food, or when we're eating, she drools. Is this common, or is something wrong with her?—T. P.

DEAR T. P.—Pavlov, the Russian psychologist, based much of his work on your dog's sensitive salivary reflex. It's quite normal for dogs to drool when they smell food, and they can be conditioned to salivate at the sound of a bell, a voice, etc. Also, cockers have pendulous lips, and this tends to make the saliva flow out and onto the floor rather than into the mouth to be swallowed.

scavenging in garbage (dogs)

DEAR DR. FOX—We have a terrible problem with our dog. She likes to tip over other people's garbage cans, eat all the leftovers, and walk off, leaving behind a terrible mess. We give her regular meals and snacks, so why does she have to do this?—P. S.

DEAR P. S.—Dogs can be perverse. They love to get into garbage because they are natural scavengers, and in the wild will eat the natural equivalent of garbage—carrion or the remains of dead animals. The smell of garbage might be perfume to a dog, and many of them will roll in it to achieve a scent. Your only solution is not to let your pooch roam free—which, incidentally, would make you a very responsible pet owner.

sharing your food (dogs)

DEAR DR. FOX—My sister has a five-month-old mongrel that's wacky. Everytime Mary drinks a beer, he sticks his tongue into the bottle for a drink too. Can this be harmful to him?—B. B.

DEAR B. B.—I see no reason why your sister shouldn't give your dog the last lick. A small dose of "suds" won't harm the dog and will make him feel loved and part of the family. Those who drink and eat together stay together. It's natural to share. If you don't, people and pets feel left out. My own pooch will even eat a few licks of hot curry sauce so as not to feel left out. But everything in moderation, please.

BATHROOM HABITS

carrying stools (dogs)

DEAR DR. FOX—We have a male and a female Lhasa apso who pick up their stools. They only carry, never chew or play with them, and we keep their yard clean. We spank the dogs and wash their mouths, but it doesn't seem to help. Why do they do this, and how do we stop the dogs from carrying on this way?—A.D.

DEAR A.D.—You should be happy that they don't eat them—many dogs do. It sounds as if your dogs have a little game going on. Your best solution is to give them some rubber toys or a knotted tube of sock or nylon stocking as substitutes. Also, clear up their droppings as soon as they drop. It is bizarre what things animals will do; boredom is a common underlying factor in many cases. More games—tugs of war and retrieve-the-ball—with your pets might also help.

doesn't lift leg to wet (dog)

DEAR DR. FOX—Our poodle (fourteen months old) doesn't lift his leg when urinating. He squats and hits his front legs and chest. I can't bathe him daily and am getting disgusted with him. How can we teach him to lift his leg?—J.M.H.

DEAR J.M.H—Some young male dogs do take a while before they learn to lift their legs. Actually, this style of urinating is affected by male sex hormones, so have your veterinarian examine your dog. He may be sexually immature or incompletely developed. A shot of testosterone, male sex hormone, may get him up on three legs and save his undercarriage and you from an unpleasant daily cleanup.

prefers cement to grass (dogs)

DEAR DR. FOX—My dachshund will only "go" on cement, probably because he lived the first five months of life in a kennel. He just will not "go" on the grass. I've tried spray repellents, drops, rubbing his nose in it, and spreading pepper all over the cement. I even tried tying him in a corner of the yard, but all he does is howl and disturb the neighbors. I cannot allow him to mess up the driveway, garage, and patio where my young children play. Please help.—J.G.

DEAR J.G.—Count your blessings. Thank your dog for "going" on concrete and not on the soil or grass. All you need are a hose and a poop-scoop for a daily cleanup. Your dog's toilet habit is much more desirable than if he were to mess on grass, lawns, etc. Dog urine kills grass, and the contaminated soil and lawn, etc., can become a source of disease for your children. I would say you have a public-minded pooch.

spraying (cats)

DEAR DR. FOX—I was really shocked when I saw my cat spraying the other day, because my cat is a *she*. Could she have learned it from her brother?—M. S.

DEAR M. S.—Female felines do "spray." Backing up against some vertical object with tail upright and trembling, they send out a jet of urine. Ethologists believe that this is more common in male cats because they are more territorial. But females will do it too, no doubt to mark their territory, to advertise their occupancy, and to warn intruders to keep away.

use of litter box (cats vs. dogs)

DEAR DR. FOX—Can you tell me why dogs can't be trained to use the litter box the way cats do? It would make life so much simpler!—G.R.

DEAR G.R.—If oranges were apples, we'd never have to worry about an apple shortage. In other words, cats are cats and dogs are dogs. In nature, cats bury their droppings, whereas members of the dog family never do. Cats accept training to use the litter tray because they have an instinct for it.

SEX PLAY

aroused by dog not in heat

DEAR DR. FOX—Our miniature schnauzer, Morning Star, was in heat when she met our friends' Labrador retriever. Naturally, Salty reacted as any male would. Ever since then, whenever Salty sees Morning Star, he acts as if she's in season, and we know she's not. Other dogs she comes in contact with will leave her alone, but not Salty—he drools and licks her. Our friends have changed our dog's name to Blaze Star. Any explanation?—L.J.

DEAR L.J.—I sometimes wonder if dogs fall in love. After being snared by the perfume of a bitch in heat, a dog may have a complete recall of sexual arousal when he meets the same dog later or possibly one of the same breed. I do not believe that Salty is sexually abnormal in any way. He may simply want, or lack, experience.

homosexual behavior (cats and dogs)

DEAR DR. FOX—We have two male cats (about eighteen months old), both from the same litter. In all seriousness, the cats appear to be homosexual. We have seen evidence of this several times. Is there a reason for their behavior? What should we do?—J.L.S.

DEAR J.L.S.—Cats, like many other animals, will often act homosexual with each other. This is not some unnatural perversion. Rather it illustrates how catholic animals can be in their tastes, which are in part shaped by early experience and rearing conditions. Hence, a cat may mount a companion cat of the same sex. But please understand that not all sexual-looking behavior is purely sexual; there are also the elements of dominance and play. I would suggest you do nothing. Adding a female cat could cause much conflict and jealousy. Your cats are harming no one. And they'll probably grow out of the behavior.

DEAR DR. FOX—This problem may sound far-fetched, but it's bothering my husband and me. Is it possible for dogs to become homosexual? Our Brittany spaniel-beagle has attached himself to a friend's husky. Both dogs are male.

It's unbelievable how devoted my dog has become to this husky. It's gotten to the point where my dog no longer associates with us and disobeys me when I call him to come or stay. My husband insists it is not normal for two male dogs to act this way. Is he right?—A.D.

DEAR A.D.—Dogs of the same sex do frequently develop a close buddy system and like to roam and play together, even sharing toys, food, and grooming with each other. Sometimes they will engage in mock fights or sex play, one mounting the other as though it was in heat. The more dominant buddy may assume the less passive male role.

This "homosexual" play is perfectly normal but usually disappears as heterosexual interests develop with sexual maturity, although occasionally they may still engage in homosexual play with a friendly dog. This is all natural, so let dogs be dogs and tolerate any embarrassment you may feel.

identity crisis (dog with cat)

DEAR DR. FOX—Ever since our poodle was neutered, he thinks he's a tomcat and that our spayed cat is available. He is six years old, and he never did anything so crazy until he was fixed. Is this normal?—D.B.D.

DEAR D.B.D.—No, this isn't normal, but it's not really normal for a cat and dog to live together, or for them to be neutered. My guess is that the operation on your dog triggered a surge of hormonal output from the pituitary gland and he found a convenient, if inappropriate, outlet via your cat. If your cat doesn't mind and you're not upset, let them be. One interpretation is that it's a form of play—not a perversion—and that it's natural, relatively speaking. An injection with a long-acting anabolic steroid might inhibit such behavior. On the other hand, such hormonal manipulations could have unpredictable side effects. I would let him be.

oversexed cat

DEAR DR. FOX—Last year I found and took home an adorable orange male kitten. This playful little tyke, however, soon became a sex maniac-rapist and it was almost impossible to keep him in the house with Gertrude, our spayed female. It got so she could not even walk from the kitchen to the living room if Chester were in the house, since he would attack her. Last week I took Chester to be neutered. Well, he's just the same. Now we have a neutered cat attacking a spayed female every minute he sees her walking by or wagging her tail. Is this what I get for being a Good Samaritan?—A.K.S.

DEAR A.K.S.—Some cats, like people, always want everything their way. Usually, they end up living alone. Get oversexed Chester off your hands, find someone who would love a spunky character like him and who has no other living thing in the house. Otherwise Chester will continue to be a pesky puss. I would not endorse tranquilizers or a lobotomy; either could make Chester into a zombie, which is just as bad as being a sex maniac-rapist—at least for him, if not for your Gertrude.

spayed dog makes advances

DEAR DR. FOX—My four-year-old spayed poodle tries to mate with just about every dog she plays with. Could you explain her odd behavior?—CURIOUS

DEAR CURIOUS—Spayed female dogs will often engage in sexlike activities, especially during play with another dog. They will mount, clasp the other dog around the waist with their forelegs, and generally behave as though they were male dogs. This may be related to a hormonal imbalance, but a more likely explanation is that this is simply a displacement of sexual behavior. Unspayed female and male dogs will also show such behavior when they're playing with other animals. Occasionally, you'll see one dog mount another in this way—not playfully, but to assert dominance over the other dog. So don't worry—you don't have a deviate on your hands!

GROOMING BEHAVIOR

dog washes like cat

DEAR DR. FOX—My toy poodle washes himself like a cat after he eats, by licking his paws and arms and rubbing them on his face. Isn't this strange behavior for a dog?—*MRS. J.E.M.*

DEAR MRS. J.E.M.—It is surprising how catlike some dogs are. I have had people suggest that their dog is a reincarnation of a deceased cat and all kinds of other odd interpretations.

Religious creationists won't like this, but there is good evolutionary evidence that cats and dogs are distant cousins (related also to bears, racoons, foxes, and ferrets). Therefore, it's not surprising that some of their behaviors are quite similar. Bobcats bark like dogs, and some dogs wash their faces like cats.

Living with another species can also affect an animal's behavior through mimicry. Some dogs, like one of mine, mimicks a toothy human grin. So are dogs related to humans? In essence, most likely, as all living things are part of the same breath of creation.

nail trimming (cats)

DEAR DR. FOX—My cat keeps chewing on her back claws so furiously that I fear she will make herself raw there and bleed. Can you tell me why she does this? She is otherwise healthy and happy, since we play with her often and give her plenty of toys.—*G.S.*

DEAR G.S.—You've supplied one important clue: your cat is not bored, so that rules out self-mutilation from boredom. Excessive chewing may indicate that there is an infection between the toes or at the root of one or more of the claws. Examine your cat carefully and see if you can detect any redness, swelling, secretion, or pain on pressure. If this is the case, then have the animal checked out by your veterinarian.

However, it is quite common for cats and dogs to trim their own toenails, and in chewing on her back claws, your cat may simply be grooming herself. My guess is she's giving herself a manicure. You might help her by trimming the claws yourself.

nail trimming (dogs)

DEAR DR. FOX—My chihuahua bites the nails on her back paws, even when they are clipped. She's not even the nervous type, as most chihuahuas are, so why the nail-biting?—*S.H.*

DEAR S.H.—Don't worry—part of self-grooming for many dogs includes gnawing and nipping toenails. Providing your dog isn't mutilating herself or licking her paws excessively (which could lead to a secondary infection), just let her alone. But make sure to give her plenty of exercise. And don't scold or reward her when she's biting her nails, otherwise this could lead to all kinds of bizarre conditioned associations.

preening (parakeets)

DEAR DR. FOX—My poor little parakeet, Ricki, is always scratching himself, even though I clean his cage often and dust him with lice power. Help!—S.B.

DEAR S.B.—Birds, like cats and dogs, scratch themselves frequently. This is quite a normal part of self-grooming, but some owners get overly concerned and wrongly apply flea or mite powder to their pets. Give him medication only if your vet confirms that your bird has feather mites. If Ricki's feathers are normal and he isn't scratching himself raw or bald, it could well be normal preening behavior that you are misinterpreting. Your bird could also be bored and need more exercise, handling, and a variety of cage toys (ladder, bell, or mirror). If your doubts persist, have your vet check for parasites on the skin and feathers.

DEAR DR. FOX—A few years ago I gave my mother my two parakeets to keep for me. Soon after, they produced three nests of eggs, which all hatched successfully. Now it seems that the other birds are picking the feathers out of the mother's head (her mate is the worst offender). Poor things! I have taken her back and put her in a cage all by herself.

She seems quite happy now, and the feathers are growing back on her head. Can you explain this cruel behavior?—A.C.

DEAR A.C.—Now you've heard of parakeet-pecking. Sounds to me like the cage was overcrowded and the mother got the worse end of the stick.

Once a bald spot appears, excessive social preening by other birds occurs because the bald spot attracts them, and they begin to use it as a toy to pull at. You seem to have found the cure yourself for now. If you do want to put the mother back once she has a well-feathered head, just make sure that the cage is big enough for the family. Crowding can make even parakeets "cuckoo."

pulling out loose nails (cats)

DEAR DR. FOX—I notice that my Siamese cat pulls out the toenails of her hind paws with her teeth. Under each nail is a fully developed nail. Is this a natural thing for her to do? My other Siamese cat never does this.—D.L.W.

DEAR D.L.W.—Some cats chew and groom their nails, others aren't so fastidious. But pulling out loose nails is quite normal—just as it's normal for a fresh one to be growing out. It is disconcerting to owners who don't realize that a cat's claws are being constantly replaced. So don't get alarmed if you see a claw "shell" on the carpet. A neurotic cat will self-mutilate during emotional stress. Excessive self-licking and claw-chewing warrants a veterinary checkup.

whisker trimming (cats)

DEAR DR. FOX—My Siamese cats' whiskers are only about a half-inch long. Is it possible the cats could be biting each other's whiskers off? What should I do?—B.J.H.

DEAR B.J.H.—You've got it. Your Siamese cats are probably trimming each others' moustachios. One of our cats fastidiously trims down the long whiskers on our other cat's forehead. Perhaps this is to tell other cats that she's married or already has a grooming partner—although, of course, we never let either of them outdoors except under strict supervision. But joking aside, this is a curious phenomenon. It may be a quirk, or it may be that cats who trim others' whiskers off need more roughage in their diets. Our barber-cat can't wait to get outdoors to eat grass. Perhaps as she keeps the lawn trimmed she'll lay off her companion's whiskers. Try yours on fresh grass, too.

HUNTING

birds attacking cats and dogs

DEAR DR. FOX—For the last three weeks two birds have been tormenting my cat. They chirp over him all day and dive at him if he makes a move. They are driving him insane. What can we do? We can't keep the cat indoors because a family member has allergies—*M.R.*

DEAR M.R.—Here's a switch—usually my letters are from people worried about how to protect their yard birds from their neighbor's cats. Various species of birds, especially blue jays, will mob predators such as foxes, bobcats, and domestic cats. They will also, when flying, dive at crows, hawks, and owls—a natural, instinctive response to predators. It's unlikely that the birds will hurt your cat and even less likely that they will drive him insane. The cat may certainly be afraid or frustrated about not being able to catch these birds. But I would simply let nature take its course, since nothing serious is at stake.

DEAR DR. FOX—I own a Brittany spaniel who is contantly chased by a mockingbird. The bird returns every spring to the same place, dives down, and pecks our dog's tail. Our dog seems to ignore the bird, but I'd like to know if this bird is actually attacking my dog.—*C.G.*

DEAR C.G.—Mockingbirds are playful and perceptive birds and will often mob a cat or dog, and sometimes even get other birds to join in. There's nothing personal about the attack—it's based on the mockingbird's instinctual reaction to predators and is a behavior intended to confuse and repel would-be adversaries.

discouraging hunting (cats)

DEAR DR. FOX—You have said several times that you love cats, yet you advise people to keep them indoors to prevent them from killing wildlife. How do you recommend this be done? I, too, love birds, rabbits, squirrels, butterflies, etc., and am terribly upset when my neighbor's cats destroy these creatures. But my neighbors insist that their cat's killing is part of the balance of nature and that cats need to be free. How do I answer their arguments?—*MRS. M.S.*

DEAR MRS. M.S.—Your letter raises some important ethical questions. My position is that domestic cats who are fed by their owners should not supplement their diet by killing various wildlife species. This can upset the balance of nature in suburban areas, where several free-roaming cats in a given locale would have a significant impact upon young squirrels, rabbits, ground-nesting birds, and fledgling birds of tree-nesting species.

It is indeed inhumane to confine a cat indoors when it has spent the earlier part of its life roaming free outdoors. But a cat who has been raised indoors does not miss going out and is quite happy to stay at home.

Two cats living together are generally healthier and happier than one alone, especially when the owner goes to work during the day. When trained early in life, many cats enjoy walks on a leash and harness, having an outdoor run, or perching on a window-sill observatory and looking out.

Cats will claw furniture whether they live in or out of doors. The cat should be trained to use a scratch post, and its claws trimmed to reduce injury to upholstery. Your neighbors' belief that a cat should be allowed to live as "natural a life as possible" is ecologically unsound and analogous to saying that human beings have a right to do whatever they want, regardless of negative social and environmental consequences.

discouraging hunting (dogs)

DEAR DR. FOX—We have a chow chow who is kind hearted in all respects except that he quietly kills cats that come in the yard. What can we do? We are very upset.—J.P.

DEAR J.P.—Some of the nicest dogs I know are like your dog—cat-killers. His behavior is not wholly abnormal; in the wild, carnivores will attack and sometimes kill smaller ones. This is one of the reasons why I insist that cat owners not let their cats roam free. By using a leash and choke-chain, you can condition your dog not to chase and kill cats. My book *Understanding Your Dog* will give you all the pointers you need. Essentially, one uses a sharp verbal command followed by a quick snap of the leash to deter the dog from chasing when it sees a cat. A running cat is a potent stimulus for a dog to chase, and such a reaction is a deeply ingrained instinct.

DEAR DR. FOX—I can't stop my Siberian husky from chasing and killing cats and squirrels. She is five years old and otherwise very obedient.—H.R.

DEAR H.R.—The instinct of prey-chasing and killing is virtually impossible to inhibit in some dogs. A course in obedience training would help you gain better control over your dog. Also, never let her roam free—she could be hit by a car while chasing a squirrel or cat across the road. Keep her on a leash at all times. A choke-chain may make it easier for you to handle her. An elderly neighbor of mine has a young dog like yours and nearly broke his neck each time he walked his dog on a harness. A choke-chain has made him feel much safer.

pack instinct (dogs)

DEAR DR. FOX—In the last few days, every time we go outside our dog starts chasing our chickens. Why does she do that? It is very weird. I'm asking this question because I want to be a vet when I grow up.—R.L.

DEAR R.L.—Your dog is showing off. Stimulated by your presence, his pack instinct to hunt is triggered. What he'd really like is for you to join him and chase the chickens. Throw him a stick or a ball to redirect his behavior. If that fails, have him on a long rope and pull it short to inhibit him with a loud "Stay" or "Sit" before you pull. Reinforce this with some basic obedience training. I do hope you become a vet—but you'll have to get good grades!

THE DOG'S HUNTING INSTINCT

Dogs have a strong natural instinct to hunt and often will chase cars, mail carriers, joggers, etc., for this reason. One way to satisfy the hunting instinct is to give a dog toys that can be prey substitutes to chase and "kill."

problems with hunting (cats)

DEAR DR. FOX—You have frequently urged cat owners to keep their cats inside the house. I cannot help but rejoice, however, when my cat Fred brings home a rat for dinner. Considering the diseases rats spread and the amount of food they devour, they are humankind's worst enemy. If two or three times a year Fred leaves a pile of feathers in the yard, he must be forgiven because of the revenge he wreaks upon humanity's greatest scourge.—W.O.

DEAR W.O.—As a regular reader of my column, you should know my reasons for not allowing cats to roam free. Aside from the fact that free-roaming cats kill wildlife like birds, your cat could bring home a rat with some diseases that could make you very ill. But there is one legitimate exception—working cats on farms and in warehouses should be free to hunt rodents, provided they receive veterinary care when needed and aren't allowed to overmultiply.

So I only half-agree with you. We created the rat problem in the first place, by storing grain and other food in poorly designed buildings and containers. Preventive rat control is better than putting out rat poison that might also kill your cat if it eats the bait or a poisoned rat.

IMPORTANT HUNTING SENSES

Until recently, it was believed that cats, like dogs, are colorblind. But recent investigations indicate that the cat's retina does have some few cone cells that are sensitive to both green and blue, and possibly even to red. But even if a cat can see colors, this ability is not used much in its everyday life. Cats rely mostly on movements and sounds to locate prey.

DEAR DR. FOX—I have a very healthy and happy four-year-old cat, but why must she hunt down little animals and then carry them home? Recently, within a twenty-four-hour time span, she brought home two mice (one was still alive) and a squirrel. Not only am I concerned that innocent animals are being killed for no reasaon, but I'm also worried for my cat's health. Any advice?—S.N.

DEAR S.N.—You are right to be concerned. There are certain diseases, such as toxoplasmosis and tapeworms, that a cat can get from mice and other prey. However, once cats get a taste for the outdoors, it can be difficult to keep them indoors. I also feel that it's not right for a housecat to be allowed to kill wildlife, including mice, which are not "vermin." If you are lucky enough to have a screened-in sun porch, your cat might enjoy that. And you could supply her with substitute prey (toys) or a paper bag to crinkle and crawl into. Next time make your kitten a homebody.

TERRITORIALITY

defending territory (birds)

DEAR DR. FOX—I placed a large, round mirror under a tree in my backyard. Now Mr. and Mrs. Red Bird spend all day fluttering and pecking at themselves in the mirror. My friend said I was wrong to do this because now the birds are neglecting their natural duties, such as building nests, mating, and laying and hatching eggs. Should I remove the mirror?—H.R.M.

DEAR H.R.M.—Yes, I'm afraid your friend is right. What you have done is set up a rival couple in your Red Birds' territory. They respond to their mirror images as though two other birds had invaded their territory. Eventually they might become habituated to the mirror, but in the interim it is going to disrupt their lives considerably, if not drive them away from your yard for good. English robins, which have red breasts, will even attack a ball of red wool hung from a tree in their territory as though it were a rival. So let's stop the experiments with nature's children and return things to their original state—no mirrors, please.

defending territory (dogs)

DEAR DR. FOX—Our four-year-old schnauzer is always barking—especially at the mailman. We have a large window in our living room, and he always runs to the window and barks wildly. I know that schnauzers were brought from Germany to be watchdogs, but this barking is too much. What should I do to calm him?—K.A.W.

DEAR K.A.W.—One reason your schnauzer barks so much is because he's confined indoors much of the time in a relatively monotonous and unstimulating environment. The mailman's coming is one daily event that breaks his monotony. The dog anticipates this with enjoyment because he can put on a show, bark, and defend his territory.

I would not try to inhibit this behavior, but instead give your dog more exercise and attention. Have him meet the mailman and try to establish a more trusting relationship (if the two will accept each other). After that, your dog won't bark quite so intensely. Dogs bark loudly to defend their territory from an intruder, but give a few yaps to greet a friend.

DEAR DR. FOX—I have a very friendly nine-year-old German shepherd-husky. I have no trouble getting her to go for two walks each night when she is in the house, but if she is in her doghouse I can't budge her. All she does is growl. I usually end up pulling all seventy snarling pounds of her out of the doghouse; halfway out, she changes into a dejected, submissive dog—ears flat, tail low, and head down. It seems she knows that she's been a bad dog. I pet her, give her a tidbit, and then say, "Let's go for a walk." Her ears instantly go up, and she prances around eagerly. Is there any explanation for this strange behavior?—J.H.G.

DEAR J.H.G—Your dog is obviously defending her territory. She may also simply not want to go out once she's settled down outside for the night. I think I'd growl too if I was anticipating being dragged out to go for a walk. Why don't you leave her alone when she growls next time and let her work it out for herself so she won't feel guilty and have to apologize halfway out? Wait for her to come to you —call her, rattle the leash, and give her a treat.

pecking (birds)

DEAR DR. FOX—For two years now, we have been visited by a yellow-bellied sapsucker who pecks persistently on our barn drainpipe. This makes quite a racket on the metal, and he has been at it for at least a month. Any ideas why a drainpipe instead of a tree?—C.N.

DEAR C.N.—The drumming sounds that sapsuckers and woodpeckers make on dead trees is not just part of their wood-drilling in search of bugs. They drum to advertise and display their territorial presence to other birds. Choosing a metal drainpipe is certainly an insightful choice.

protecting owner (dogs)

DEAR DR. FOX—My dog has this crazy habit, and it really bothers my folks. He won't let them come into my bedroom when I go to sleep. I feel bad for them. What should I do? I am eleven years old.—G.B.

DEAR G.B.—Only you can rectify this situation. The dog obviously sees you as its master, and it is being protective of you. Next time he growls at your mom and pop, tell him that it's OK for them to come in while you reassuringly pet him. Keep up the propaganda. By the way, your dog is not crazy. It happens often that a dog gets very attached to a young member of the family.

DOMINANCE AND SUBMISSION

crying (dogs)

DEAR DR. FOX—We have a two-year-old German shepherd-Doberman mix. When one of our female dogs walks in front of him, he cries. If we try to comfort him, he snaps or bites us. What can we do to break him of this bad habit?—T.S.

DEAR T.S.—Why is it a bad habit for your dog to cry when one of your other dogs walks in front of him? Maybe he's expressing his affection, excitement, or submission. Let him do his thing—no need to comfort him. And if you let him do his thing, maybe he won't snap at you. He wants to be free to communicate to other dogs. Having him neutered may calm him down, but I would advise obedience training for starters.

leader-subordinate interaction (dogs)

DEAR DR. FOX—Our springer is pitiful. He follows our nine-year-old neutered cocker-poodle everywhere. He rests his head on the cocker, cleans him, and drives him so crazy that the cocker will bite his nose ten times in a row.

But that only makes the springer stick even closer. The cocker is not fond of the springer and makes his feelings known, although on rare occasions they do play together. The cocker's teeth are not sharp, so we have no real problem. We just want to understand.—D.S.

DEAR D.S.—I first saw this kind of behavior when I was studying wolves and detailed it in my book *The Soul of the Wolf*. At first sight it looks like a sadomasochistic relationship. Yes, the subordinate wolf or dog actually solicits being dominated and snapped at by the leader.

In reality, this is less a display of aggression (or of sadomasochism) than it is one of allegiance to the leader, an affectionate bond where the leader does not injure the subordinate but responds to its obedient puppylike submission like a lord and master.

DEAR DR. FOX—We have a three-year-old male Shih Tzu, and whenever my father calls the dog to sit in a chair with him, he always goes to my mother instead. Nonetheless, he shows affection to all members of our family, including my father. Any idea why he does this?—L.S.

DEAR L.S.—My interpretation is that your dog is intimidated by your father and goes to your mother for protection. The dog probably sees your father as the "pack leader," and to be invited to sit so close to the leader could be a little too much for a subordinate pooch. It's also possible that the dog could have been sat on or scared off the chair by your father once—or even ordered to get down. Either live with the situation or tell your dad to go on a campaign to win your dog with plenty of tender loving care.

DEAR DR. FOX—We recently bought a female standard schnauzer puppy as a companion for our older dog., The new pup gets along fine with the older dog and is affectionate to my wife, but is leery of me. She won't let me pet her or even hold the door for her when she goes out. I've never had this happen with our previous dogs.—*R.B.*

DEAR R.B.—You may be misinterpreting your dog's behavior. She may be showing submission toward you as the dominant pack leader in the house. Does that make you feel any better? However, she may well be scared or jealous of you. If you begin to take charge of walking and feeding her, gradually she might develop a stronger dependence on you.

MIMICRY

copy-cats

DEAR DR. FOX—Our cat, Nuisance, is proof that cats copy their owners. Nuisance observed us washing our faces at the basin. When the faucet was left running a few days later, she put her paw under the drip and washed the side of her face.

One day when I was going to leave the house, she ran to the door, stood on her hind legs and spread her front legs across the door. She also puts on a great gymnastic show on her padded bar to entertain our guests.—*D.E.L.*

DEAR D.E.L.—Sounds to me as though you have a very bright feline in your family. The expression "copy-cat" is probably related to the fact that cats do frequently copy each other. Kittens copy mother's actions and through observational learning quickly acquire skills to hunt and kill live prey in the wild.

The survival value of such remarkable behavior is greatly reduced in the safe domestic environment we provide our cats. Still, the need and ability to mimic surfaces in many cats. Thanks for the insightful anecdote.

ADOPTING OLD SOCKS AND OTHER STRANGE ACTIVITIES

crawling into cars (cats)

DEAR DR. FOX—How can one keep stray cats away from parked cars in open carports? Homeless cats come in out of the cold to use the warmth from automobile engines, and, at the same time, they leave their footprints all over dark-painted cars. It is very exasperating.—*J.A.T.*

DEAR J.A.T.—Acid rain will cause more damage to your car's paint work than all the pussy paws in paradise. So fight acid rain—that's a real environmental concern. However, do keep your windows up, because cats will spray inside open cars to mark their territory. And do make a habit of tooting your horn or looking under your hood before you start the engine. More than one cat has been chewed up in the fan or fanbelt. The whole problem would not exist if all cat owners were responsible and did not let their cats roam free.

dropping toys in food dishes (cats)

DEAR DR. FOX—After playing with their toys, why do cats deposit them in their water and feed dishes? I thought perhaps you could enlighten me. All my wondering doesn't come up with much that's logical.—*M. MAC.*

DEAR M. MAC—I'm afraid you've got me stumped on this question, too. I have not heard of other cats doing what yours do. One of your cats may have started this idiosyncratic behavior and the others followed suit.

It's rather like hoarding and retrieving: keeping everything handy in one place, food, water, and toys conveniently in one spot. Or the toys could be like tokens, with the cats being rewarded for putting them in their bowls by your removing them and giving your cats fresh food and water. But explanations and theories notwithstanding, your cats are just cats, and, like most, are unpredictable nonconformists.

reaction to perfume (dogs)

DEAR DR. FOX—My Yorkie has the strangest reaction whenever she smells perfume. She will bark and growl at the offending bottle, rub her nose and the sides of her head along the carpet for ten minutes, then proceed to roll over the bottle several times. Is this normal? Also, she loves to bury her nose in pillows and shoes. Why does she do this?—*E.T.*

DEAR E.T.—Dogs have a sense of smell possibly a million times greater than ours, so they can detect various components of perfume that we can't. As a result, they will react strongly. Many perfumes contain animal musk, which could make your dog bark and growl as though a strange animal had come into her territory and left its mark. Dogs roll in some odors often out of pleasure, perhaps to "wear" the odor on their bodies just like people enjoy wearing visually appealing clothes. Let your dog enjoy her perfume occasionally, but avoid expensive perfumes that contain the musk of endangered species.

rolling in foul smells (dogs)

DEAR DR. FOX—Can you give us one good reason why all dogs, including our snow-white poodle, love to find something really foul smelling, and roll and roll until they get as much of the stink on them as they can? Ginger is a real darling, except for this silly business.—*N.K.*

DEAR N.K.—All dogs, no matter how well bred, trained, trimmed, bathed, and cuddled, will roll in foul-smelling things. They do it instinctively, and I think they enjoy it—in spite of owners' reprimands, which they often know will be forthcoming. My theory is that dogs like to "wear" strong odors as we, and more visual species, enjoy wearing certain colors and patterns. We get rewarded—people notice us. A dog, too, certainly catches the nose of other dogs after a good roll in something unprintable and untouchable.

DEAR DR. FOX—I have a toy poodle and a Yorkshire terrier who cannot enjoy the yard because there are two cats next door who are allowed to roam and use my grounds for their litter box. I am seventy-four years old and live alone and have to stay with my dogs the whole time they are out. Could you advise me what to do about my dogs rolling in and eating the cat excrement?—*FRUSTRATED*

DEAR FRUSTRATED—Other than asking the neighbors to keep their cats indoors, you might consider leaving your dogs out as much as you can to drive the cats off your property. An "anointing" under the chin with some perfume or cologne may well deter them from rolling in the cats' waste, since it will satisfy their desire for some new, exciting aroma. This trick is often quite effective and is better than keeping your dogs cooped up all day.

rubbing (dogs)

DEAR DR. FOX—Our small spayed Chihuahua has developed an inexplicable habit—she puts her head to the carpeted floor and rubs it back and forth, snorting and scratching at the carpet with her front feet. She does this several times a day at no particular time. Could she have pain in her head or perhaps her ears?—D.Z.

DEAR D.Z.—Dogs pick up all kinds of odd habits—rubbing various parts of their bodies against furniture, bushes, carpeting, and so on. But it's always important to rule out irritation or infection first. Do check your dog's teeth and gums, because she may have a chronic inflammation that leads her to rub her head back and forth to alleviate the discomfort. On the other hand, it could simply be a sudden idiosyncrasy; all dogs occasionally acquire new tricks. Don't rule out that the behavior could be comforting to the animal, much like people stretch or scratch their heads when they feel relaxed.

shredding books (cats)

DEAR DR. FOX—Am I right in assuming that when my cat, Salome, shreds my books, she is jealous of the paperwork I do at home? When I give her more attention, though, she still doesn't stop.—M.B.

DEAR M.B.—A spouse could be jealous of your books, but not a cat. More likely, Salome considers playing with your books an entertaining diversion. Try giving pussy a variety of toys, such as a big fluffy rabbit or a cat mobile of hanging strings with fluffy birds on the end. You may end up jealous yourself when these interesting playthings prove more attractive to your cat than you!

sleeping in flower beds (dogs)

DEAR DR. FOX—We need help. Our German shepherd thinks the flower beds are the only cool places to sleep in the summer time. How can we break her of this habit?—A.G.

DEAR A.G.—Sensible dog. Flower beds are nice and soft and cool—cooler still when, with canine common sense, your pooch digs the top soil up to expose the cooler earth beneath. So you must give your dog an alternative—a soft bed in cool shade. That and a running line so she can move around but not get to the flower beds, or a barrier of bamboo canes around the lower bed if you don't want to tie your dog up. Of course, she may be just as happy indoors during the summer, provided, of course, she has a soft rug, air conditioning, regular exercise, and an occasional bone to chew on. No flowers, please!

tail-chasing (cats)

DEAR DR. FOX—My thirteen-year-old cat has recently developed an interesting habit: chasing her tail. She will stalk it cautiously and then run in circles, swatting and pouncing. She will also watch her tail for several minutes at a time, with a fierce, predatory expression, waiting for any slight movement or twitching, the signals for attack. She scorns cat toys. Is she crazy, or just bored?—*S.P.*

DEAR S.P.—It just goes to show you that old pets can acquire new ways. No, I don't think your cat has gone crazy. It sounds just like the kind of healthy behavior one sees in kittens and in playful adult cats. It's also an indicator that cats have active imaginations.

I wonder if your cat is becoming more infantile as she ages. If the tail-chasing becomes very intense and the tail actually gets bitten, then a brain abnormality— a tumor or hemorrhage—might be the cause. She may scorn toys, but perhaps not if you encourage her to play with you and the toy. It might be worth a try.

transporting objects (cats)

DEAR DR. FOX—Every night after we go to bed, our cat starts meowing and goes into the laundry room where I keep a basket of unmatched socks. She takes the socks out, carries them into the living room, and puts them on the floor. Can you please explain this very odd habit?—*F.M.*

DEAR F.M.—My Burmese cat does exactly the same thing during the day. Carrying socks around and depositing them in one spot could be a displaced maternal behavior of tending for kittens. It could also be a form of play behavior related to retrieving prey. My cat will sometimes attack her socks as though to kill them. Instead of discouraging your cat, play with her and give her other toys. Life as a domestic pet can be unstimulating. Your cat is trying to adapt and to find an outlet for her pent-up instincts and desires. Listen to the message.

DEAR DR. FOX—Your column sure has saved us vet bills, and we thank you. Now, our problem—our cat is driving us crazy. During the day, she carries everything in her mouth downstairs—letters, photos, bills, even clothes in plastic bags. At night she carries it all upstairs again. Now her kitten has picked up the habit. My children are grown and gone, and here I am now picking up after *cats!*—*C.S.*

DEAR C.S.—Look at it this way—you have a very active, intelligent cat who needs to be busy during the day, and she has found herself an ideal activity for herself and her offspring. Personally, I would live with this feline's idiosyncrasy. She has found an outlet for some of her instinctual needs, and to try to block this would cause even more undesirable behavior. You could put a variety of her own toys in a box for her to pull and hide. It might be interesting to see if she takes them upstairs and downstairs, too.

DEAR DR. FOX—We would like your interpretation of our calico cat's evening antics. Nightly in her own privacy she will take one of her stuffed toys in her mouth and proceed to walk around with it—usually in a darkened room, making funny noises as though she were talking to her toy. It always amuses us, but we feel sure that there is some meaning for her behavior.—*O.M.*

DEAR O.M.—Cats will naturally do natural things in unnatural settings, like your cat calling to her kittens to come and get the "prey" she has caught for dinner. We often forget that our pets live unnaturally deprived lives, devoid of contact with their own species, with prey, and so on. The more we can compensate for such deficits, the less deprived our pets will be. Give her plenty of toys (as prey to kill and carry and as kittens to carry and protect). Also another cat for companionship is beneficial, but read up first about how to make such changes in your cat's life.

EVERYONE'S A CRITIC: HOW ANIMALS
REACT TO MUSIC AND TELEVISION

enjoying music (cats)

DEAR DR. FOX—When one of us starts to hum or sing, Littlebit, our calico cat, will rouse from a sound nap (even in another room), come to where we are, look at us as if she wants to join us, then start to meow.

We've had pet cats for thirty years but never experienced anything like this. What is she trying to tell us?—E.M.D.

DEAR E.M.D.—I've heard before of such a reaction in cats whenever they hear their owners whistle, hum, sing, or play certain musical instruments. But when I play my shakhuachi—a Japanese flute—my dog howls in harmony while my cats do the opposite; they run away, and I can't blame them. My interpretation is that cats enjoy the sound and will chorus in—much as when they congregate outdoors and "caterwaul" together. I believe that, like wolves howling together, cats caterwaul not only out of sexual rivalry but as a social activity. So enjoy your cat's opera. (Any other readers have similar experiences with singing pets and musical beasties?)

DEAR DR. FOX—I read in the Sunday paper that you would be interested in hearing from your readers anything about cats and music. Well, my cat is an avid Elvis Presley fan. Whenever I put his music on, whether it be his ballads, gospel, or rock songs, she will plop herself down right in front of my stereo, and lie there in a contented trance. I am positive that cats can and do relate to music—at least mine does.—M.S.

DEAR M.S.—It is surprising that your cat likes all of Elvis Presley's different styles, since animals generally tend to prefer gentle ballads or classical music to rock 'n' roll. Music appreciation is certainly not limited to human beings.

Both humans and animals get enjoyment and relaxation from music. I wonder if animals, like their owners, sometimes feel something spiritual as well. I like to entertain that notion when I play my flute and my wolf sings-howls with me.

DEAR DR. FOX—You recently mentioned a musical cat in your column. Well, our cat gets absolutely turned on by music—but only if someone sits down to the organ or piano to play. When my son plays piano, Pumpkin will come from anywhere in the house, jump on his shoulders, purr, and rub his nose all over my son's neck and head. It ends up with Philip cradling Pumpkin, the cat with his feet in the air, purring for all he's worth.—L.T.

DEAR L.T.—What a delightful story—"Pumpkin, the Piano Lover." Cats certainly have as many idioscyncrasies as people.

I received a letter from a reader whose cat repeatedly flushed the toilet, and another about a cat who waits patiently by the door for the mail to come through the mail slot and then runs away as though terrified.

The likes, dislikes, and quirks of cats adapted to the unnatural conditions of our homes (compared to their original desert origins) can give us added insights into their psyches and show us how they satisfy instinctual needs in a relatively bland and artificial world in which they live. Keep on playing for cat's sake—he obviously enjoys it immensely.

enjoying music (parakeets)

DEAR DR. FOX—Have you ever heard of a parakeet who loves country-and-western music? Well, now you have. My Larry loves it so much that if I put on anything else, he fusses like crazy. His vocabulary also contains more than 2,000 words and increases every day. He can hold a conversation with you. People don't believe me until they meet him. Have you ever heard of such behavior?—B.R.W.

DEAR B.R.W.—It sounds as if you have a wonderful bird. Isn't it remarkable how attuned parakeets can become to us? I wish more people would realize just what wonderful companions they do make, and how easy they are to care for.

Birds are animals, and like cats and dogs they can suffer and show affection and playfulness. So let's support animal rights—including birds—and help everyone learn to respect all creatures, be they feathered or furry.

enjoying music (pigeons)

DEAR DR. FOX—We had a pet pigeon named Molly who loved music. If I just began playing the piano, in seconds she was at the door. Then in summer, she would come in and sit on my shoulder. She loved to run her bill around my ear (very gently) and coo softly all the time. Sometimes she would land on the floor, puff out her chest, spread her tailfeathers, and do sort of a running strut as though dancing to the music. Is this unusual?—E.S.

DEAR E.S.—No, dogs, cats, birds, deer, and a host of other animals, wild and tame, are known to enjoy music. Musicians playing in the wilds have attracted, to their surprise, deer, lizards, foxes, and various birds. Birds sometimes seem to respond or sing in chorus, and dolphins are certainly attracted to musical sounds broadcast underwater. Orpheus tamed the beasts with his harp, and, of course, Pan played his pipes for all creatures. Even in today's satanic factory farms, confined pigs and cattle have Muzac piped in to soothe them. In my book *The Soul of the Wolf* I theorize that we can have communion with animals; certainly, as you confirm, music is one very potent way.

excited by whistle (cats)

DEAR DR. FOX—I believe I have a unique cat. If I sit in my chair at night and whistle a tune, she becomes very excited, jumps up on the chair, and bites my arm quite hard. Sometimes she cries while she is biting. Could this whistling be affecting her hearing, or annoying her in some other way?—J.K.

DEAR J.K.—Your cat is unusual but not unique. I've heard of other cats who get very excited when their owners whistle. Several years ago, behavior researchers in France found that cats are "turned on" by certain tones—one tone in particular even arousing them sexually. There may be something in your whistling, some particular note or tonal quality that is acting as a trigger or release for your cat to be aroused and perhaps confused, because he ought not to act aggressively or sexually toward you. Your whistling could contain elements of a cat's specific call to mate or to come out and fight.

DEAR DR. FOX—Every cat I have ever had has climbed up in my lap and rubbed its face around mine, purring loudly, when I whistle. One in particular would come from anywhere in the house, even if she were sound asleep! They seem to enjoy a melody, and the higher the pitch the better. I thought this might interest you.—J.L.A.

DEAR J.L.A.—You may have trained your cat to come for food when you whistle, and now she comes any time you whistle. Being attracted to human whistling without any such food reward is a curious behavioral phenomenon. It may be related to the birdlike "trill" call that cats give as a social signal to their own kind.

Since so many people say their cats respond positively to whistling and music, we might be on the threshold of creating entertaining music for our pets to make their bland lives indoors more stimulating.

DEAR DR. FOX—Whenever someone whistles, my cat will perk her ears up and waken if she's asleep. She then looks frantically around and starts to meow low in her throat. If the whistling is continued long enough, she becomes violent and aggressive, and she's usually a very docile animal. Why this strange response? —*A.H.*

DEAR A.H.—Cats, like dogs, can often be conditioned to respond to sounds, such as whistling, and learn to come when called. Many cats enjoy the sound of whistling. The bizarre reactions of your cat most likely are a result of some negative situation which contaminates the conditioned approach of your cat to your whistling. For example, your cat could have been accidentally trodden on when someone was whistling. Or, it's possible that a sound frequency is setting up a negative reaction. Some cats do find certain pitches distressing. Have your cat's ears checked to be sure there is no physical reason for her unusual behavior, and in the interim, don't whistle.

interest in television (dogs)

DEAR DR. FOX—I am thirteen and I would like to know if dogs can see in the dark. Also, can they see colors? Can they see TV clearly? I thought that since their eyes are different from human eyes, they can't see those things.—*M.S.*

DEAR M.S.—Good thoughtful questions. Dogs are colorblind, but they are extremely quick to detect anything moving. They see well in the dark, but not so

---

A NEW BREED OF CRITIC

Some time ago I asked readers to write in describing their pets' reactions to watching television. The responses have been fascinating.

From the examples sent in, it seems that dogs are more responsive than cats. One cat watches only animal shows, and a particular Siamese "chases" football players. One poodle bites at the screen when there's a pet-food commercial to get at the animals. A mutt named Brownie enjoys watching *Boomer*, although his favorite stars are Sha-Na-Na; Brownie gets very agitated, however, when actors fight. Willie the dog runs to the TV when he hears any commercial that has music, cocks his head, barks, and howls. Another dog has to be put out of the room since she growls so much when a particular local newscaster appears on the screen.

I have an idea—why not have cable TV programs especially for pets? That way the set could be on while the owners are out at work, and the pet's life would be enriched and less lonely.

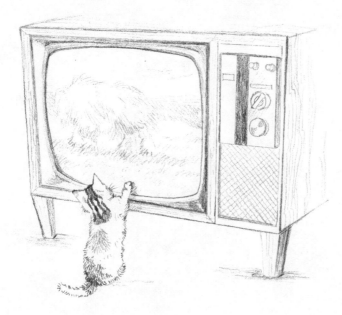

well as cats, and they cannot see in total darkness. But they still do very well at night because of their keen senses of hearing and smell.

Dogs can see TV, but most are sensible enough to show little interest in the general run of shows and few ever become TV addicts. Some dogs like to watch certain programs (possibly mimicking their owners), and others show fleeting interest in shows with animal sounds. But then, like people, dogs are individuals and there can be exceptions. Let's hear from readers about how TV affects their pets—other than keeping cats warm who sleep on top of the set. We'll publish the answers.

whining or howling during music (dogs)

DEAR DR. FOX—I love my Labrador-shepherd, but I have one problem. If music is on the radio or TV, he whines like a baby. The veterinarian told me the dog has sensitive ears. What am I supposed to do? I like to listen to music, and so many commercials have music in them. Any suggestions?—R.D.

DEAR R.D.—Your dog may have hypersensitive ears, and high-frequency radio waves distress him. But that should not cause any permanent damage. From the tone of your letter, I get the impressioin that he's a much-loved and possibly overindulged dog.

Does he whine when music or TV is playing if you're not in the room? He just may be wanting your undivided attention. If that's the cure, some discipline is in order. Also, leave the radio or TV on while you are doing chores around the house, so that he gets habituated. A last resort would be to put some cotton-wool plugs in his ears, or teach him to sing along, since some whining is not a sign of distress but a preliminary to having a good howl.

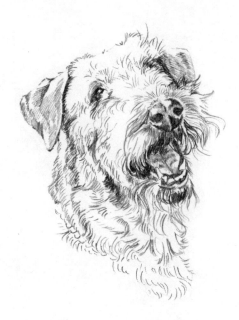

DEAR DR. FOX—Whenever our dog, Shadow, hears high-pitched notes from a harmonica or an alto saxophone, he starts howling. I was under the impression from a recent letter in your column that these sounds didn't hurt dogs' ears, but a teacher at school says they do.—*D.R.W.*

DEAR D.R.W.—Your teacher may be thinking of high-frequency sounds, which can, indeed, be irritating to animals (and people). In fact, any intense, high-pitched, or ultrasonic note will actually drive animals away. But it is unusual for a musical instrument such as a saxophone or harmonica to reach sufficient intensity to hurt a dog's ears; if it did, few people could stand the music. A dog is not likely to howl when his ears hurt. Your dog's howling is a social response to certain musical sounds—much like a wolf howling across the hills in response to a companion.

12

They're Trying to Tell You Something

VERBAL COMMUNICATION

animal sounds (incorporated in music)

DEAR DR. FOX—Recently, I heard about a musician who imitates animal sounds and can communicate with whales, wolves, and other creatures. Is this really so—or fake?—S.R.

DEAR S.R.—Really so! But the musician in question does not claim to communicate with whales and wolves, but rather he incorporates their sounds into some of his group's compositions. His name is Paul Winter and his Consort group has performed to a full house at New York's Carnegie Hall.

His music is undoubtedly most original and inspiring and is attracting a large following, especially among nature lovers and those concerned with conservation. His latest album is called *Misa Gaia*. For more information write to Paul Winter's Living Music Foundation, Box 72, Litchfield, CT 06759.

barking and howling (dogs)

DEAR DR. FOX—What are some of the reasons a dog barks? Is it inhumane to keep a dog outdoors all day and let it bark? Isn't this considered noise pollution? With so many dogs in the neighborhood, what can be done to stop this nuisance?—M.S.

DEAR M.S.—Wild dogs keep silent in order to catch their prey, but domestication has changed the dog's natural vocal behavior. Dogs bark for many reasons: out of sheer excitement, for attention, to let other dogs know where they are, to challenge intruders. It's not inhumane as much as socially irresponsible to leave a dog outdoors barking constantly. Dogs can be trained not to bark incessantly. Many municipalities have ordinances regulating noise pollution. So have a word with your neighbors, and if they won't cooperate, call your local authorities. Of course, some people are hypersensitive about the slightest noise, and that's just too bad. But I regard any dog that persists in yapping for fifteen minutes at a stretch to be a public nuisance. The dog's owners should be notified to correct the problem.

DEAR DR. FOX—At what age does a puppy start to bark? I bought an eight-week-old Boston terrier, and the first few nights he gave one small bark but since then not a sound. He's fine in all other ways. Do some dogs never bark?—R.W.A.

DEAR R.W.A.—All dogs can bark except the African basenji, which can make a variety of other sounds. Many pups have a quiet adolescence during which they rarely bark, but as they reach maturity, barks may "pop out" when they feel a challenge (as by someone knocking on the door and invading their territory).

I've actually seen young pooches around four to five weeks of age act startled after they have barked—as though they were surprised at what they could do. You can try barking yourself—this could set your dog off soon. Animal behaviorists call this "social facilitation."

DEAR DR. FOX—When my German shepherd wants something, she barks like a little puppy, but if she hears something at night, she barks like a fully mature dog. I don't understand it.—J.L.B.

DEAR J.L.B.—You have made an excellent observation. Not all pet owners take the time or make the effort to notice how their pets try to communicate with their body-language signals and variable vocal repertoire. Getting to know this language can be both rewarding and fascinating.

Your dog will act more like a puppy when she is feeling playful or is soliciting your affection or indulgence with her favorite food. People, too, will whine and sometimes act childishly in certain contexts, and then behave maturely, as your dog does, at other times—for instance, when she barks like an adult to scare off would-be intruders at night.

DEAR DR. FOX—Our two-year-old Labrador-?-mix is beautiful, shiny black, and lovable, but she very rarely barks. We have no way of knowing when she wants to go out or come in, or whether she's hungry or not. We've managed by anticipating these things, but is there any way we could train her to make her needs known?—A.Z.C.

DEAR A.Z.C.—Not all dogs communicate their wants by barking. I wish my own pooch didn't bark so much! What you must do is reward your dog for barking. (That's a switch!) One technique is to get your dog to mimic you as you look out the door or window and bark at a passing stranger or dog. (Never mind what the neighbors think—don't they act crazy sometimes?) Your dog's interpretation of your behavior will be that you are vocally defending your territory, and she will probably imitate you. The other technique is to teach your dog to say "woof" before she gets a treat. However, you should really be counting your blessings —you have a sweet dog who wouldn't say "woof" to a wolf.

DEAR DR. FOX—Can you help me? My grandmother has a one-year-old Boston terrier who is smart in every way but one: when the doorbell rings, she runs to the door but never barks. She does bark, however, when she's outside with other dogs!—*DISAPPOINTED*

DEAR DISAPPOINTED—While some dogs need to be trained not to bark, others need to be trained *to* bark. Your grandmother's dog is still young and perhaps not mature enough to be motivated to defend her territory by barking. Intimidation may help, either by someone barking and growling on the other side of the door when they ring the bell or even your grandmother barking and encouraging her dog to bark when you or a friend ring the doorbell. It is surprising how well this kind of training works. Give it a try.

crowing (roosters)

DEAR DR. FOX—Is there any way to stop a rooster from crowing, other than surgically caponizing him? This fellow's cock-a-doodle-doo is driving me crazy.—*MRS. B.*

DEAR MRS. B.—The best way to stop a rooster from crowing is to change his sex by giving him a hormonal implant. This is safer than surgically caponizing him. A veterinarian can give the implant, and within a few weeks you should see a marked change in the rooster's behavior, provided the implant is releasing sufficient female sex hormones.

discouraging barking and howling (dogs)

DEAR DR. FOX—My five-year-old schnauzer barks loudly and fiercely, and it takes a long time to shut him up when company visits. But I found a squeaky toy that shuts him up immediately. I don't use it much because it makes him so meek. Should I use it? Will it make him too scared? I don't want to change his whole personality, because I really love this dog.—*MRS. J.K.*

DEAR MRS. J.K.—It seems as though you have found your own remedy. A squeaky toy will not cause any damage to your dog's ears, but it is sufficiently intense to make him shut up.

If, over time, he grows accustomed to it, you can condition him by squirting water at him from a plant-spray bottle. Most dogs detest this. Two seconds before you squirt him, squeak the toy. This way he will associate the squeak with an

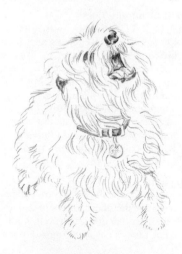

unpleasant squirt of water, and after a few sessions a squeak alone will shut him up.

discouraging whistling (cockatiels)

DEAR DR. FOX—My cockatiel is a darling, but he doesn't want ever to leave me, even to eat. He sits on me by the hour. He won't eat sunflower seed at all, but must have a sample of everything I eat or drink—even my highball. The biggest problem is his whistle. He starts in at 6:30 A.M. I'm afraid my neighbors will gripe. Is there any way to break him of whistling?—G.A.

DEAR G.A.—Your cockatiel is imprinted onto you, and it looks like he will only be happy if you are in his cage with him. Go easy on sharing your food and highballs with him. Get him a gymnasium-type perch to sit, climb, and play on, and a light chain to go on one leg. Then he will be safe to take outdoors on your shoulder, too.

As for his whistling, I would buy a radio-clock that goes on around the time he starts to whistle. It will act as a sound screen and should help your neighbors sleep. A low radio plus screeching whistles is less obnoxious than sudden whistles out of a silent void. As you know, I'm against people owning wild "exotic" pets such as cockatiels unless they've been bred in captivity, since the exotic pet trade is decimating wildlife population. A cage mate might quiet him down if he's not too imprinted upon you to accept one.

growling (dogs)

DEAR DR. FOX—My seventeen-month-old male rottweiler has been an aggressive puppy from birth and has "talked" (low and medium growling) since he was eight weeks old. I am concerned that the angry talking when a stranger extends his hand to pet the dog will someday go a step further—and result in a bite. Can you give me any insight or suggestions regarding the "talking" described above?—N.H.H.

DEAR N.H.H.—There are different kinds of growls: one while greeting (dog's body language is friendly), while being petted (dog is relaxed), or when meeting a stranger (dog is tense, tail not wagging). If your dog fits the latter, look out. Obedience training is a good idea, either way.

growling at phantoms (dogs)

DEAR DR. FOX—I was awakened one night by the growling of my dog, and found I was involved in a seance (contact with a spirit). I won't elaborate on this, but I might add that dogs are like babies; you don't deceive them. I've had other dogs who, when apparently looking at nothing, started growling. A dog like this might be branded neurotic, but I don't believe so.—B.P.

DEAR B.P.—Thank you for your letter. No, your experience is not unique. There are many cases of cats, dogs, and horses responding with obvious fear when near some "haunted" spot or when apparently face-to-face with some invisible force or phantom, which humans present may also see. A pediatrician friend in Kentucky had a poltergeist in his home for years who was on friendly terms with his dogs.

meowing (cats)

DEAR DR. FOX—My cat will be sixteen years old next month. He has had an irregular heartbeat for about a year now and finds it hard to get up steps, but otherwise he's doing very well. Four months ago he started meowing quite loudly a few times a day for no apparent reason. Do you have any explanation?—E.C.

DEAR E.C.—Your cat may be in pain, psychologically distressed, or in need of attention. When he meows, see if extra tender loving care will quiet him for longer periods. He may just want to be stroked or let outdoors or taken to his litter tray. If all your attentions fail, you may have to see a vet.

purring (cats)

DEAR DR. FOX—What makes my cat purr? I asked my mom, and she said to write you.—B.C.

DEAR B.C.—Cats purr when they feel—or even anticipate—pleasure. Thus, they will purr when they approach something they like, see someone they like, are being petted, or when they are just downright contented. Purring is first associated with nursing. The kitten purrs while it is breathing in and out and momentarily stops between swallows. As a cat matures, purring becomes a signal of friendly approach.

What causes the purr? The cat sets up a resonant sound in its larynx or voice box, in such a manner that it can be maintained as it breathes in and out. I think purring is very relaxing for cats—a way of stroking each other with sound. However, some cats rarely, if ever, purr—and so far, there has been no satisfactory answer for that. But one thing you do know—you have a contented cat.

CONVERSING WITH YOUR CAT

Who says cats don't talk? Although normally they "speak" with body language, we all have heard the cat's purr of contentment and hiss of anger. Also, cats will purr or meow if they're outside and want to be let in. A cat owner gets to be able to distinguish his or her cat's voice from others.

Tonal qualities vary from cat to cat; so does the degree of conversation. Siamese are very talkative, so much so that their owners often complain. If your cat is normally quiet, talk to it repeatedly, and you may get it to answer.

DEAR DR. FOX—During its first two months our kitten always purred. But in the last half-year we noticed that he doesn't purr any more. He's healthy, curious, and otherwise normal. What could be wrong? I notice my kitten's mother meows quietly. Any connection?—A.S.

DEAR A.S.—Some cats, like yours, simply quit purring altogether for no apparent reason, and others never purr. It's an idiosyncracy. Interestingly, though, some cats that live with a more dominant cat will let the leader do all the meowing and purring. Perhaps in this case mama cat is boss. However, I know of some cats who purr nearly all the time, but the sound is so faint that it can hardly be heard. The purring is revealed by attaching microphones to their collars. Try feeling your cat's throat when she's being petted. You may be able to feel a purr, but not hear it. And if you feel nothing, don't worry. Your cat isn't abnormal, isn't suffering, and isn't doing it on "purr-pose."

DEAR DR. FOX—My sister has a part-Persian cat who does not meow—except if you step on her paw. Previously, she had a male Persian that would meow when he was hungry and also when he wanted to go out. Does purring have anything to do with the cat's gender?—*S.F.*

DEAR S.F.—Nice try, but you're way off the mark in your guesswork. Some cats, regardless of sex, hardly ever meow (or purr), while others, notably Siamese, are very talkative. My interpretation is that some cats are simply more outgoing and vocal than others—noisy extroverts—not unlike some people I know. Also, there are many cats who are ambiverts and meow when they please. Our pets are more like people than we dare think.

purring (dogs)

DEAR DR. FOX—As I was massaging the back of my sister's Kerry blue terriers, the dog made a sound that resembled a definite purr. I mentioned it to my sister, and she laughed at me until she listened too. Can a dog make a contented sound that is similar to a cat's purr?—*E.R.*

DEAR E.R.—Funny, isn't it, what pet owners miss because they tend to take their animals for granted? I bet your sister's dog has made contented purrs before that weren't heard, because "dogs don't purr." We often perceive only what we expect. On the other hand, your sister may not have given the dog such pleasurable massage stimulation before. Either way, dogs do make grunts, low growls, and long purring-growls as signs of contentment. The purr is an indicator of the close evolutionary link between cats and dogs; supposedly, they have a common ancestry. Try my massage book for animals, *The Healing Touch*; it will give you many insights into something you have discovered yourself—that massage is good for man and beast alike!

purring (guinea pigs)

DEAR DR. FOX—We've noticed that occasionally our guinea pigs make a low rumbling sound. Is this a happy, sad, or angry sound?—*L.B.*

DEAR L.B.—Guinea pigs have a vocal repertoire of several sounds including clucks, squeaks, whistling tweets, staccato tut-tuts, and deep purrs. The purrs are probably the deep sounds that you noticed, and they are a friendly signal probably indicating a desire to maintain contact—to be petted or groomed, as the case may be. Try mimicking back some of these sounds. Or play them back on a tape recorder and see how your pets react.

rabbits' noises

DEAR DR. FOX—My rabbit is a fabulous pet. He can be walked on a leash, is trained to the litter box, and is always very well behaved. But I have never heard him make a single sound. Can you tell me why?—*RABBIT LOVER*

DEAR RABBIT LOVER—Yes, indeed, more and more people are beginning to realize (and many through my column, I'm glad to say) that rabbits are very intelligent, respond well to people, and can be trained—even to do tricks. As for your silent bunny, no cause to worry. The only sound I've heard rabbits make is a scream when they are in intense pain, as when caught in a cruel steel-jaw trap.

DEAR DR. FOX—In a recent column, you said that a rabbit can scream only when in pain. Our pet rabbit Flopsy makes grunting noises and nasal sounds when we play with her. She gets so excited at times, it seems she is talking to us. Flopsy also growls occasionally, and when we pet her, she makes soft little sounds like a meowing kitten.—*P.L.R.*

DEAR P.L.R.—Thanks for the additional insights about the rich vocal rabbit repertoire. The nasal grunting tones are not true vocal sounds—I was referring to vocal sounds only, the scream being the most common, and a grunting noise, almost like a bark, when alarmed or threatened. I've never heard of soft meowing sounds in rabbits.

DEAR DR. FOX—Take it from someone who has been associated with rabbits for years: they have a variety of voices. If they are kept in cages you rarely hear them, but if allowed house privileges (they are as easily house-trained as a cat), they have quite a repertoire. They can warn dogs away, ask for food, romp almost noisily with our small dog. Unfortunately, they have one unpleasant habit—they love to taste wood—any wood.—D.W.R.

DEAR D.W.R.—Thanks for sharing with us some further insights about rabbits. They certainly aren't dumb bunnies. The rabbit I owned as a kid used to make friendly or contented snuffling sounds and had a very clear bark, a sharp expiratory grunt, that was an alarm or threat signal. As a point of interest, rabbits are not rodents. They are classified as Lagomorpha. Try that on your friends some time.

singing (birds)

DEAR DR. FOX—I bought a ten-month-old crested canary in October. He was a singer, but for the last three or four weeks he hasn't sung a note. He is active—eats well, chirps, takes a bath. I even play a canary record to stimulate him, but he won't sing. What should I do?—R.P.A.

DEAR R.P.A.—When a bird stops singing, you should be on the lookout—it could be coming down with a disease. But not all changes in behavior mean your pet is off-color. Singing is influenced by internal hormones, sunlight (or lack of it), and social contact. A mirror might help provide the latter. And as spring returns, your bird should start to sing again, if there's nothing physically wrong with him. He could just be off-season rather than off-color.

squeaking (gerbils)

DEAR DR. FOX—I have five gerbils. Very often when they're grooming each other, they squeak. Does this mean they are happy or unhappy? Are they in pain?—N.Z.

DEAR N.Z.—I'm glad you are so observant of your gerbils' behavior. You might want to check my book *Understanding Your Pet* for more general information on gerbils—they are fascinating and have a rich repertoire of behavior patterns and communication signals. Yes, gerbils do like to groom each other (so do pet mice), so it's not right to keep them alone without companions. Their squeaks are most probably signals of pleasure and excitement and help maintain closeness, perhaps not unlike a cat's purring. Louder squeaks could mean "Ouch, that hurt" or "That's fun, let's play fight-or-chase," so you must now closely observe what happens when they make certain sounds and what follows just afterward.

"talking" (dogs)

DEAR DR. FOX—Our Scottish terrier "communicates" with us, not by barking or growling, but by making sounds like a Scotsman rolling his r's! "Hello" sounds like "herro"; "no" is "ro"; our daughter Laura is "Ra Ra." What do you think of that?—A.G.

DEAR A.G.—Some dogs do have greater vocal abilities than others, being able to produce specific howllike sounds for specific occasions, like "hello," "out" or growling gravelly noises, as your dog does. I'd be interested in hearing from other readers of "talking dogs"—and especially in receiving a good tape recording of any dog who is supposed to talk. I received one of a malemute that could clearly say "Oh my God" and make other human sounds, too.

talking (parakeets)

DEAR DR. FOX—During my early teen years I had canaries as pets, usually a male for his singing. My father bought a female because she cost only a few dollars, and we put them in separate cages. Soon the female began singing and we thought we had a bargain—a second male at a low cost. Not long afterward she laid two eggs. What we had was a female who sang beautifully!—B.N.B.

DEAR B.N.B.—It's always good to hear there are exceptions to the rules of life. I have heard from other owners of canaries whose females were able to sing. Usually singing is triggered by male sex hormones, but with selective breeding for singing ability, there may well be a genetic change in females as a consequence of human manipulation. Experimental treatment with hormones can make female birds sing like males. This means that female birds know how to sing but are not usually turned on, as males are, to perform.

DEAR DR. FOX—I breed parakeets for a hobby and have chosen one out of the clutch to tame for myself. I'm trying to teach it to talk by repeating the phrase "Hello, Bridgit." Would hearing the other parakeets in the house affect his learning to mimic the human voice? He hasn't had any contact with other birds for several months and is rather attached to me.—T.B.

DEAR T.B.—According to bird experts, the general rule to follow if you want a talking bird is to give the bird as much human contact as possible, so the books say, from as early an age as possible, and keep it out of sight and sound of other birds. Parenthetically, I think that is inhumane deprivation, and I see nothing wrong with allowing your bird some time each day with its own kind. A happy bird is more likely to talk. I know of a bird who was deprived of the company of parakeets and exposed to two dogs, who now prefers to bark rather than chirp or talk!

DEAR DR. FOX—I just received a parakeet as a present. I'm dying to start training it to talk. Any precautionary measures? I don't want to do the wrong thing.—L.V.

DEAR L.V.—Restrain yourself. Your bird needs to settle in before you can start training it. It needs, first of all, to lose its fear of you and get to trust you. You'll win it by gently talking to it and, after a few days, offering it food from your finger.

As you talk to it, gently scratch its head. After a few weeks go by, let it fly around the room. By that time, it'll be so close to you that you can start your vocal lessons.

DEAR DR. FOX—In a recent column, you suggested that owners of talking animals share their good fortunes. I am enclosing a list of sayings our parakeet, Midgie, delights us with: "ABCDEFGHIK" . . . "Happy birthday to you" . . . "Good morning to you" . . . "Midgie go bye bye" . . . "See you later, alligator" . . . "I love you" . . . "Bill's home" . . . "Midgie super bird" . . . "Hello, stinky pants" . . . "Dirty bird take a bath." —MRS. W.H.S.

(Note: This is only a sampling of Midgie's self-expression. Thirty other short sentences were included with Mrs. W.H.S.'s letter.)

DEAR MRS. W.H.S.—This must be an all-time record for a parakeet: more than thirty phrases. But people may ask if your bird just mimics what you say or if she is aware of what she says, using phrases appropriate for the context.

For instance, when Bill is home, does she spontaneously say "Bill's home"? One also could argue that it's simple conditioning. While we may never know what animals think, we can know how they feel, and your bird must feel happy and loved to be such a chatterbox.

BODY LANGUAGE

biting (cats)

DEAR DR. FOX—Why, without apparent reason, does my cat bite me on the legs or arms when I am sitting or walking beside her at home? She does not bite when I wear long sleeves or stockings.—*J.A.S.*

DEAR *J.A.S.*—Your cat is either giving you a playful feline "love bite" or using parts of your anatomy as substitute prey to stalk and pounce upon. The love bite is an affectionate play-soliciting gesture (which can sometimes hurt). I would advise you to get a ball of wool or strip of fur on the end of a long string that you can pull on the ground and swing over her to catch and kill.

All cats enjoy some outlet for their playful instincts—better a toy than your arms and legs. As for why she prefers your bare arms, do you like to kiss someone through a veil? One of my books, *Understanding Your Cat*, describes your cat's behavior in detail.

biting (parakeets)

DEAR DR. FOX—My parakeet is the cutest little bird; he is very active and talks all the time. Of late, however, he bites my fingernail polish. He seems to chew what he can chip off with his beak. Is this harmful to him? Also, when he is in his cage and people come over, he'll run to his mirror, flip it over him, and sit behind it. Is he scared, or what?—*J.R.T.*

DEAR *J.R.T.*—Give your parakeet a little box around one end of his perch (it could be of cardboard or plywood). He seems to want a safe "roosting" place. That's why he hides behind the mirror. When dry, fingernail polish is not very toxic, and if your bird is simply flicking it off and not swallowing it, then just accept the social preening graciously. He's showing you he likes you.

clinging and rubbing (cats)

DEAR DR. FOX—I have a new tabby kitten about six months old, and he seems to act like I'm his mother. He clings and nibbles on my neck. My family thinks the cat is "sexy," but I think he's just affectionate for his master.—*M.K.*

DEAR *M.K.*—Many people mistake a cat's intimate social behavior as being weird, if not perverse. Yes, cats will cling and even sit up and hold their front paws out to be picked up, just like a child. When they rub you with their bodies, especially with the sides of their bodies or the sides of their faces, they are actually anointing you with their own scent. This social anointing ritual leaves the cat's odor on you, and although the scent is too subtle for our noses to detect, it is obviously important to cats—akin perhaps to a "love mark." The clinging and nibbling is kittenish nursing behavior—a quite natural response since you are regarded as a parent figure.

ears laid back (rabbits)

DEAR DR. FOX—I recently bought a rabbit, because I heard they make such good pets. But sometimes Thumper lies low with his ears back and his eyes half-closed looking at me. What does that mean?—*C.L.*

DEAR C.L.—You are describing a friendly, submissive gesture. Your bunny likes you. On the other hand, if he should suddenly jump to face you and thump his hind foot, also grunting sharply, then he is being threatening. Rabbits, like all animals, communicate via body language. After some time, you'll recognize his signals.

fin movement (fish)

DEAR DR. FOX—Maybe this is a silly question, but do fish have emotions? Do they have any way of communicating?—A FISH-LOVER

DEAR FISH-LOVER—If you are really a fish-lover, you must be a fish-watcher. If so, observe carefully, and you will note that, yes, fish do have certain clear likes and dislikes. Some are bullies, some timid, and there is a pecking order among them. They will raise or lower their fins to express threats or submissiveness, and a few, when they become emotional, will change color the way we blanch or blush. The "kissing" of gouramis is a ritual form of combat, while a lowered head in some fish is a threat display.

licking (cats)

DEAR DR. FOX—My Siamese cat is very affectionate. When she's in my lap she wants to lick my hands and arms. Does she do this because she loves me, or is it, as my "catty" friend says, because "she has a craving for salt"? She gets a well-balanced diet, which includes salt.—MRS. A.C.

DEAR MRS. A.C.—Your "catty" friend is way off course (even though your salty arm might well taste very yummy). What your cat is doing is giving you the feline equivalent of a massage—a very relaxing superficial grooming. One cat will do this to another. It helps maintain a close bond and is a very clear expression of affection. Some people don't like it and try to discourage their cat from grooming them. Poor cat . . . Hence, in such cases I advise people to have two cats rather than one.

FELINE BODY LANGUAGE

To show affection, cats will often touch their foreheads to a human. They'll also rub up against their owners' legs when they want attention. If they don't get it, they may jump up onto a table or chair. Spitting is a cat signal. A cat will usually spit when it wants someone or something to stay away. Mother cats protect their babies from intruders this way. Watch out if the cat arches its back or its fur rises while it's spitting—that means attack is imminent!

Observe your cat's eye and ear signals for insight into its attitude toward what's taking place around him. If his ears point up and his eyes are at rest, he's probably just being watchful. If his ears are directed forward and his eyes open wide, then he may be on the warpath—warning another animal away from his territory. If the pupils are dilated and his ears are twisted backward, you will know he's afraid.

raised rear end (cats)

DEAR DR. FOX—I have a cat that keeps getting into this strange position. She puts her back legs up as high as she can and the front part of her body all the way down to the ground. It looks like she's stretching, but I know that's not it. What is she doing?—*T.H.*

DEAR *T.H.*—"Tail up, head down, rump high, shoulders low"—that is the way Kitty says, "I like you." This is one of the cat's basic body-language displays that I describe in full in my book *Understanding Your Cat*. Often, when being stroked, the cat will raise its hind end, and at other times it will bow low and rub its head or lip on the floor or against your hand. This is a friendly way of marking a companion with its scent, because cats do have scent glands on their heads. It's too bad that most people have no idea what their cats or dogs are saying. Neither cats nor dogs are "dumb" creatures; they can "talk" with their bodies and express their emotions and intentions very clearly. It's we who are dumb. But the fact that you asked about your cat shows that you are attuned to the possibility that she is trying to communicate something. Congratulations! And keep on observing.

"smiling" (dogs)

DEAR DR. FOX—Whenever I come home from a long trip, my dog, Scuffy, will come to greet me. At these times, he raises both sides of his lips like a smile. Is that common for a dog?—*C.K.*

DEAR *C.K.*—Dogs give two kinds of smiles or greeting-grins. The first is the typical canine grin, where both sides of the lips are pulled back. (Dogs with very pendulous lips have problems displaying this expression.) Then there's the mimic of the human grin, where the lips are retracted to expose the front teeth, and it almost looks as though the dog is snarling. I believe these expressions respectively reveal that dogs have emotions not unlike our own, and that they are very aware of our emotional expressions and can learn to mimic them somewhat.

sticking tongue out (dogs)

DEAR DR. FOX—Why does my dog stick his tongue out when he sees me? I know he's not being fresh, but I'm concerned.—*G.R.*

DEAR *G.R.*—Dogs will "extrude" their tongues toward a person or another dog as they approach as a sign of friendliness. It's not unlike blowing kisses. Then, when contact is made, they give friendly licks. Thus, the extruded tongue signals the information that the approaching animal has friendly intentions. However, when a dog sticks its tongue out and then curls it back toward the nose as though it were anxiously licking itself, beware. That is a signal that the dog is apprehensive and ambivalent. It's particularly common in so-called fear biters, who, if cornered, may turn and snap.

thumping (gerbils)

DEAR DR. FOX—I don't know the age of my gerbil, but I've already had him one year. Just lately his nose developed sores on it, and sometimes his left leg thumps. The pet shop can't help. Can you?—*T.M.*

DEAR *T.M.*—The thumping that gerbils do with one hind foot does make it seem as though they have a nervous disorder or perhaps some irritant on the foot that they're trying to dislodge. Actually, this behavior is a threat signal—a form of communication. Remember Thumper the rabbit? As for the sore nose, a small hole, sharp edge, or rough corner somewhere in the cage is the most likely cause of those "cage nose" sores. Some gerbils thump so violently, that they actually fall over. This is a form of epilepsy that's quite common in these rodents, as it is inherited.

wing spreading (birds)

DEAR DR. FOX—Whenever my husband goes near our canary's cage, the bird perches on a stick and spreads his wings as if he's ready to fight. Also, when my husband raises his finger, the bird follows its movements. For me, he only chirps, and when I talk to him he just stares.—MRS. W.

DEAR MRS. W.—Wing-spreading is a social display that some animal behaviorists interpret as a sign of submission. It may have overtones of courtship. It is surprising how birds do behave differently to owners of the opposite sex, but the difference may be due to your husband behaving in a different way from you rather than being attributable to the bird discriminating that you are a female and your husband is a male. Your husband might try mimicking how you interact with your bird and see if the bird changes its behavior accordingly.

MANIPULATIVE BEHAVIOR

barking and whining (dogs)

DEAR DR. FOX—My little poodle barks so much that our landlord wants to put us out of our apartment. I am seventy-seven years old, and he is my darling companion. How can I stop him from barking at every little thing?—E.B.

DEAR E.B.—Some poodles are very bright and can have their owners trained to do just what they want. I remember one that barked continually until her owner picked her up and petted her. Like you, the owner wondered why she barked so much, not realizing that picking her up actually rewarded her for barking. So check out what you do every time your dog barks. Perhaps you shouldn't give in to him, but ignore him. Other times he might well require some discipline, especially if he ever nips at you to get what he wants. One must sometimes be "cruel" to be kind, and as you have learned, being too kind can mean you finish up with a spoiled brat. Change his "cupboard-love" to respect and affection by being firm and letting him know what you want, for a change. It's a dog's life when you let a dog run your life.

DEAR DR. FOX—Our five-year-old dog is spoiled to the point where she barks for something to eat whenever we sit down at the table. Even when she has just been fed, she'll come up to our chairs and bark for a snack. How can we stop this?—E.O.B.

DEAR E.O.B.—By not feeding her from the table. You have obviously given in to your dog, and now your pooch has you trained to feed her from the table. Keep her out of the room until you have finished, or, conversely, hang in there and let her bark. After a few days of being totally ignored and being given no leftovers as soon as you finish eating (which will only encourage her to bark more) she should, if she has two grains of sense, stop barking. You are describing a frequent problem of pet owners who are too softhearted and gullible.

midnight disturbances (cats and dogs)

DEAR DR. FOX—Our cat is driving us crazy. Kit gets us up sometimes as often as three times a night, insisting on being fed. She meows unmercifully and jumps on things if we try to ignore her. We leave her dry food and water before we go to bed, but she still gets us up and insists on canned food. Sometimes she gets sick right after we feed her during the night. Our vet says she's fat and that we should decrease her portions. We've tried that, along with scolding, but to no avail. Help!—B.M.

DEAR B.M.—Your cat has you trained and twisted around her manipulative little tail. You must firmly reestablish who's boss and break your overindulged cat of her expectations. Lock Kit out of the bedroom. Give her moist food just before you go to bed. Such a change in routine will help break your cat's habitual expectations. Do not give in. If you get up and feed your cat after she has yelled and jumped in protest, you will only be again rewarding the behavior you deplore.

DEAR DR. FOX—My cat flips things—anything—books, magazines, newspapers. The problem is he does this around 4 A.M. and won't quit until I get up and feed him. Feeding is the only thing that will stop him. I haven't slept through a night in two years. Help!—S.C.

DEAR S.C.—It's quite common for cats to knock things over, walk heavily over their owners, and disturb their sleep. Unfortunately, you have rewarded your cat by feeding him.

You'll have to keep your cat out of the bedroom or simply starve him out and have a few sleepless nights until he stops disturbing you in your sleep and accepts, like any civilized cat should, having his breakfast at a normal time. I'm sure I don't need to remind you that clever cats can train their owners, and yours has you wrapped around his tail. I wish you luck.

DEAR DR. FOX—Our one-year-old miniature schnauzer refuses to go through the night without prancing around our bedroom until one of us is awakened out of a sound night's sleep to let him outside to relieve himself. How can we cure this insensitive canine? This dog was completely housebroken when he was a pup.—B.R.W.

DEAR B.R.W.—Your dog has trained you, clever little manipulator that he is. Take him out just before you retire and soon after you get up. When he starts acting up, shout "No" and give him a squirt in the face with a plant spray-mister. Hang in there for a few nights to break him of his willful expectations. If this fails, put him in the basement or in a holding cage when he starts to act up and wants out. This should soon break him of the disturbing habit that he has so artfully conned you into satisfying.

INTELLIGENCE

dreaming (dogs)

DEAR DR. FOX—Do dogs have nightmares? Sometimes while my dog is sleeping, she starts shaking and whining. I have heard tests performed on humans proving that a sudden wakening from a dream can be harmful. Is this also true of dogs, and am I damaging my dog in any way when I wake her?—E.S.

P.S. I am concerned over the rights of animals and would like to volunteer some service—time, not money. Which organization could use my help the most?

DEAR E.S.—Dogs *do* dream, at least insofar as they have brain-wave patterns virtually identical to those of humans when they dream. Judging from their behavior, like us, they certainly do seem to have nightmares. It's not advisable to wake your dog up in the middle of one. Let nature take its course. Some owners have been severely bitten while waking their dogs up from a deep, severe, or violent nightmare.

The rights of animals are receiving a great deal of media exposure of late. My recent book, *Returning to Eden*, explores animal rights and human responsibilities in depth. For more details on the question of animal rights and how *you* can help, write to The Humane Society of the United States, 2100 L St. N.W., Washington, D.C. 20037.

DEAR DR. FOX—Tommy, our puppy, whimpers, shakes, and makes queer noises in his sleep like he's having terrible nightmares. Will he outgrow this when he gets older? Is it harmful, and is there anything we can do to help him?—*E.C.*

DEAR E.C.—Your puppy is dreaming but not necessarily having nightmares. He could be dreaming of chasing another puppy or eating grass—or whatever. We have no way (as yet) of knowing what dogs dream, but research and studies show that they have dream stages similar to ours. Also, like people, puppies will "talk in their sleep" and whimper, whine, growl, make running movements, and jerk, and twitch. Just leave your dog alone and hope that he is having pleasant dreams.

dreaming (hamsters)

DEAR DR. FOX—I noticed recently that my teddy-bear hamster made loud noises in her sleep. She was also squirming. Could she be dreaming?—*L.L.*

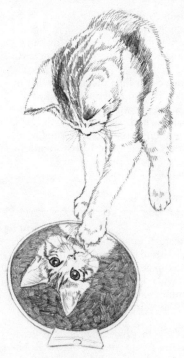

DEAR L.L.—Yes. Just like humans, hamsters have two sleep phases, one of quiet, dreamless sleep and the other of so-called activated or rapid-eye-movement (REM) sleep. During this latter phase, humans dream, twitch, roll their eyes, and sometimes talk in their sleep. We only know by inference that hamsters and other animals have dreams, since like us, when they are in REM sleep, they will twitch, roll their eyes, and make noises. So, similar to us, animals probably have an inner mental world.

kinship among animals

DEAR DR. FOX—I agree with what you say in your book *Between Animal and Man* that people shouldn't kill or mistreat animals for profit or enjoyment. But I must disagree with you about our "kinship" with animals. Humans are different because they have souls. Doesn't that make sense to you?—R.L.

DEAR R.L.—All creatures, including us, are part of the same creation. Those who contend that animals don't have souls conveniently separate themselves from being responsible and compassionate to the rest of creation. Such a belief, which I cannot support from an ecological and evolutionary perspective, can lead to irresponsible abuses and exploitation of animals.

DEAR DR. FOX—Why is it believed that only humans have souls and animals don't? I find this thought obnoxious.—G.R.

DEAR G.R.—Early Christian mystics believed that all creatures, including humans, have souls. Ecclesiastes stated that it was vain to think otherwise. Aristotle contended only humans have immortal souls, and this idea was later incorporated into Christianity. Such is human arrogance. I believe we and animals are all part of the same creation, and that we should treat animals humanely and respect the divinity within all.

memory (dogs)

DEAR DR. FOX—About a year ago we gave away our dog to a family who lives in another state. We plan to visit them this summer and are wondering if she will remember us—if not by appearance and sound of voice, perhaps by scent.— L.K.L.

DEAR L.K.L.—Chances are that your dog will go crazy when she sees you. Dogs do have long-term memory, especially for those whom they love. Be prepared, though, for a momentary initial reaction of indifference until the dog remembers your smell and the sound of your voice. Then look out; you may well be knocked over by your joyous pooch.

reasoned behavior (cats)

DEAR DR. FOX—In answer to your recent request to readers for a report on their feline's idiosyncrasies, here this: Our dear little calico-mix female cat (now four years old) discovered some time ago that she could hurry up her feeding time by pressing the bar attachment to the electric can opener. If the resultant buzz does not get proper attention the first time, she continues "buzzing" intermittently until successful!—A.F.

DEAR A.F.—This only goes to show where the word "copy-cat" comes from. Yes, cats are adept observational learners, which harks back to their wild nature. Kittens learn much from their mothers, especially through observation—how to hunt, kill certain prey, etc.

This destroys the myth that all animal behavior is instinctual and automatic.

Many animal species can reason. They have imagination and possess insight and intelligence, in spite of claims to the contrary by those people who contend that animals are unthinking machines.

reasoned behavior (dogs)

DEAR DR. FOX—Some people say that dogs only hear the tone of your voice, not the words spoken. If this is so, then how come, when you call your dog by his name, he comes, even from far away?—N.C.

DEAR N.C.—Some people think dogs and other animals are simple, mechanical things that respond unthinkingly and can't reason or think. This is rubbish—and another example of how people demean animals. Dogs respond to words just as you or I in terms of how the words are said, or the emotional tone of the conversation. They also respond to specific words that have symbolic meaning for them and us, such as their names and words like "out", "down," "leash," "ball," etc. Simple conditioning? So what! Most of what we do, like driving a car, is also based on simple conditioning. That dogs can discriminate different words means that they possess the power of reason.

reasoned behavior (parakeets)

DEAR DR. FOX—I must boast about my unbelievable parakeet, Daffodil! She is two years old, and we got her at age two weeks. She not only talks with human expressions, she seems to join into our conversations. She makes sentences from the words we teach her, such as, "Oh, hello, pretty baby girl," plays peekaboo with us and when we stop playing, says, "Come on, come on."

She even laughs at jokes before we do. Her favorite toys are two penguins—we really believe she thinks they are her babies. If we remove them from the cage, she panics. When she plays with the penguins, she'll corner one, holding it with both feet, and sit on the floor of the cage on her bottom, shaking back and forth. Is she special? A genius? Normal?—MRS. P.K.

DEAR MRS. P.K.—Your bird is special and intelligent. Having been raised with you from an early age, she is especially responsive to you and has learned to mimic your voice and play elaborate games. Without such a strong bond, your bird's talents wouldn't be revealed.

Many skeptics think such birds merely "parrot" their owners, but so often birds talk and act spontaneously and appropriately for special occasions that it implies a degree of awareness far beyond simple mechanical conditioning.

I believe birds, like other animals, are aware, and that they feel and often think (reason) much as we do. Though they can't express ideas in words, they can "tell us" without words just how they feel, and those that can mimic human speech often say the right thing at the right time.

How aware they are is part of the great mystery of life, which, as Albert Schweitzer urged, demands our respect and deep reverence.

unhappiness (dogs)

DEAR DR. FOX—Is it true that dogs cry? We had a little mixed-breed dog who wept real tears on occasion. In fact, she was so sensitive that we had to shield her from hurtful situations. (I think this must be a sign of extremely high intelligence.) She was crying for us in her cage at the humane society after we had spoken to her and then gone to look for an older dog. When we came back, we couldn't resist her tears. If she made a mistake on the carpet, we would find her

---

ANIMAL BULLETIN: PIGEONS TO THE RESCUE

This U.S. Coast Guard Search and Rescue Division has begun a program using trained pigeons riding in helicopters to spot people lost at sea. Their visual acuity is far superior to any pilot's.

Pigeons are first trained to peck a response key for food whenever they see an orange flag—the standard sea-rescue color of life jackets. Later, the bird will signal to the helicopter pilot whenever it detects an orange-colored object in the sea.

---

crying when we came home. On the day we moved, I closed her off in a room in the new house so she wouldn't bark at the moving men; an hour later I found tears on her face and also on the floor.—*E.S.*

DEAR E.S.—Some dogs seem to cry but, in fact, they have defective tear ducts that don't function properly, so the animal only *seems* to be crying. However, your report is not unique. I have heard of two others dogs that did shed tears suddenly and obviously when they were upset. Perhaps this behavior is learned by mimicking their owners, or perhaps some dogs have this capacity naturally? But so far, no studies of dog behavior—wild or domestic—have described such lachrymal behavior.

13

Making Adjustments

HELPING A PET ADAPT TO YOUR HOME

move to a new house (cats)

DEAR DR. FOX—Charlie, our five-year-old male cat, is staying at our vet's until we hear from you. We moved two miles away a few months ago, and Charlie wouldn't accept the new house. He keeps going back "home." The family that bought our house finally adopted him—since he had already adopted them. But now that he's scratching their new car, they want us to take him back. We've tried, but he walks around howling and sometimes disappears for days. Please help.—B.D.

DEAR B.D.—Some cats suffer considerable disorientation when moved to a new home. I would prescribe confinement in the new home for at least two weeks. Then take Charlie for walks on a leash and harness, and have your veterinarian prescribe a mild tranquilizer such as Valium for ten to fourteen days. Such medication has helped many cats through the difficult transition time that yours is facing.

DEAR DR. FOX—Recently I retired and am planning to move shortly. I have two cats. Would you recommend anything special to get them used to their new surroundings?—W.N.

DEAR W.N.—First, keep your cats indoors for at least ten days once you get into your new home. They are likely to get lost if they get outdoors. Try to arrange the furniture much the same way as it was laid out in your old home—in at least one room—and keep the cats there. Stick to regular routines of feeding, grooming, play, etc., and all should be well. Be sure your cats quickly learn where the litter tray is—being disoriented and anxious in a new home will cause a cat to become unhousebroken.

relocating pet with another family

DEAR DR. FOX—We have two cats—one eight years old, the other one year old. We're moving overseas next July, and my son is upset at leaving his pets behind. I know the older cat will have a difficult time adjusting to anyone new because of her disposition. I have considered putting her to sleep, because most people don't want an old cat. I can't bear the thought of bringing her to the shelter. Can you help me?—*J.L.*

DEAR J.L.—Don't jump the gun—some people may be most willing to take both cats. The one-year-old might be upset if separated from the older one. Advertise in your local newspaper and ask around the neighborhood. The people who may be buying your house may well want your pets.

Make every effort, for your son's sake as well as the cats', to avoid separating them and destroying the older one. Have you considered taking the cats with you? Some countries have no quarantine restrictions. If you can't find any solution, help your son with his tears by sharing his grief.

training to sleep in garage (dogs)

DEAR DR. FOX—We just bought an eleven-month-old Brittany spaniel, and we are trying to get him to sleep in the garage at night. But he cries and yelps so loud that our neighbor came over at 2:30 A.M., pleading with us to quiet the dog. So we let him sleep in the house, and he was fine after that. How can we train him to sleep in the garage? If we continue to let him in at night, won't it be hard to break the habit?—*J.L.*

DEAR J.L.—The first few nights with a new pup are usually difficult, and more so when neighbors are disturbed. Considering the circumstances, I would let the pup sleep indoors until he's settled down, and then after a couple of months put him in the garage with his *own* blanket, basket, and box or kennel. Leaving a radio on nearby may help. Advise your neighbors to bear with you for two or three nights because the dog will probably yelp and whine somewhat, but much less once he's settled into your family. Always feed him in the garage, too, so that he associates being in there with some reward.

INTRODUCING ANOTHER ANIMAL INTO THE FAMILY

mixing cats and dogs

DEAR DR. FOX—I have two fantastic cats, aged three and four. I now want to get a dog. What are the chances of them all getting along?—*A.D.*

DEAR A.D.—Your chances are pretty good if you don't get a fully grown dog. The cats will have difficulty adjusting to it, especially when it becomes excited and chases or even attacks them.

Generally, different species get along if they are raised together when young. But failing this ideal situation, you should make sure that the species you introduce is very young. I suggest you get a large-breed dog while it is still a puppy.

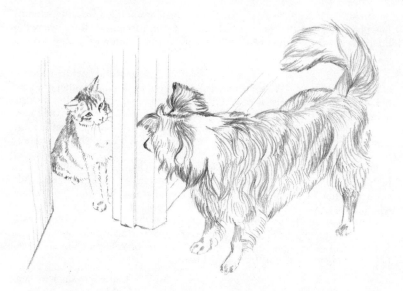

Your cats will discipline the puppy and teach it "manners," and as the puppy gets bigger (even ten times their size), they'll still be dominant overlords.

DEAR DR. FOX—Two years ago, I brought home a five-month-old female poodle and introduced her to my twelve-year-old male cat, and it was love at first sight. The cat now brings the poodle his catches, which I refuse to let either of them have. He also holds her down by the hair on her ears, so he can wash her face and neck. She seems to love the attention. Is this unusual?—M.S.

DEAR M.S.—I'm not surprised to hear about the happy "mixed marriage" between your cat and dog. It is remarkable how well cats and dogs communicate and take care of each other. Your pets are showing you how animals enjoy each other's company. That's why I'm in favor of people keeping not just one pet, but a pair. Such pets are generally healthier and happier and, as a rule, cope better when left alone for any length of time.

DEAR DR. FOX—Scooby, our nine-year-old dog, is getting used to my neighbor's cats. So I'm wondering if it would be all right to get a kitten. Do you think our dog would get along with it?—J.A.

DEAR J.A.—I can understand your wanting a kitten, too. And it's fun to have a two-pet menagerie. But you do have to take some careful steps. First, remember that a small creature like a kitten could mean prey to some dogs, so have your dog held safely on a leash when you make first introductions. Be especially alert to those times when kitty runs, as running can release the prey-chasing response in Scooby. If you see that he looks ready to chase, don't hesitate with some corrective discipline. Also be sure at the same time to give your dog extra love and attention, because the other serious problem that can loom is jealousy or sibling rivalry. Kitty may hiss and claw until she settles down, but if both are handled right from the start, they could be friends for life.

neighborly love (dogs)

DEAR DR. FOX—I have an eight-year-old, fourteen-pound Bichon Frise, and now that my neighbor has acquired an adorable Chihuahua, we would like them to be friends, but don't know how to go about it. My dog is a little on the rough and sexy side, while her dog is trying to be brave, but isn't. Any suggestions?—*G.S.*

DEAR G.S.—I appreciate your warmhearted idea of getting your dog together with your neighbor's, but be warned: although Chihuahuas might not appear so, they are not only very brave, but assertive, and because they're so small, they can get into trouble with a larger, rougher dog.

You and your neighbor should arrange to meet on neutral territory, such as a park, with both dogs leashed. Let the animals meet, sniff, and go through the usual canine rituals. After three or four meetings like this, chances are they will become friends. But there should be at least six meetings on neutral territory before putting them together on the edge of your property line. On home base, you may have less of a problem with your dog defending his territory when the neighbor's arrives and vice-versa. Keep the animals leashed just in case they scrap and have to be pulled apart. But don't hold them on the leash indoors, or you may confuse their territorial sense.

older animals with new companions (cats)

DEAR DR. FOX—We'd like to get a kitten companion for our four-year old cat, who is unable to have kittens of her own. Would she accept or reject it?—*B.Y.*

DEAR B.Y.—You just can't tell. But give it a try. First, get a kitten of the opposite sex, around ten weeks old, and have the two meet on neutral territory such as a friend's garage, backyard, or kitchen, where your resident cat won't feel her territory is being invaded. Let them investigate each other for a long time, and then take them home. Give the older cat plenty of extra attention so she doesn't feel jealous. Don't worry too much if she hisses now and then and runs off. She's just establishing who's who, and that often takes a few days. Unfamiliar smell can trigger aggression, so anointing both cats with a little of the same brand of perfume for two or three days may help.

DEAR DR. FOX—I have a twelve-year-old neutered Siamese who has been top cat since his step-brother died a year ago. Rama, who is Mr. Friendly with most cats and all people, hisses and arches his back and growls at my new, three-month-old kitten. The kitten is frightened but hisses and arches his back in return. The poor kitten wants to play, but Rama will have none of it. We have tried holding them, talking to Rama, and punishing him, but it does no good. Any suggestions?—*D.B.A.*

DEAR D.B.A.—You are experiencing what many cat owners know—the solitary side of a cat's nature. Some prefer to live alone after the death of a companion cat, and no amount of extra attention or discipline will help make the survivor accept a newcomer. But it's always worth a try.

Put a collar and leash on your Siamese and let him be with the kitten, even "attack" and dominate it. Use the leash to pull him away if he starts to bite hard. He may not. Very often a cat just wants to dominate rather than injure or kill its rival. Once it has established its dominance, peace and harmony will return. If he does actually attack, then little kitty needs another home.

DEAR DR. FOX—We've had two Siamese cats for more than five years. Recently a black Balboa cat joined our family. We had all the cats "fixed," but the younger Siamese has still not accepted the new cat and still hisses and hits at her. How long will it take? This war has lasted over four months.—R.B.F.

DEAR R.B.F.—It takes anywhere from one to two months for a new cat to settle into an established cat family, and sometimes it never settles in. Often the established cat family undergoes social stress and changes in relationship with old friends, even becoming enemies. I don't generally advise people to add more cats to an established family of two or more cats. More often than not, trouble ensues and things never settle down. Also, there is the risk of introducing disease; cats are walking virus factories. My advice is to find a good home for the newcomer as soon as you can. While I know of several large and happy cat families, your two Siamese have been together perhaps too long now for them both to accept a new cat in their midst.

older animals with new companions (dogs)

DEAR DR. FOX—I have been considering obtaining a companion dog for my two-and-a-half-year-old beagle-cocker. The problem is that she is so spoiled she's jealous if I even pay attention to another dog in the neighborhood. Would she ever accept another dog, or should I forget the whole idea? If I do get another dog, what type would be best?—M.S.

DEAR M.S.—Two dogs are often better than one, keeping each other company and healthy and active through games together, etc. Some grouchy and very jealous old pooches have been rejuvenated by a new puppy in the house. Others have their noses and tails really put out of joint and never seem to recover, going into a permanent state of jealousy, depression, or frustration, with snappy behavior and even neurotic overeating and house-messing. So if you can, try a new pup *on approval*, and see how things work out. Have the two meet first on neutral territory—a quiet side street or park—and give your older pooch plenty of extra attention. Then, let the pup "follow" you home. Chances are they will be friends for life.

DEAR DR. FOX—How can I get two male German shepherds to get along? Our five-year-old, who has been a watchdog for our business, will not tolerate the presence of our new one-year-old on the premises. When they tangle, there is bloodshed. I now keep them on opposite sides of the shop, but would love to see these two on good terms.—DOG LOVER

DEAR DOG LOVER—You have, unfortunately, broken two golden rules. The first is to get your dog between six and eight weeks of age, since this is the best age for it to become attached or socialized to you. Also, a pup is much more likely to be accepted by an old-timer than a new adult dog. Second rule: Be sure the new dog is the opposite sex from the one you already have. If these two rules are broken, then bloodshed from fights is the rule rather than the exception. Your solution—find a good home for one of them, ideally the new one. Chances are that even with discipline and you acting as boss, your two males will never make a truce.

DEAR DR. FOX—My husband and I have a great yen for a puppy, but we're concerned about our dog, aged thirteen. He has never gotten used to being around male dogs. Would it make sense for us to get a female puppy?—D.Mc

DEAR D.Mc.—From what you say, the chances are that your dog will be extremely jealous and distressed by a newcomer to his territory, regardless of its sex. The simplest answer is to wait until your old dog has gone on to doggie heaven before getting another dog. However, it sometimes happens that a youngster rejuvenates an old dog. I would suggest a trial run. Bring the pup of your choice home when it's about six weeks old. Be sure to give old Fido lots of extra attention. If he accepts the pup, then take the pup to the vet for a checkup and required shots when it's about eight weeks old.

outcast in a group (parakeets)

DEAR DR. FOX—We have four parakeets that all get along with each other. The fifth, however, bites and stays by herself. Sometimes she lies on the bottom of the cage. I am eleven years old and asked my mommy if I could take the birds to the animal doctor, but she says vets don't take care of birds. So I want to ask you— is my bird sick?—R.R.S.

DEAR R.R.S.—You have a pretty normal, social group of parakeets. These birds usually live in large flocks in Australia, their proper name being Australian grass parakeets. In almost any social group of captive animals, you find one member that's an outcast. In the wild it could escape and perhaps join another group. So I would give the outsider its own cage and perhaps put a male bird in the cage with her. This way you will liberate her from the social stress of being an outcast, and she will be able to perch, preen, feed, and drink whenever she likes.

By the way, there *are* veterinarians who examine and treat birds. If the vet you call doesn't he or she should be able to recommend one who does.

raising natural predators and prey together (dogs and rabbits)

DEAR DR. FOX—Cocoa, our two-and-a-half-year-old Netherland dwarf rabbit, is wonderfully housebroken and has been our family pet all her life. Now we're contemplating buying a puppy, preferably a husky or a wolf hybrid. We know Cocoa is afraid of dogs, even of their scent. What do you see as an outcome? Possible or not?—L.A.S.

DEAR L.A.S.—Several studies have been done on the question of raising natural predators and prey together, such as dogs and rabbits, and cats and mice. Surprisingly, it can work. A puppy can be raised with a rabbit and disciplined when it plays too roughly (and the rabbit may discipline it, too).

The older rabbit should soon get used to the pup and lose its fear. But look out—as your rabbit learns to trust the dog at home, it may fall prey to the dog next door. You'll have to decide whether you want to take this risk.

BABIES AND ANIMALS

introducing pets to babies (cats and dogs)

DEAR DR. FOX—I am expecting my first baby in February. I have a five-year-old spayed tabby Persian and a two-year-old unaltered Maltese dog. Both animals get a lot of attention and love. How can I help the animals adjust to less attention, maybe before the baby comes?—K.D.

DEAR K.D.—You are obviously a sympathetic pet owner and a potentially great mother. Good luck with motherhood! Your pets will be curious, so let them

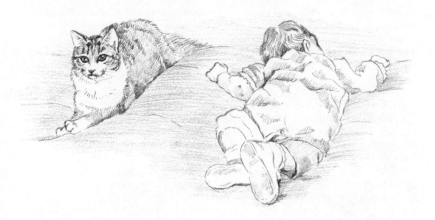

sniff and see the baby while you reassuringly talk to them. Never leave them with the baby while he or she is unattended. If you give them plenty of extra attention so they won't feel jealous and neglected, all should go well. The time to be protective of both baby and pets is when the child is crawling and grabbing on to things —otherwise one of them may get hurt. Many people forget that children can hurt animals, too.

keep leukemic cat at a distance

DEAR DR. FOX—We are expecting our first baby in a few weeks, and our cat Spooky is already sleeping in the crib. Even though I spank him and force him out, I find Spooky right back in the crib every morning. I'm afraid that when the baby comes, he will try to sleep with it. Also, Spooky has leukemia—is this a danger to our baby?—D.S.

DEAR D.S.—Who said cats are dumb animals? They like warm, soft places too. Keep the cat out by shutting the nursery door, or by putting a net over the crib. You can dangle baby toys from the net to entertain baby, too. Getting your child in and out will be no problem once you've become accustomed to the net.

While there's no evidence of a connection between feline and human leukemia, I would not allow Spooky to have any close contact with the infant.

preparing for baby's arrival (cats)

DEAR DR. FOX—A couple I know are expecting their first child. They now live in an apartment with more than ten cats. Couldn't this possibly be a danger to the new baby?—P.G.

DEAR P.G.—Ten cats in an apartment does sound like a houseful, doesn't it? However, if the cats are healthy, all should be well. I would have all the cats checked for toxoplasmosis and ringworm and put the baby's father in charge of cleaning out the litter boxes.

A net over the baby's crib to keep cats out is a good idea: Cats won't suck out a baby's breath—that's a myth—but some will play with a baby and might accidentally scratch it. If the cats ever get outdoors, I would also be concerned about them bringing in fleas that can bite the baby and produce welts—often confused with chicken pox.

puppies and babies

DEAR DR. FOX—We are expecting a baby and would like to get a Doberman pup before then. My husband is worried that the pup might hurt the baby. We are not going to train him to be an attack dog, just a family pet. What do you think?—*D. & B.*

DEAR D. & B.—I would be very leery about getting a puppy so close to the time when you expect to have your baby. Pups can be rough and sometimes jealous of babies. The ideal situation is to have a mature dog in the house before the first baby is born—a dog that is obedience-trained and that can be trusted and reasoned with. Another alternative is to defer getting a puppy until your child is four or five years old and can be instructed on how to handle the pup with gentleness and some understanding.

CHANGES IN ATTITUDES

different odor causes attack (cats)

DEAR DR. FOX—Our male cat always had full respect for our female cat, who was virtually queen of the household. When we had eight cats at home, none of them would even walk in her path, although any one of them could clearly demolish her. When we had her declawed and brought her back from the hosptial, the tomcat suddenly attacked her. We kept him outside for a few days, but when we reunited them they both hissed and howled. Do we have to get rid of him? What caused this unusual behavior?—*S.C.W.*

DEAR S.C.W.—It was the change in your female's odor that triggered the tomcat's attack—some smell that came back with her from the vet's or the surgery. Put a little perfume on a warm, moist sponge and wipe it all over both cats. After that, put them together and separate them only if they fight and make physical contact. Repeat the odor-anointing a few days later. If all this fails, keep the female in one room and the tomcat in an adjoining room. They will sniff each other under the door and get used to each other's odor again. Patience and understanding are your prime tools.

different odor causes attack (mice)

DEAR DR. FOX—I own two mice. When I went on vacation recently and left them with neighbors, one of the mice got out of the cage for a while. Since we got them together again, they've been fighting. What should I do?—*T.E.*

DEAR T.E.—Mice will fight when they don't know each other. When your mice were separated, the one out of the cage acquired a different odor. Smelling like another mouse, he was attacked when put back into the other's territory. (Cats are like that, too.)

To introduce a new mouse, put it into a small cage and then put the small cage inside the resident mouse's cage. That will protect the stranger until they get used to each other's odor. After five to seven days, the animals will be ready to interact freely. This is also a good technique for introducing a new cat into a cat's home.

incompatible mates (finches)

DEAR DR. FOX—My finches are having a bloody war with each other. I have two males and two females. One of the males was injuring the other so severely that I took him out and put a female in the cage with the injured male. They liked each other for about six months. Now the female is viciously picking at him. What's causing all this hatred for that one poor male bird?—D.C.

DEAR D.C.—While birds of a feather flock together, finches don't always pair off well when their marriages are arranged. Who knows—you may have selected the wrong female! When fighting breaks out, try to ascertain which is the trouble-maker, and then remove it from the cage. If the group doesn't settle down then, you must remove the "omega" or lowest-ranking victim. Some finches seem to prefer having their own cage, especially when the colony cage is too small—pro-vided, of course, they can see and hear each other. You must experiment and find which are "groupies," which make compatible pairs, and which, if any, really want to have a cage all to themselves. Any way you slice it, life in a cage isn't natural, so you are bound to have some problems with birds who don't adapt.

learning friendliness (parakeet)

DEAR DR. FOX—Our two-and-a-half-year-old parakeet, Sam, has always been standoffish, even though we talk to him, give him toys, and allow him to fly around the room. Since we got Bailey, a friendly basset hound, Sam has become very friendly. He's especially interested in Bailey, lands on her back, and "talks" to the dog, touching his beak to her nose. Do you have any explanation for this change in behavior? Our dog has just gotten over being in heat—could that have anything to do with it?—J.M.

DEAR J.M.—I think it's sheer coincidence that your bird became more friendly toward your dog during the time she was in heat—but who knows? We do know that parakeets are not sexually aroused much by odors, so it is unlikely that your Bailey's "heat aroma" had any effect on Sam. My interpretation is that with all the tender loving care he has been given, your bird has at last learned to trust his companions and relate to dogs and humans with affection, just as he would to his own kind. He may even try to "court" and "bill and coo" with you. In a good environment, parakeets will live for fifteen to twenty years, so enjoy!

love triangle (parakeets)

DEAR DR. FOX—We have three parakeets named Jaye (male), B.B. (fe-male), and Blue (female). Before we got Blue, Jaye and B.B. were really fond of each other. When we got Blue, Jaye got attached to her, B.B. became grouchy and selfish. Whenever Jaye or Blue would go to the tray to eat, B.B. would peck them away. And B.B. seems to think the whole perch is her territory. Is this nor-mal? What can or should I do?—K.O.

DEAR K.O.—You have a triangular situation of jealousy and emotional dis-tress from a broken relationship. What you saw and described is just as true for birds as it is for humans. You owe it to B.B. to get her a mate. Two's company; three's a crowd. Some people—scientists, theologians, and others—claim that animals don't have feelings and do not suffer emotionally as we do. Your very clear observations prove them quite wrong. I wish more people really "observed" and appreciated animals as you do.

struggle for dominance (cats)

DEAR DR. FOX—About four years ago, some people moved out of our neighborhood and left behind a sick tomcat. We took him to the vet, and he's now healthy and beautiful. Then we found a young kitten had joined our cat. It was so wild that we couldn't get within four feet of it. However, the tom accepted and bathed the kitten. The kitten is now four months old and tame, after much love and patience. But now the tom has changed. He hisses and growls whenever the kitten gets near him. What's the problem?—*N.B.T.*

DEAR N.B.T.—Isn't it wonderful how the old tom adopted the wild little kitten? He's more humane than those sick neighbors who abandoned him.

The kitten is maturing sexually and has become a social rival to your tom. Neutering the kitten may help, but there's no guarantee. Toms are often great with kittens, but they just don't get along well with adult cats. You could also consider neutering your big tomcat—he's less likely to want to roam, get injured in fights, and spray the house when he feels he needs to mark his territory. And he may then accept the other cat better. But face it—chances are you will have to find a home for the latter.

struggle for dominance (dogs)

DEAR DR. FOX—I own two Shih Tzu dogs. The oldest dog is cranky lately and can't stand for anyone to get close to him. He growls at the other dog and at my husband and me. My two dogs have grown up together, but now I'm afraid they'll start fighting and have to be separated. What could have brought this on, and what can we do to get him out of it?—*D.B.*

DEAR D.B.—Your young male is reaching the age when he is ready to assert his dominance and establish himself as the top dog of your household pack. Obedience training to establish yourself as leader may help. Having two males can be a problem if one refuses to submit to the other. Disciplinary intervention helps, but only if you are perceived as the leader. Neutering both males is your final solution.

MOURNING THE DEATH OF AN OWNER OR COMPANION ANIMAL

loss of companion (cats)

DEAR DR. FOX—I raised two kittens, brother and sister. They were inseparable; they romped together and curled up in one ball at night. At six months of age, one got out the door when my children were coming in and was killed by a car. Now the sister hardly eats and seems to have forgotten how to use the litter box. Will she get over her grief? How can I help?—*B.S.*

DEAR B.S.—Your tragic account demonstrates how affectionate and strong the social bond can be between two animals. The surviving cat is showing obvious signs of mourning and depression, although some people still insist animals don't really have emotions and that my interpretation is anthropomorphic.

Cats, dogs, and other animals are more similar to us in their emotional needs than they are different. There are cases of animals mourning the death of an owner, too—and even dying of heartbreak.

Give the survivor plenty of extra attention, and consider adopting a young cat of the opposite sex as soon as possible. Have your vet check out the new cat for any infectious diseases. Be sure the surviving cat also is vaccinated against the common feline viral diseases before you introduce her new companion.

loss of companion (dogs)

DEAR DR. FOX—We have five dogs, and one of them has heartworm. She is past help. She has a two-year-old pup that's been with her constantly since birth. We're worried about what will happen to this pup when the mother dies. Is there anything we can do to make it easier on the pup?—*K.T.*

DEAR K.T.—I respect your sensitivity and concern. Animals often do suffer emotionally from the loss of a companion, becoming withdrawn, depressed, and disinterested in food and in life in general. You will have to give the bereaved survivor extra love and attention. After two or three weeks, consider getting a companion pup.

It is surprising and heartening to see how a lonely pet will take renewed interest in life when given a new companion. But you must take care not to get the first pet jealous. With your sensitivity, I'm sure you will not err in judgment.

DEAR DR. FOX—A week ago our family had to put our twelve-year-old German shepherd to sleep. Since that time, our other dog, a fourteen-year-old mutt, has been listless and has hardly eaten. Is it possible for a dog to be depressed?—*M.G.*

DEAR M.G.—Yes, dogs, just like people, suffer from depression, and one of the most prevalent causes is the death of a companion. Very often, the survivor expires not too long after. An antidepressant drug such as thorazine may help your dog during the period of mourning, plus lots of extra attention, grooming, and walks outdoors. Your experience with your dog serves to remind us that animals can and do suffer emotional problems and that they are, in many ways, more similar to us than they are different.

Some religious fundamentalists have publicly criticized these views as being heretical, yet I consider it a heresy to contend that animals are unfeeling automatons created for our own amusement to exploit as we choose. For more insights, and an introduction to animal-rights philosophy, see my book *Returning to Eden: Animal Rights and Human Responsibilities.*

loss of master (dogs)

DEAR DR. FOX—My husband died of a stroke two months ago, and my boxer mourns him twenty-four hours a day. When I ask for his toy he brings it, lays it down at my feet, and goes off in a corner to lie alone. When he comes across something that has my husband's odor, he races through the house hunting him. My veterinarian suggests adding a puppy to the household, but I'm not sure that Beau would tolerate an intruder. Any suggestions?—*H.E.H.*

DEAR H.E.H.—You must simply be supportive of your dog while he goes through the heartbreak of mourning the loss of his beloved master. It would also help if you cleaned out all your husband's things, or at least stored them out of your dog's reach so the odor would not trigger the dog's sense of loss.

With older dogs, adding a new pup to the household can create more problems, and your animal doesn't also need to feel jealous or insecure. Try to stick to the routines your dog had while your husband was alive.

reaction to owner's grief (dogs)

DEAR DR. FOX—My dog whined the night before my dad passed away. The same thing happened the night my husband passed away. How do you explain this?—*M.N.*

DEAR M.N.—Dogs are extremely sensitive and observant and will easily detect any change in their owners' moods. When you feel and act sad, a dog who is attuned to you will whine and mope around. However, sometimes dogs will react to the death of a person (or animal) some distance away, before anyone in the house is even aware of the event—and sometimes at the precise moment of death. Indeed, enough cases of animals' psychic powers have been documented for experts to conclude that our pets are more psychically developed than we are.

14

Handling and Training

PROPER HANDLING TECHNIQUES

best age to start training (dogs)

DEAR DR. FOX—How old does my German shepherd have to be before I can start basic training? At what age should I have her spayed?—*MRS. L.K.E.*

DEAR MRS. L.K.E.—Any time after a pup is ten weeks old, you can start calling it by name to come and teaching it to sit and to follow properly on the leash. Consult your vet about spaying. Most vets like to do the operation when the pet is around six months old.

easily trained cats

DEAR DR. FOX—My cat, Omar, gets on my husband's lap and lets my husband brush him on one side. When my husband says "turn over," so he can brush the other side, Omar does. After that Omar gets a reward for being so good. Thought you'd enjoy this story.—*V.N.*

DEAR V.N.—Your cat clearly demonstrates how easily trained some cats are. Given the right understanding and respect, plus patience, cats can be trained to do a variety of tricks. In my massage book for cats and dogs, *The Healing Touch*, I describe how easy it is to make a pet lie on one side and then roll over for massage on the other side. One of my own cats, when it has had enough brushing or massage, rolls over to present the other side without my telling it. Then it'll roll over again for more.

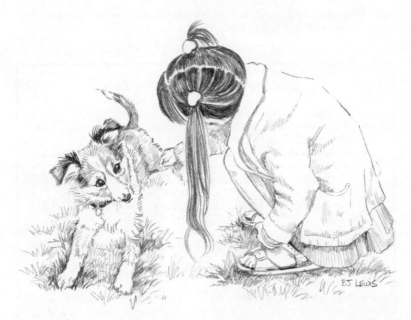

right way to handle (dogs)

DEAR DR. FOX—The other day I took my dog to a low-priced animal clinic to get her a parvo shot. I was struck by how bad the place smelled, even though it looked clean. But worse—while there, I observed a large dog being lifted by the skin on his back. The dog was crying in pain. When I questioned the vet, he assured me that this is the proper way to pick up a dog. I don't agree, do you?—*B.H.*

DEAR B.H.—First, animal hospitals often have strong odors because scared animals will occasionally evacuate their anal glands. Second, lifting a dog up without support under its chest and abdomen is wrong, You have every right to question the vet. Such treatment can so scare some animals that they will release their anal glands out of fear. Perhaps the vet was scared of the dog.

Large dogs often need two people to handle them and get them onto the examination table. Trying to do it alone is risky and may necessitate grabbing the animal's skin to lift it—but only in emergencies. What you saw may be the way to handle sacks of potatoes, but not dogs.

DEAR DR. FOX—My family and I own a two-year-old beagle. I have noticed ever since she was a pup that her front legs are bowed. I once read that picking up pups by their underarms can cause loose shoulders and bowed legs. Could this be the reason?—*J.B.*

DEAR J.B.—No, no, no! Don't blame yourself. Blame bad breeding that has resulted in your beagle having a basset hound's front legs. It's a common breed deformity in beagles. Even so, one should not pick a puppy up by its front legs, because this could cause injury or hurt the puppy momentarily and make it touch-shy. Pups should be "scooped up" with one arm around their legs and the other supporting their undercarriage. No pup should be picked up by its front legs, shoulder scruff, collar, or ears.

CHILDREN'S SAFETY REMINDER

Give this advice to your children on handling their pets.
- They must wash their hands after handling a dog, cat, or caged creature—especially before sitting down to a meal.
- Although they think they are comforting a young animal by taking it into bed with them, they are really running risks: (1) of making the pet too dependent; and (2) of the kitten or puppy falling out of the bed and hurting itself.
- Showing affection to an animal is necessary, but no kisses on the mouth, please!

Give this advice to your children, verbatim, on how to behave around a strange dog.
- If its owners are there, ask to be introduced, and then ask if it's OK to pet the dog.
- If the dog is off the leash or the owner isn't with it, don't show you're scared. Stand still; don't stare at the dog, but say quietly; "Hi, dog, good boy, nice to see you."
- If it approaches, don't run off. Stand still and let it sniff you. If you try to run off, it may chase and nip you.
- If you're out running (or jogging) and you see a dog, stop and talk to it, then walk or back away slowly. The dog isn't likely to chase you then.

DEAR DR. FOX—Eighteen months ago, I acquired a 125-pound rottweiler who'd spent his entire life in the kennel. He is timid but gentle. My teenaged son recently started to play with him.

He picks the dog up, puts him on the couch, and rubs his stomach. The dog remains rigid. My son will sometimes chew on Derek's cheek. Derek growls, and my son takes this as "play" noises, because our five other dogs react this way. The other night Derek nipped my son. As a result, my son needed sixty stitches in his upper lip. What do you think—should we keep Derek?—MRS. A.A.

DEAR MRS. A.A.—Some dogs simply cannot tolerate too much handling. They don't have a sense of humor. Your son should be aware of this, and you should be thankful the dog did not do more damage to him.

Your son was behaving with the best intentions in mind, but his actions were too much for the dog to take. Most dogs are not innately vicious, but they cannot tolerate too much stimulation.

Encourage your son to let the animal be himself and come over to people when he feels like it. Avoid getting the dog in situations where he might feel the need to defend himself.

right way to handle (guinea pigs)

DEAR DR. FOX—When I pick up my guinea pig, he runs to my chest and up to my neck. Then he bites my neck. Can you help me?—*T.P.*

DEAR T.P.—You must learn to handle your guinea pig correctly. Right now, what you're doing is stimulating your guinea pig to nuzzle and root onto your neck, so little wonder that he nips. Get him used to being in your lap or between your legs while you are sitting on the floor. He will enjoy being groomed, too, once he gets used to it. Sometimes guinea pigs nip when they get scared, so the more confident and competent you are about handling your pet, the happier it will be and the less likely to nip you.

right way to handle (parakeets)

DEAR DR. FOX—I recently purchased a blue parakeet, and he is a nipper! At first, I thought he was just upset at the big change from the pet shop to my home, but now I don't know. The worst time is when I let him out of the cage for exercise. It takes me an hour to get him back in, and I have to wear gloves to protect my fingers from his pecks. Any advice?—*K.K.*

DEAR K.K.—Some parakeets are difficult to handle because they haven't had much handling when young. This is a problem when you buy a fairly mature bird from a pet store. The older he is, the harder he will be to train and to get him to become attached to you—just like a puppy. You'll have to put in time and patience and at first handle the bird inside his cage. Let him perch on your hand and hand-feed him. He needs to get used to you. After a couple of weeks, let him out to exercise on a regular basis, but persevere with the in-cage handling.

right way to handle (rabbits)

DEAR DR. FOX—I give my rabbit the most wonderful care, but if I touch her, she scratches me. Why?—*SCRATCHED-UP*

DEAR SCRATCHED-UP—Bunny rabbits will scratch, especially with their hind feet, if they are frightened while being handled. I suggest that when you handle your bunny, you sit down so if the rabbit slips out of your arms, it won't fall and get hurt. Put on a thick jacket to protect your arms and just keep picking up the bunny and holding her as long as you can. Don't let her go until she remains quiet. Talk to her in a reassuring voice, and eventually she will become more tractable as she gets used to being held. Fear is difficult for all of us to overcome.

HANDLING AND TRAINING DEVICES

accustoming pet to collar and leash (dogs)

DEAR DR. FOX—We cannot keep a leash or even a flea collar on our thoroughbred sheltie. When we put so much as a string around her neck, she goes crazy trying to get it off. When she can't get it off, she will crawl into a corner and not move. We've never punished her in any way. Please help.—*D.E.B.*

DEAR D.E.B.—Your dog has a very obvious phobia reaction to contact around her neck. I suggest that you take her to your veterinarian, who will weigh her and prescribe a mild tranquilizer, or give her an injection with one. Once your dog has been given her Mickey Finn, put on the collar (not the flea collar) and keep it on. The tranquilizer should help in the desensitization process. Repeat the medication, then put a leash on the dog and let her get used to a little pressure while under the influence of the drug. If this fails, get a reliable dog trainer to work on your dog.

DEAR DR. FOX—I was recently given a darling five-year-old Lhasa apso who was never trained to a collar or leash. I've tried every way I know to get her to accept the leash, but have had no luck. Can you help?—J.P.

DEAR J.P.—Let your dog wear the leash and collar around the house so she gets used to it. Pick up the end of the leash occasionally and let the dog feel a little tension, then drop it. Keep repeating this process. When the dog is good and hungry, gently pull on the leash and coax her to feed from your hand. Repeat the process over several days and, holding the leash, just follow your dog around house and yard, going wherever she wants to go. Then call her to you with a gentle pull, and pet or feed her. She will gradually learn to associate pleasure with the leash and should allow you to make her follow you. This will give you both a new "leash" on life.

choke collars (dogs)

DEAR DR. FOX—Please use this true incident to alert your readers to the danger of using choke collars unwisely. My neighbor recently saw what seemed to be a slaughtered goat dangling from the back of an open truck. Then he realized it was a sheepdog caught by a choke collar and anchored leash. The dog had evidently been tossed free of the truck. His legs reached the pavement and were being scraped. My neighbor was able to signal the driver, and the two of them spent some time reviving the dog. The journey was resumed with the dog on the front seat.—M.A.O.

DEAR M.A.O—There are two morals to this tragic story. First, never travel in a pickup truck or a car with windows down, unless your dog is tethered or secure in a cage. I have seen dogs fall out of cars and tumble off trucks as the driver stops or turns suddenly. Second, there is no doubt that choke chains can be lethal, causing dogs to get hung up on fences, tree stumps, etc. Choke chains should be left permanently attached to the leash and should be on the dog *only* for training purposes and for control when out walking. A dog should *never* be tethered with a rope or chain attached to a choke chain.

shock collars (dogs)

DEAR DR. FOX—Where can I purchase a shock collar for my dog? And how do they work? Is there a good training book on this subject?—F.S.

DEAR F.S.—Shock collars that give the dog an electrical shock from a remote-control unit operated by the trainer should be outlawed! In inexperienced hands a dog can suffer, and in cruel or impatient hands, the dog could become a nervous wreck. Even in sensitive hands, some dogs will go crazy anyway. Such devices should be used only by qualified certified trainers and dog psychologists. Any book that recommends using shock collars should be burned.

using leashes and harnesses (cats)

DEAR DR. FOX—I know you recommend that cats be kept on a leash when outdoors. However, please pass along the warning to cat owners—to make sure that the leash is securely tied. My cat was too fast for me, and while I was untying her, she broke away, ran up the nearest tree, and came very close to hanging herself on a limb.—A CAT LOVER

DEAR CAT LOVER—I hope everyone will take note of your warning. I can also recommend using a harness for those cats who may get frightened by leashes.

The harness goes around the cat's chest and through its front legs. When properly fixed, the harness doesn't slip off and seems more comfortable than collars for some cats.

using leashes and harnesses (dogs)

DEAR DR. FOX—Our seven-year-old unneutered Cairn terrier pulls on his leash whenever he sees a loose bitch in our neighborhood. I try to pull him away, and often this chokes him. Can this cause permanent damage to his neck organs?—F.T.

DEAR F.T.—It is sensitive of you to write about this worry, and I'm surprised how rarely readers ask this. Yes, a sudden hard jerk on the leash, especially if the dog is wearing a choke chain instead of a collar, could cause damage to the neck vertebrae and larynx or voice box. Many dogs will pull until they are blue in the face and never harm themselves.

What one has to worry about is losing one's temper and snapping that leash too hard in order to make the dog obey. For a leash-puller, I would advise a choke chain. Then the dog is less likely to pull you off your feet.

using leashes and harnesses (monkeys)

DEAR DR. FOX—What is the best type of collar or harness to put on a small squirrel monkey? We've been told that these creatures have very frail necks and that regular collars were dangerous. This little fellow was about a year old when we got him, neglected, mistreated, and afraid of everyone. Now, he's so playful that we'd like to take him out with us—if we have the right kind of leash.—J.W.S.

DEAR J.W.S.—Your squirrel monkey would probably be most comfortable wearing a harness around his chest—a miniature version of what people put onto their children when they are learning to walk. Yes, the leash or reins attach to the back of the harness, but give your pet time to get used to the harness before you take him out. Chances are he will soon be trying to put the harness on himself—that's if he really enjoys going outdoors.

Personally, I don't like to see monkeys and other wild creatures being kept as pets. So, readers, don't rush out and buy a squirrel monkey even if they do look cute. Wild animals have the right to be wild and free and are healthier and happier in their own environment.

SPECIFIC BEHAVIOR PROBLEMS

barking and howling (dogs)

DEAR DR. FOX—Our dog has a loud, frequent bark. I want her to bark to warn me of impending danger, but once I have assured her that everything is all right, I would like her to stop. All my disciplinary methods have failed. Any suggestions?—M.G.T.

DEAR M.G.T.—Noisy dogs are a pain to live with. My own mutt, Benji, always seems to manage to bark right in my ear every day. The only solution is very consistent discipline. Basic obedience training—"come, sit, stay"—will give the dog a feeling that you are the pack leader and in control. Hyperactive dogs, especially, need such training. To control the bark, always give the verbal command *before* the punishment—a sharp "Shutup," followed with a snap of the choke chain, a rap under the chin, or a squirt in the face with a water pistol. Soon the dog will learn to respond to the verbal command and won't require punishment every time. Be consistent, and never let her get away with it. Reward her only after she has quieted down.

DEAR DR. FOX—We have a six-year-old cocker spaniel who is friendly, well-mannered, and healthy. The only problem is that he howls like a wolf. This is annoying to neighbors, to say the least, and bothers us too. Since we give our cocker spaniel lots of attention, time, and exercise, we're wondering if a female dog in heat in the neighborhood could be the cause of the problem.—S.L.

DEAR S.L.—Howling is part of a dog's natural repertoire of communication. Dogs howl when they are stimulated by some sound, like a police or ambulance siren or even another dog's howl. Dogs will also howl when they want to go out or when they are in love. Try to figure out why and when your dog howls. If it's caused by an outdoor noise, then you might try leaving a radio on inside as a sound barrier. If it's when he's lonely, perhaps you should get him a companion pooch. Two pets are often healthier and happier than one. Just pray that they won't start to howl together.

DEAR DR. FOX—For the past six months, our eight-year-old English pointer has been howling, whining, and barking almost incessantly. When we reprimand him, he quiets down for a few minutes and then starts again. I will add that he is on a run in our backyard, has a doghouse, and has never shown this kind of behavior before. Any light on the subject?—MRS. H.A.

DEAR MRS. H.A.—I appreciate that you wrote to me, but I find it hard to believe that you have simply lived for six months with a dog that has been "howling, whining, and barking almost incessantly."

He may well be in great pain. A veterinary examination is needed at once. Part of the dog's problem may be you. He may want some love and attention. Dogs howl, whine, and bark for a reason, and merely reprimanding the dog for bad behavior is ignorant, if not callous, indifference. I opt for the former in your case, and only wish that more pet owners would listen when their pets try to communicate.

DEAR DR. FOX—We own a large black dog that we love dearly. Our problem is his loud barking, and in our neighborhood the houses are close together. Before we go to work each day, we tie him on a long rope in our backyard. The police came by and told us that the dog barks every second we're away. If we don't tie him up, he will jump the fence. Help!—WORRIED

DEAR WORRIED—Your problem is a tough one. It may help to use a running line away from the fence, so your dog can move more freely. Dogs that are tied up generally tend to bark more. You could try some training: secure him in the yard as you do during the week, then walk off, come back when he barks, shout "No, quiet, boy" and throw a can of water at him. Many dogs soon learn not to bark with this simple water-training method. However, a companion dog may do the trick—your pet is probably lonely.

biting (horses)

DEAR DR. FOX—My pony is always trying to bite people—even when I mount him. Is there any way I can prevent him from doing this?—K.A.

DEAR K.A.—Some ponies are nasty biters. I would suggest this method of handling yours: Get a friend to help you. Then get a thick old glove or jacket sleeve and put some Tabasco on it. Have your friend let the pony bite the glove or sleeve. Hold the pony's reins and look out. (And for God's sake, don't sit on the pony, he may buck.)

Have a bucket of water on hand so he can cool off. Such aversive conditioning is worth a try and better than physical punishment, which many horse experts seem to endorse without seeking more humane alternatives.

digging holes (dogs)

DEAR DR. FOX—We were "gifted" with an adult Bouvier because we have property to accommodate a large dog, but we are now looking our gift dog in the mouth, so to speak. He *continually* digs *large* holes around the outside of the house. It is unsightly, to say the least, and takes at least a wheelbarrow full of dirt to fill each one. Help!—*MRS. J.A.G.*

DEAR MRS. J.A.G.—Hole-digging is a favorite game of many dogs, and my mail is full of letters like yours. Why do you think your dog digs? Is he bored? Is he making his own comfortable pit to lie in, especially in hot weather when there's no shade? Does he have toys—sticks, balls, bones, and the like to play with? He is telling you that he needs exercise and activity.

You could put down some chain-link or chicken-wire fence material and cover it with a few inches of soil. Your dog won't dig through this. The wire can be snipped in places to let trees and bushes come up. Some people also claim success with magic-store crackers. These let off a loud but harmless bang when they are subjected to pressure. Pop a couple of these in a freshly started hole, or throw one in hard as the dog is digging. Repeat as needed.

digging, urinating around plants (cats)

DEAR DR. FOX—We have two three-month-old kittens, one male, one female. The female digs in the larger floor plants, despite all our efforts to discourage her. Is there anything we can do to keep her out of the plants?—*M.C.*

DEAR M.C.—One solution is to buy yards of string and make macrame hangers for your plants—or simply repot them in hanging pots. Another solution that we have adopted in my home is to wedge some decorative rocks in the pots. As an alternative, you could use cut bamboo stakes and place them in the pots, and give your cat her very own pot to play in. Accommodation is often the best and most humane remedy.

DEAR DR. FOX—I am desperate to keep our cats from using my (very hard-worked-for) herb garden as a litter box. A box is provided, and they also have several acres at their disposal. But gravel pathways and soft dirt in the garden are irresistible. Commerical sprays advertised to repel them attracted them instead, and red pepper suggested by the local extension service did not seem to work either. Help!—*B.M.Z.*

DEAR B.M.Z.—One of the many come-ons of entrepreneurs is the claim that compound X will keep cats away from gardens. They don't work—like the ultrasonic flea-repellents now on the market. Your best bet is either a dome of chicken wire over your herbs or a zig-zag barricade of bamboo stakes. The latter is visually more attractive and will certainly keep your cats from getting into your herbs. Grow some catnip in one corner of your garden just for them. It will divert them.

eating feces (dogs)

DEAR DR. FOX—My German shepherd has the disgusting habit of eating feces. My veterinarian told me to add meat tenderizer or pineapple juice to the dogfood. I've done this, but it hasn't stopped my dog. Can you advise?—*L.B.*

DEAR L. B.—There are many remedies for this habit, such as feeding the animal a little raw liver or brewer's yeast every day. More often, however, the dog grows out of the habit rather than responding to the remedy. This behavior may in some cases be related to a nutritional deficiency, but most cases simply seem to be a nasty habit.

Consistent discipline, and even a muzzle at times, may be your best solutions to deter the dog. Tabasco sauce or hot-pepper juice sprinkled on the stools is also worth a try, though passers-by may think you a little odd if they see you spicing the bait.

eating from table (dogs)

DEAR DR. FOX—Our Great Dane has the infuriating habit of eating from the table when my back is turned. She even puts her front feet on the kitchen counter and pulls food out of the cupboards. Last week I set a cake out to cool and left the room for a minute. When I came back, most of it was gone. Please advise.—*HUNGRY*

DEAR HUNGRY—You have a big dog with a big problem, and it's not going to be solved easily without very consistent training. First, put a choke-chain collar on your dog and attach a leash. Then put some human-type food on the table or counter and when she dares to go for it, shout "No, bad girl!" and firmly snap the leash. After several repetitions for a week or so, she should learn. If this fails, you could buy some mousetraps (the snap kind) and set them to go off at half-strength. Put them near the food counters that the dog normally tries to reach. These should cure her habit.

housebreaking (cats)

DEAR DR. FOX—Until two years ago our cat gave us no problems, even though he was usually alone in the house all day. Then he suddenly began to urinate in various places around the house. Our veterinarian finds no physical causes for this behavior. We tried keeping a kitten to provide companionship, but our cat hissed and screamed until we got rid of it. We walk him daily on a leash. We promptly clean the areas where he sprays, so that he won't be attracted to them again. But nothing deters him. We also notice that he howls and runs from window to window when neighbors' cats are outside. What's the story?—*E. and E. W.*

DEAR E. AND E. W.—Your cat is most likely marking his territory because he feels invaded by neighbor cats, who are probably spraying around your house. Hormone injections may help. As a last resort, let your cat out briefly to spray around outside your house. But be alert for cat screams—prelude to a fight—and intervene immediately. Better to run the risk of a few bite wounds than to get rid of your cat. Ten minutes outside morning and evening may well do the trick.

DEAR DR. FOX—We have two male cats and one female. One will not use the litter box for any of its functions, but instead uses the floor, plants, furniture, etc. Is there any nontoxic dye or substance we could feed them to trace our "problem child"? And is this problem physical or psychological?—*M. M.*

DEAR M. M.—It often happens that when cat becomes an outcast from a group such as yours, it becomes unhousebroken. If you can feed the animals separately you have a chance of finding the culprit. Cut up some thin colored plastic tape or wrapping into tiny, TINY pieces and add them to your cats' food—

a different color for two of the cats and none for the third. The plastic is inert, won't hurt your cat, and will be a marker. Once you detect which is the disturbed cat, you should consider finding a good home for it—providing, of course, there's nothing physically wrong. It could, for example, be constipated or have blocked anal glands or an inflamed bladder—all of which can lead to litter-box aversion.

DEAR DR. FOX—Over the years, our Siamese cat has frequently urinated on the bottoms of our floor-length dining-room draperies, and neither vinegar, mothballs, nor all-purpose ammonia cleaner has diminished his compulsion.

I had a similar problem with the family-room draperies, and when I replaced them with sill-length drapes, he did not urinate there. I would prefer not to replace my custom-made dining-room draperies. Help!—M.K.V.

DEAR M.K.V.—Unwanted urination, as distinct from spraying, is a common behavior problem in housecats. Some will show such behavior when they are suffering from cystitis. It is also a sign of frustration, cured in some cases by simply allowing the cat to spend some time outdoors, either on a leash or in the backyard under a watchful eye.

Veterinary treatment with hormones, such as megesterol, can be effective in certain cases and is certainly worth considering as a potential solution for your cat. As for your cat's preference for floor-length drapes, I would suspect it's simply more convenient to go on the floor than on the windowsill. So why not, in addition, take your drapes up a few inches off the ground?

DEAR DR. FOX—I promise to do whatever you say, if only you can help me. My beautiful Siamese cat insists on urinating everywhere but in his litter pan, and in particular on the shag rug in our TV room where we spend our evenings. Now we discover that he is using the sawdust pile in my husband's workshop as well as the laundry basket that's ready for the washing machine. This morning Mr. Kitti was outside, but did he urinate in the grass? No. A few minutes after coming back into the house, he used the rug instead of his pan. Please, please help, or I may have to put him to sleep, as much as I adore him.—K.H.

DEAR K.H.—If you only knew how many people write me anguished letters like yours! Unfortunately, an unhousebroken cat is a difficult problem for which there's no simple solution. First, rule out the possibility (at the vet's) of a possible bladder infection. Also, is he constipated? And if he hasn't been neutered, neutering may help. Your cat may simply have developed the vice of using certain parts of the house instead of the litter tray because, somehow, he got away with it as a kitten. One way to break this is to keep him confined in a large cage or in the bathroom, with litter tray, blanket, food, and water, for about two weeks. Let Mr. Kitti out for play and exercise but only under constant supervision so that he won't mess anywhere while he's out. Good luck.

DEAR DR. FOX—My housecats have always used a litter box, but they have developed a bad habit of sometimes using the guest-room bed! The litter box is located in a corner of the guest room away from the bed. We've tried various types of reprimands to no avail. Can you imagine how embarrassing it would be to have company discover a big surprise on the guest bed?—V.R.

DEAR V.R.—Yes, I can imagine how embarrassing it would be to have a guest wake up to the aroma of cat on the bed. But what about the smell from the litter tray? Presumably when guests come, you take the litter tray out. But why are you keeping the litter tray in the guest room—so it will be out of sight? You're paying for that luxury. If I were you, I would put the litter box in another convenient place and close the guest-room door to keep the cats out. This will probably break their habit of using the guest bed.

DEAR DR. FOX—My eleven-year-old cat has taken to using the bathtub instead of the litter box. I can't understand what prompts her behavior. What do you suggest I do?—MRS. E.J.N.

DEAR MRS. E.J.N.—Many cats will use the bathtub as an alternative to their litter box. Usually it's out of sheer laziness or convenience. You have two options. If you stop her from using the tub, she may go elsewhere in the house, and that would be harder to clean up. A bathtub is easy to clean. You also could try putting a litter tray in the tub. If you want her out of the tub entirely, simply keep an inch or two of water in the bottom. You may then have to retrain her to use the litter box.

DEAR DR. FOX—Recently I acquired a kitten who had been well trained by her mother to use the litter box. She had been sleeping in a sheltered spot in our screen porch, but when the weather turned unusually cold, I shut her in one of the rooms in the house. That's when the problem started—she will not use the litter pan. What can I do now to retrain her to her litter box, short of leaving her outside in the cold?—V.R.

DEAR V.R.—Cats can thrive in very cold weather, provided they are healthy and have good coats. Don't think it's the winter that is affecting your cat; it's the fact that you locked her up. She's venting her frustration by not using the litter box. One of my cats deliberately piddles by the front door in the summer if we don't take her for a walk in the garden so she can dust-bathe and eat grass for a few minutes.

DEAR DR. FOX—Suddenly our cat started to urinate all over our carpeting, and when nothing we tried seemed to stop her, we considered having her put to sleep. But spring came just in time, and she became strictly an outdoor cat. My question is this: can a former housecat survive a severe winter outdoors with her only protection being an unheated garage?—J.E.S.

DEAR J.E.S.—We had a similar problem with our female cat. Unless we gave her some time in the garden (always under strict supervision), she urinated in absolutely the wrong places. A cat will urinate out of its litter box if it is emotionally upset, sick with cystitis, or frustrated. So check these possibilities out. Meanwhile, you could try training your cat to a leash and harness and taking her outdoors regularly. Or build a cage-run that goes outdoors but allows your cat to come indoors as she wishes for warmth. You can build a flap-door into a window-frame. Cats enjoy living in wired-in outdoor pens and can remain healthy provided they just have a warm place to sleep.

housebreaking (dogs)

DEAR DR. FOX—I received a peekapoo as a gift when she was about nine months old. She was supposed to be potty trained, but much to my chagrin, I discovered this wasn't true. When I find evidence in the house, I show it to her, pick it up with tissue, tell her she's bad, spank her, and take her outside to show her where to go, but she doesn't catch on. What do you suggest?—B.H.

DEAR B.H.—Continue with your disciplinary procedures and add the following aversive technique. When she does make a mess indoors, take her to it, scold her verbally, put some white vinegar on her gums and take her straight outside.

Dab some vinegar on the spot she has messed after you've cleaned it up. The smell of vinegar should deter her eventually from using such spots in the future, since she will have a negative association between the smell of vinegar and its very unpleasant taste, which will cause her no harm.

Be sure she isn't going "potty" indoors because she's going "batty" when you go out. Many dogs make a mess in the house because they are frustrated and lonely. Keeping her in a large pen or holding cage while you're away may be the final solution.

DEAR DR. FOX—Whenever my four-month-old Doberman becomes excited she wets. This can happen when someone comes to the door or even if we're just playing with her. Will she grow out of this?—*L.P.*

DEAR L.P.—You're describing a common problem. Young dogs will urinate when they are very excited, afraid, or displaying submission while being petted or when greeting their owners. So do not punish or reprimand your dog in any way, since this will confuse her and possibly aggravate the problem.

Avoid exciting or greeting the dog on the best living-room rug. With time, she will grow out of it. A little rough play (tug-of-war with an old towel) may help her gain more confidence.

DEAR DR. FOX—Our two-year-old cocker spaniel has suddenly begun using two chairs in the living room as if they were fireplugs. Our vet thinks he is "marking territory" and wants us to get a urine sample to rule out infection. I find this impossible to do after many unsuccessful tries. Any suggestion?—*A. F.*

DEAR A. F.—Keep your dog indoors for several hours and give him his regular food at the usual time. Then, instead of allowing him out, keep him in two or

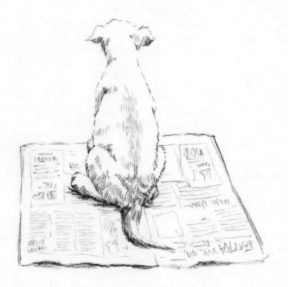

three hours longer than usual under strict supervision, so that you are sure he contains himself. Then let him out on the leash and use an old frying pan to catch the urine. Pour it into a screw-top jar. It's hard sometimes to get the sample directly from dog into narrow-mouthed jar. Your dog's waterworks are probably in top condition. My guess is that he's growing up and is now marking his territory. Castration will help eliminate this behavior. He might also grow out of it provided he's disciplined and is never allowed near the places he's marked without someone being there to inhibit him.

DEAR DR. FOX—Ever since my husband passed away my dog has been wetting wherever he chooses to lift his leg. It's driving me crazy—I've had to recover the chairs and clean the rug. The dog is two years old and I love him. What shall I do?—MRS. F.H.

DEAR MRS. F.H.—Your dog could be suffering from the loss of his master. Being insecure, he "marks" his territory more, so as to feel at home. Another possibility is that because he has now reached sexual maturity he is motivated to mark his plot. The trouble, of course, is that indoors is not the right plot. I advise you to keep him confined in a holding crate or on a short leash in one room to help break the habit. Take him out regularly and praise him for doing the right thing in the right place. When and if he raises his leg in the house, put him back in the crate or on the short leash. If this fails after a couple of weeks of confinement in the house, castration may help. Sounds cruel, but this will eliminate the sex hormone that could well be responsible.

DEAR DR. FOX—In the past few weeks Amy, my Pekingese, has begun to wet her bedding instead of the paper. What could cause a model puppy to resort to this behavior? She wets not only her own bed, but the bed of our old dog. I'm trying not to let her behavior change my feelings for her, but it's becoming difficult.—J.L.D.

DEAR J.L.D.—Be patient and look for a reason. First, have your dog thoroughly examined by your veterinarian to rule out the possibility of a bladder infection or a form of diabetes that is making her drink and urinate excessively.

If she has been spayed, it's quite probable that she's suffering from a hormonal imbalance, which has led to a weakening of the pelvic muscles so that she has difficulty retaining urine. Treatment for this is sex hormone replacement—and continued loving affection.

DEAR DR. FOX—In my dining room, I have a lace tablecloth on the table and a vase with artificial flowers. When I go out, my dog gets on the table and wets the artificial flowers. How do I get him to quit?—MRS. G. W.

DEAR MRS. G. W.—How do I get pet owners to ask themselves why their pet does such and such? There's usually a good reason. Your dog is no doubt frustrated at being left alone and finds the upright flowers an ideal target to anoint.

How often do you take him out? The more often the better. And if you must leave him at home, hide the flowers or put them on the floor by the door under a few layers of newspaper. Then he will have a way of expressing himself and you won't have much to clean up either.

DEAR DR. FOX—I have a part poodle-part spaniel who is impossible to train. The weird thing about him is that the people he was living with used to get him drunk on whiskey. Do you think that's why he so untrainable?—D.T.

DEAR D.T.—My guess is that people who will get their dog drunk for their own amusement are not very responsible or understanding pet owners. They probably never bothered to put in the necessary time to train and housebreak your dog. You'll have to keep the dog under close supervision while he's in the house. At night, keep him tied up or in a holding pen. He won't urinate where he has to lie, and he should learn what is expected of him within a few days. Let him outdoors first thing in the morning and give him plenty of praise.

An outdoor kennel and run are an alternative. Some male dogs seem mixed up and mark their territory inside the house. Having the dog neutered does help in some such cases.

housebreaking (rabbits)

DEAR DR. FOX—We bought our children a dwarf Netherland rabbit as a pet. They enjoy cuddling and petting her, but if she can, she gets away and the chase is on. Could it be that the children frighten her when they get excited? Also, I have heard that rabbits train themselves to "go" only in one spot, but that's not true of ours. Help!—C.H.

DEAR C.H.—A rabbit's favorite games are chase, hide-and-seek, and catch-me-if-you-can—all in sequence and not necessarily in that order. Your rabbit may be engaging in just such a game.

Young children do excite and sometimes frighten animals when they get excited themselves. It is important that the children be educated to remain calm and quiet and not shout, scream, or run around, especially with young bunny rabbits.

For housebreaking, try a cat litter tray or a stack of newspapers. Put a little soiled paper or urine and droppings in the litter; it may attract the rabbit to using the litter tray regularly.

hyperactivity (dogs)

DEAR DR. FOX—I found a puppy last year, but she's hyperactive and I can't seem to calm her down. Is it true that there are medicines to calm an animal? —HYPER DOG OWNER

DEAR HYPER DOG OWNER—Your veterinarian could give your dog a tranquilizer to calm her, but would you really want a drugged animal as a companion? I wouldn't. Hyperactive pets require (1) plenty of exercise, (2) obedience training, (3) discipline.

They should be disciplined, for example, not to jump up or race around, which they often do for attention. When that happens, ignore the dog and simply say "No." Then pet her when she has responded to your command. Some hyperactive dogs seem to calm down when given a cup of strong coffee with a little milk first thing in the morning. As your dog reaches full maturity at about one to one-and-a-half years of age, she may naturally begin to calm down more. So patience is the word.

DEAR DR. FOX—My daughter's puppy will in no way let people show affection toward it. It will not hold still and continuously wants to gnaw or bite on you. She is at her wits' end trying to make the puppy behave, as she loves it dearly. Is it possible that it will be a vicious animal later in life?—B.H.J.

DEAR DR. B.H.J.—Your daughter's puppy may have a naturally hyperactive temperament, which will take some adjusting to. While some pups will be quiet when handled, others want to chew and play all the time. The answer is plenty of exercise and games, such as pull-the-towel, hide-and-seek, and fetch-the-ball. When the puppy is four months, your daughter can start basic obedience training —stay, sit, come, etc. With the right handling, the pup will gradually relax, but love alone won't help.

DEAR DR. FOX—Our two-year-old English sheepdog is super hyper. She won't leave company alone when they come; she licks constantly and barks a lot. She's a big, lovable pain. Is there anything we can do to calm her down? Obedience school has not helped.—D.O.M.

DEAR D.O.M.—Congratulations! You are one of thousands who own a "perpetual puppy." Some of the signs are continuous puppyish activities, such as solicitous behavior, hyperactivity, pawing, licking, yapping, panting, tail-wagging, and fits of near hysteria when left alone.

Dogs were once bred for various work-related functions. Your dog's breeding was originally directed toward protecting sheep. Now bred to be pets, these sheepdogs seem to be more infantalized and dependent. Quite frankly, these animals aren't dogs; they are better termed *doglets*—sweet, innocent, and basically mindless, or at least irrational and emotionally hypersensitive. Some people like to indulge such doglets as substitute children. The cure is in improved breeding and rearing, which includes obedience training. Ignoring, not rewarding, infantile solicitous behavior is the way to start.

DEAR DR. FOX—We have an eleven-month-old Doberman male who comes from good bloodlines. He becomes extremely panicky when left alone even for short periods—pacing, whining, crying, and howling the entire time. When I return, he runs and jumps all over me, his tongue is foamy, and his eyes are glazed. He is not destructive, but we're going crazy nonetheless. Is our dog becoming a neurotic?—A.A.B.

DEAR A.A.B.—Your dog is already neurotic, overdependent, and hyperactive. Some of these perpetual puppies are so attached to their owners that they go berserk when left even for a short period. I advise either a short course of tranquilizer therapy under veterinary supervision or trauma therapy. This will involve leaving your dog at a kennel for three or four days with other dogs, and repeating such a separation about four times over a period of two or three months. He may then outgrow this problem. Somewhere in the breeding procedures, there must have been some failure in quality control. Actually, it's more usual for dogs to wreck the house when left alone.

DEAR DR. FOX—Our six-month-old dog born of a purebred bloodhound (father) and a purebred English pointer (mother) is becoming hyperactive. Is this because of the cross of the breeds? Should we give her a relaxant?—J.H.D.

DEAR J.H.D.—It's not usual for an adult dog to show a change in temperament and become hyperactive. Possibly you have overindulged her and not given her sufficient obedience training. Also, you may be rewarding her hyperactivity by giving her attention whenever she barks and acts up. Some nutritionists believe that hyperactivity may be related to certain adulterants in food, particularly coloring materials and preservatives. Try your dog on a different brand of pet food, or prepare your own diet from nonprocessed foods. Your dog may want more activity and playful interaction with you. She might respond well to having a companion dog. You might consider getting her a puppy, ideally of the opposite sex.

DEAR DR. FOX—In my thirteen years of breeding dogs, this is a first—a hyperactive bulldog. He is easily excitable and prefers being outside, even in the coldest weather. I have heard that hyperactivity in children can be helped by removing artificial coloring and preservatives from their diet. Could you give me a balanced diet for a sixty-pound dog that would eliminate the above?—L.E.H.

DEAR L.E.H.—Most likely, your hyperactive bulldog is that way because of his temperament, and you should not even consider breeding him unless he "cools down" by the time he's two years old. Many health-food stores carry "natural" preservative-free dogfoods. Or you can make your own by baking sugarless whole-meal cookies (whole-wheat flour, salt, shortening or vegetable oil) and a stew based on rice, onion, potatoes, and other vegetables plus ground beef or chicken parts. You can get by with as little as one-quarter part of meat scraps in the stew. Keep the stock in your refrigerator. Try this for about four weeks, and if there's no improvement, go back to regular dogfood and consider having your dog neutered.

DEAR DR. FOX—You are always saying in your column that a high-strung dog may need some tranquilizer medication to calm him. Well, our dog (part shepherd-part collie) is almost two-and-a-half years old, and two vets said that he would outgrow being high-strung by the time he was two. He hasn't. So how do I go about getting tranquilizers if the vet won't give them to us?—B.J.M.

DEAR B.J.M.—I agree with the other veterinarians with whom you have consulted. We do not endorse the continuous use of tranquilizers to calm a dog who has a hyperactive temperament. Such drugs are best used for special emergencies.

Prolonged use can cause liver damage and other complications. You can't change your dog's temperament with drugs without harming the dog. Try obedience school and plenty of regular exercise. A diet of homemade food, low in meat and high in rice, without any preservatives and adulterants such as dyes, may also help.

DEAR DR. FOX—Toro is a small part terrier-part pit bull who lived in the mountains for years and now lives with me in an apartment. When we're out, if Toro smells or sees a dog, he starts jumping and barking so violently that I can hardly cope with him on the leash. If we're inside, he runs to the windows and goes into the same tizzy. Would neutering help him?—M.B.R.

DEAR M.B.R.—Your pet is "dog happy." He probably wants to investigate and play with his own kind, rather than defend you from them. A choke collar may make it easier for you to control him on the leash. Snap it harshly with a loud "No!" when he starts to act up. A course at a local obedience school may help both of you cope better. If there is a park nearby where you can let him loose to run with other dogs, so much the better—provided, of course, he isn't a fighter. This pit-bull terrier background could be a problem, and, yes, neutering may be the final solution.

jumping up (cats)

DEAR DR. FOX—Our cat likes to get up on our table and plant stand. We discipline her by squirting her with our plant sprayer, but after we do this she goes right back up. Any suggestions?—M.D.

DEAR M.D.—Some cats are resistant to straightforward discipline, even to plant sprayers with the nozzle set to give a sharp blast at pointblank range. Sure,

TRAINING TIPS

Always give the verbal command ("No," "Down," "Come," or whatever) before you give discipline, be it in the form of a pull on the leash or a tap on the nose. Very often people get the conditioning sequence the wrong way around, and this confuses the pet. The animal will learn to anticipate that discipline will come after the verbal command, and eventually it will respond to the word and won't need to be punished.

Giving mild punishment before the verbal command means the animal will never learn and will always have to be punished. A well-trained dog or cat will readily respond to verbal rebuke or control without ever having to be hit. Always praise verbally or with a pat on the head for good behavior.

the cool cat will get out of the way, but she will be back into mischief soon after. You must be sure that you are conditioning your cat correctly before you give up and accept the fact that she has a stronger will than you. Shout, scream, and jump about one or two seconds before you squirt your cat. Make a big deal out of it. After only a few such trials, one yell and no squirt will probably suffice. Also, build your cat a jungle gym to play on. It sounds like she needs plenty of stimulation. Putting some mousetraps, bent to snap loudly but not harm the cat, under a sheet of newspaper on the table and plant stand may also do the trick.

jumping up (dogs)

DEAR DR. FOX—Is there any way to get a French poodle not to jump all the time? I guess they are high-strung. As soon as someone comes in, the dog starts jumping.—C.K.

DEAR C.K.—Poodles are "jumpers" who love to be the center of attention. Small dogs seem to need to jump up to make face contact. I would advise basic obedience training. Find a good school nearby, and train your dog to "sit" and "stay" and only pet it when it is in the "sit" position. Never pet your dog when it jumps up: Either ignore it or, once it knows the commands, make it "sit" and "stay."

neighborhood dogs use lawn as toilet

DEAR DR. FOX—We recently moved into a new house and received a welcoming present: all the neighborhood dogs use the area in front of our garden gate to relieve themselves. I don't want to harm these dogs, but I do wish they'd find another spot. Any suggestions?—R.A.

DEAR R.A.—Dogs do have to doo-doo somewhere, and it's their owner's responsibility to see that they don't do it on other people's property. Soak the area with a strong solution of ammonia or vinegar and, when the ground has dried off, put down a liberal powdering of cayenne pepper. Repeat this for several days. Then hope the dogs will find a more pleasant-smelling area to do their duty.

pecking on window (birds)

DEAR DR. FOX—There is a robin who pecks on our window incessantly. This is the third year this bird has come back. It's always the same window—and

I'm quite sure it's the same bird. He pecks most of the day and sometimes after dark when the blinds are drawn. Sometimes he pecks so loud that our dog barks, thinking someone is rapping at the door. What makes this crazy bird act like this? And how can I discourage him?—*E.H.*

DEAR E.H.—All things could be just right to stimulate this bird to return frequently to the same window and tap out his crazy tattoo. For instance, there could be a convenient ledge to perch on, or the right reflection to give the robin the illusion that it is seeing a rival in the windowpane in his own territory. You can discourage the bird, if you must, in various ways. Put a pan of water on the sill, or put up a wire screen covered with a sheet of cardboard. Animals are creatures of habit, and once their routines are disrupted, habits are often repatterned or inhibited.

running off (dogs)

DEAR DR. FOX—My dog is always running into the road, and I don't know what to do. Any suggestions?—*D.R.*

DEAR D.R.—Operation leash-control! You need to put a choke-chain collar and a long leash on your dog and then let him run out toward the traffic. Then, give him a loud verbal reprimand—"Stop!" or "Stay"—and pull him up short. Also, teach him to sit on command and not get up until you say so, using the chain and leash (held short) to control him. There's probably an obedience school in your area, and if I were you, I'd sign up at once. Obedience training will not only help save him from being hit by a car, but also make him a more enjoyable pet, after he's educated.

DEAR DR FOX—We live on a farm, and our dog has plenty of room to run. However, since she became acquainted with our neighbor's children and their dog who live up the road, she wanders off to visit them unless we keep her tied. How can we train her to understand that she belongs here?—*MRS. H.S.*

DEAR MRS. H.S.—Let's face it: it's probably more fun at your neighbor's house with the kids and the other dog than being tied up at your place. Perhaps you shouldn't have let your dog roam free in the first place. If you want to try training her to stay at home now, let her free only in the late afternoon, either every other day or two or three times a week. You could also keep her restrained on a long rope with plenty of running room, and walk her over to play with the neighbors every now and then. It's a good idea to make life more fun for your dog, with extra play and special treats.

spraying (cats)

DEAR DR. FOX—Shortly after my cat was neutered he started spraying on everything and anything he could get near. No matter what I do, I cannot break him of this habit. This problem is particularly aggravating as I live in a mobile-home park and have to keep the cat inside most of the time. Also, he seems healthy except that he doesn't like being touched on the stomach. Is it possible the neutering was not done correctly?—*J.R.*

DEAR J.R.—The sensitive spot on your cat's tummy has nothing to do with the operation. Many cats can't bear to be touched there and will bite or scratch when they are.

The spraying has many possible causes, but hormone treatment with Ovoban, prescribed by your vet, may help. Cage confinement or keeping the cat in one room for ten or fourteen days may also break the habit. If not, often it is wise to have any cat who sprays checked for cystitis—bladder infection—which makes many cats unhousebreakable.

DEAR DR. FOX—There's a cat in my neighborhood who sprays on my car's windshield. The spray goes down into the grill of the hood, and when I turn the motor on it smells as if the cat urinated right in my car. I've tried many repellents, but none work. The owners of this cat say they can't keep it in the house and that I can do whatever I choose to—whatever that means. Do you have any suggestions?—D.L.

DEAR D.L.—I sympathize with you. And with winter coming and all the more need to put on your car heater, you're certainly not in for any pleasant rides. I suggest that you purchase some mousetraps, lay them on top of a sheet of newspaper, and hold the newspaper down with a couple of stones. When the cat gets onto your car, the traps will go off, making a very loud noise.

If you bend the wire to soften the impact of the trap, I doubt the cat will be hurt even if it does accidentally get caught in it. The loud snapping noise should suffice to scare the cat away. An alternative is to lay over the front of your car a sheet of plastic, held down with some weights. This way, at least, the cat will not be spraying right into the windshield-wiper well, contaminating the interior of your car. Good luck!

won't sleep alone (cats)

DEAR DR. FOX—My kitten is perfectly normal except that she insists on sleeping around my face. She loves to curl up to my head and affectionately rub her face all over mine. I have tried pushing her off, but she keeps coming back for more. She's a good cat, but this 3 A.M. love affair has got to end.—MRS. W.McW.

DEAR MRS. W.Mc.W.—Cats often like to sleep close—so close as to touch noses and share the same breath. Make a routine of petting and grooming your cat every night in her spot at the bottom of the bed. Then whenever she tries to crawl beside your head, shout "no" and put her back at the bottom of the bed.

She will learn that this is her place once she realizes that sleeping by your head is unacceptable. Consistent discipline and a few sleepless nights are the cost for imposing your own way. Don't be afraid of losing your cat's love. One cat will hiss at another to tell it to sleep somewhere else. Be a dominant cat yourself and show affection at the right time and right place—at the bottom of the bed.

won't urinate outdoors (dog)

DEAR DR. FOX—Last Christmas, we gave our mother a mixed-breed puppy who was remarkably easy to paper-train, but it appears we did the job too well. She refuses to relieve herself except on the paper in the basement. Even in the backyard for hours, or on long walks, she waits to use the papers for her toilet. How can we retrain her before cold weather starts?—R.W.C.

DEAR R.W.C.—It is often a problem to get an indoor-paper-trained pooch to go outdoors. Take the paper outdoors, with a little urine on it to give her the right idea. Gradually, reduce the amount of newspaper until she is conditioned to go outside without it.

If she isn't too big, you might try her in a cat-litter tray lined with newspaper. It would be easier to clean up, and might be your solution if she never takes to the outdoors. As she gets older, she may start to urinate outdoors to mark her territory —then your problem should naturally and quickly cure itself.

won't use doghouse

DEAR DR. FOX—What can be done to encourage a young Geman shepherd female to use the doghouse built for her? She absolutely won't have anything to do with it. Even in winter, she remains outside.—W.G.

DEAR W.G.—Some dogs seem just too dumb to get under cover out of the rain. Others, given a nice doghouse, are afraid to go in or else they feel that it's a kind of punishment—hence the expression "in the doghouse."

So try to make it rewarding. Coax your dog inside with some meat scraps, and get her to associate being in the house with pleasure and praise. Otherwise she may well think she's being separated from you as punishment or react with distress when separated and perceive the house in a negative way. Some wooden slats in front of the kennel where she can lie down and keep dry will help. Many dogs enjoy lying outdoors and can take quite low temperatures provided they have a good coat.

DEAR DR. FOX—How in the world do you get a dog to go into a doghouse that once belonged to another dog? I've tried everything, but my cocker spaniel refuses to enter.—M.K.

DEAR M.K.—Did you ever hear the expression "He's in the doghouse"? Well, some dogs won't go into the doghouse because they look at it as a punishment. So what you must do is make it rewarding, either by putting some particular delicacy inside the doghouse that your spaniel likes, or rewarding your pet after it has gone inside—with a beef knucklebone, for instance. Positive associations with the house will give your dog a positive attitude about using it. But don't lose patience. It may take some time to overcome your dog's prejudice.

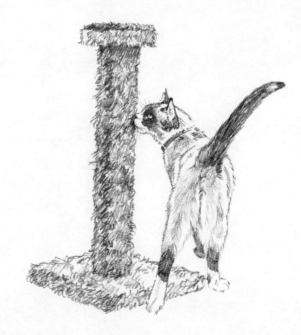

won't use scratching post (cats)

DEAR DR. FOX—How do I train my cat to use his scratching post? We don't seem to be getting anywhere.—A.S.

DEAR DR. FOX—Tack or clip a strip of carpet against the side of the sofa. Then buy some catnip and make some "tea" out of it. Pour the tea onto the cat's scratching post and let it dry. This helps attract the cat to the post. Put the cat up against the post and sink its claws into the surface and encourage your pet to scratch and make clawing movements against it, even demonstrating the process yourself. It may sound corny, but cats are great observers. Be patient, persevere, and use a water pistol to squirt at your cat to discourage it from scratching in the wrong places.

15

Animals Can Have Emotional Problems, Too

JEALOUSY

cannibalism (dogs)

DEAR DR. FOX—Why would a female dog kill and then eat her pups when they are six weeks old?—*C.M.*

DEAR C.M.—Cannibalism in dogs is not that unusual, especially when a mother gives birth to a sick or dead pup. But for a mother to kill her six-week-old pups—that's a crazy canine. The half-dozen or so cases I have encountered were all in very dependent, overindulged bitches, and I believe they killed their pups out of sheer jealousy because their owners were paying less attention to them and more to the pups.

new baby in house (dogs)

DEAR DR. FOX—My daughter, who lives with us, expects a child soon. I'm fearful that Buffy, our dog, will be jealous. He's lovable and sweet, and used to a lot of affection, but he has snapped at children. Is there anything we can do beforehand to prepare him for the baby's arrival?—*MRS. S.L.*

DEAR MRS. S.L.—There's little you can do ahead of time. After the baby arrives, give Buffy extra attention and extra treats—especially when the baby and he are both in the room together. That way, he'll come to associate reward with the baby's presence. Introduce them gradually; let Buffy sniff the infant first. And never leave the two together unsupervised. After all, Buffy feels it's his turf. With time, Buffy will probably become quite protective of the baby—perhaps too protective, and you'll be writing me for more advice.

251

status in "family pack" (dogs)

DEAR DR. FOX—My girlfriend and I have two beautiful, wonderful Aire-
dales. Max is thirty-two months old and has decided that he is "Daddy's boy."
When I stick my face down to his, he will lick me no end. When my girlfriend,
Donna, does the same, he will lick her only on occasion. On the other hand,
Minnie, our bitch, adores "Mommy" (Donna). She loves me, too, but not as
much. Max is increasingly hostile to Donna, and last night he attempted to bite
her, but I smacked him. How can I get Max to behave?—D.R.S.

DEAR D.R.S.—Max is jealous of Donna and wants to be No. 2 in the family
pack. You must let him know that such behavior is totally unacceptable. Advise
your girlfriend to avoid conflict with him, and when he does threaten her, to back
away submissively. That should stop him from acting more aggressively.

DEPRESSION

excessive sleeping (parakeets)

DEAR DR. FOX—My one-year-old parakeet sleeps almost all the time. She
has excellent care, but we do not permit her out of the cage. Is this sleeping a sign
of oncoming illness? Also, she is not friendly and snaps all the time.—S.M.

DEAR S.M.—Yes, long periods of sleeping can mean your bird has a chronic
illness—or that she's simply depressed. But if she's eating well and not losing
weight, I'd say it's psychological, and she's not to blame for being snappish, rather
her environment is! Why not put on some gloves and try to lure her out to your
hand? Social interaction, especially among parakeets who are highly gregarious
in the wild, is healthy. Also, be sure she has toys and a mirror in her cage. Even
strips of paper to play with could make her more responsive.

need for companionship (fish)

DEAR DR. FOX—Do fish have feelings? Sometimes, staring into my fish
tank, I swear that my goldfish looks depressed. Am I imagining things?—G.T.

DEAR G.T.—Do you have one goldfish? If so—yes, it's probably depressed.
Goldfish are social and like the company of other goldfish. Many tropical fish will
change color when they're afraid. And some species will act unresponsive, stop
eating, and look dull when a companion fish dies! We humans have no monopo-
ly on emotions.

LONELINESS

destroying house when left alone (dogs)

DEAR DR. FOX—I am an Irish setter and only one year old. My owners put
me in the cellar when they go to work from 9:30 to 2:30, and I'm alone there until
the children take me for a run after school's out. When I'm in the cellar I tear it
apart. When they chain me outside, I bark till the neighbors complain. Hitting
me with a newspaper doesn't help, and dog obedience classes were a flop. I just
don't want to be alone and I'm good only when I'm with people. Please, help me.
My owners have tried everything—even getting another dog, but he barked even
more than I did.—T.S.

P.S.: Please, don't tell my owners to get rid of me.

DEAR T.S.—You seem to be smarter than your loving owners. So ask them to arrange things so that it's fun to be alone for a while. They could leave the radio or TV on for company, and leave you some bones to chew on and some toys to play with.

I hope they don't overstimulate you when they come back. When owners act cool and don't make a big deal about coming and going, it seems to help. They could also play a "game" with you—slipping out quietly and then coming back after varying periods of five, ten, or twenty minutes. You would get confused, no doubt, but you'd also get the idea that no matter how long they are gone they will be back because they love you.

But you owe them something, too. So grow up and stop acting like a spoiled, overdependent pup or else you will make your owners into neurotic, overanxious parents, which they seem to be already. As you say, they've tried "everything." If they make life pleasanter for you in the cellar and you still don't cooperate, some strong discipline may be their next step. You don't want to be known as a spoiled brat—do you?

DEAR DR. FOX—Someone gave us a Lhasa apso that had been lost for some time. He is very well behaved so long as someone is in the house with him, but the two times we left him alone, he tore up the wall-to-wall carpeting and barked loudly and constantly to the irritation of our neighbors. Since then, we take him everywhere with us, which is not easy. We hate to give him away because he is a beauty, but what can we do?—MRS. C.

DEAR MRS. C.—Previously abandoned or lost dogs and/or those who are overdependent will act up when left alone in the house. There are a few remedies to try. Leave a radio or television on. Keep the dog in a room that he cannot wreck or in a holding pen. Get another animal—pup or kitten—to keep him company. There's no simple solution, and giving him away will only pass the problem on to someone else and probably intensify his fear of being abandoned. If all else fails, I guess you'll have to go on taking him with you, in which case you'll have to discipline him not to bark or jump at people, or you may find your social life being curtailed.

DEAR DR. FOX—I have a solution to a serious problem that I want to pass on to your readers. Our whippet hated being alone; whenever she was, she would tear up the house. Then we bought her a superlarge cage. We put her bed and blankets inside the cage and left the door open. The cage is in the kitchen where her bed was previously located. She learned to nap in the cage. Then we began locking her inside when we went out. We're all much happier now because when we arrive home there's no destruction and no need for punishment.—B.B.

DEAR B.B.—Many people think that keeping the dog in a large cage when they are away is cruel. But it's certainly a better alternative than getting rid of a house-wrecking dog, especially when done gradually as you described. A cage may give the dog a sense of security, provided being put in the cage isn't associated with punishment. Playpens also help in coping with a puppy before it's housebroken and when an owner is holding a litter of puppies after they've been weaned, prior to sale. Mousetraps can also be used, especially under newspaper, to deter dogs from jumping on forbidden sofas and armchairs.

need for new mate (ganders)

DEAR DR. FOX—I have a one-year-old gander, and since my goose died at the same age, the gander has been climbing on family members and trying to get on top of their heads or nibble on their necks. George will also honk extremely loudly in the middle of the night if he is not put in his pen, or if somebody raises his voice. Why is he acting so strangely?—P.O.

DEAR P.O.—George is seeking out you and your family members as an outlet for his frustrated social and sexual needs. You can either accept this with good-humored understanding or get him a lady companion. I would opt for the latter, since after all, what's a gander without a goose—or without a gaggle of lady geese, for that matter? Keep the new lady goose in a cage for few days so George won't drive her off at once. He should get used to her and realize that a goose can be a more satisfactory companion than a two-legged, featherless human-bird substitute!

too young to be left alone (puppies)

DEAR DR. FOX—My dog is three months old, and every time I go out, he tears his paper to shreds. Is it right to hit the dog after he does this, or not? Should I keep him locked up in the kitchen after he does this?—M.K.

DEAR M.K.—Your dog is only a puppy, and he is too young to be left alone. He will tear things up, bark excessively, and perhaps become unhousebroken because he is bored, lonely, and frustrated. A pup needs to be taken out frequently and have plenty of human contact. I wish more people who go out to work would think twice before getting a dog. Many such dogs turn out to be sad, confused animals and end up at the pound to be destroyed. Cats are more adaptable to your life-style—especially a pair of them.

In answer to your question, though, I don't think you should hit your dog or lock him up. Give him some tender loving care and some toys, play with him as much as possible, and, if all else fails, consider putting him in another home where he will not be alone all day.

FRUSTRATION

boredom (dogs)

DEAR DR. FOX—I would like to know why my seven-month-old German shepherd digs holes in the yard. Also, is it safe to feed my dog gunpowder to make him mean? If so, how much?—B.G.

DEAR B.G.—To make your shepherd really mean, you should feed him about one pound of gunpowder per ten pounds of body weight, and then ten minutes after he's been fed, light his tail. If this doesn't blow your head off, at least I hope it will blow away the myth that feeding gunpowder to a dog will turn it into a mean protector of home and family. It won't, and don't make your dog sick trying to see if it might work.

Your dog digs holes in the yard because it's fun and he's bored. Why not get him another dog for company?

going "stir crazy" (parakeets)

DEAR DR. FOX—Recently, our parakeet started screaming and poking at both her wings, as though something were biting her, so I have been treating her with a commercial spray for mites and lice. But it has not helped. We also give her cod-liver oil supplement. We'd like to let her fly around because she keeps trying to get out of the cage, but when we let her out she chews up everything—curtains,

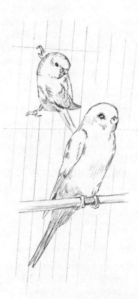

trim around windows, lampshades, books. My vet is stumped. Can you help?—
J.B.

DEAR J.B.—Since your vet obviously found no evidence of feather lice in your pet's wings, then I would conclude that the bird has a behavior problem. She's telling you that she wants to be free, so give her a space that she can fly in and wreck. Some birds do go cage-crazy, and pulling out their feathers is one of the first symptoms. Not all birds adapt to the privation of cage living—which is why I don't like the idea of raising birds for life in a cage. Get rid of that commercial spray—it could make your bird really sick. Be sure the cod-liver oil is fresh and kept in an airtight container, once it gets old and oxidizes it can be lethal, destroying vitamin E in the body.

DEAR DR. FOX—My parakeet keeps kicking her food out of her dish. Do you know why?—M.M.

DEAR M.M.—She's probably bored. Many birds spill things over or play soccer with their food, gravel, and water because they like to be active. Imagine being inside a small cage most of the time. Intelligent and curious birds will often go cage-crazy. A hooded no-spill food container would be your solution. You should also give your bird exercise (is she allowed to fly free?) and plenty of toys, perches, and other things to enrich her caged existence.

going "stir crazy" (parrots)

DEAR DR. FOX—Our African gray parrot seems healthy, but he continually pulls feathers out, especially from his tail. Can you tell me why? He looks terrible this way.—W.C.P.

DEAR W.C.P.—Feather pulling has a variety of possible causes, from boredom and mite infection to cage frustrations or some emotional stress (such as losing a companion or being worried about a neighboring cat who has taken to sitting on the windowsill outside.) Give your bird plenty of extra attention, toys in the cage, and exercise. Also, fitting a collar around your bird's neck for three to four weeks to stop him from reaching his tail may help break the habit. But first, do consider whether there's a possible psychological reason for this self-mutilating vice. Prevention is the best medicine.

separation from mate (dogs)

DEAR DR. FOX—I am a breeder of miniature dachshunds. I have a problem with my three-year-old, ten-pound stud. I use him only once or twice a year. When separated from his mate, he is so unhappy that he chews the end of his tail, which bleeds and is now one-half inch shorter. How can I stop this habit?— MRS. C.E.F.

DEAR MRS. C.E.F.—Try keeping your dog with a female companion. Then he won't be so frustrated and will probably leave his tail alone and chase hers instead.

SHYNESS

developing more confidence (dogs)

DEAR DR. FOX—My dog, Curly, seems to be sad all the time. Her posture, her eyes—everything seems to suggest it. Yet she has everything she needs, especially our love. She is healthy, too. What do you say?—L.P.

DEAR L.P.—Many dogs that seem sad, like Curly, are really timid. You have to handle them gently and reassuringly to help them ovecome their fears. Such dogs may also show submissive behavior—flattening their ears, dropping their tails, and lowering their bodies when they see a person.

It is their way of being friendly and can be misinterepreted as a sign of sadness or an indication that the dog was once abused. I hope this makes you feel better about your dog, who obviously has your love, which is the best remedy.

DEAR DR. FOX—Recently, I adopted a year-old Doberman. I expected this ferocious female to be a superb watchdog. However, my Doberman is a real chicken.

She sees strangers and runs under the table. Before I send Rosebud to the glue factory, can you help me? She is so beautiful and affectionate. Is there something I can put in her diet to make her more aggressive?—S.P.

DEAR S.P.—Your dog may have a basically gentle and shy temperament and never become more protective. But you can try to make her more extroverted by playing games with her—especially tug-of-war with a towel. However, be patient, she's still young. And for dogdom's sake, don't add to her diet any gunpowder, tabasco, or other quack junk that many people use to make their dogs "mean." It doesn't work, but one vet claims that increasing the amount of raw meat in a dog's diet helps make the animal more aggressive, provided the amount of dry, cereal-based food is reduced. Many people would be happy having a dog like yours—a sweet and gentle companion. A burglar-alarm system may be what you need now, and I bet as your dog matures—around two to three years—she will be quite a protector.

ALOOFNESS

possible causes (cats)

DEAR DR. FOX—Ever since my cat, Sneaker, was a baby, she has not liked to be held or petted. Touch her and she cries or nips you. The only time she is affectionate is when she's hungry. I love her very much, but am just curious. Why is she so standoffish? (She's part Persian.)—C.H.

DEAR C.H.—Just like people, certain cats don't like to get too close. They become scared, afraid of being smothered or whatever. Often, this is because the animal wasn't handled early enough as a kitten. But even so, there are cats who have had plenty of tender loving care as kittens and still protest when held or even petted. I put it down to temperament—an inborn trait. I advise people not to breed such animals—the trait may well be inherited and passed on to the offspring —and why should another animal-lover feel slighted as you do?

DEAR DR. FOX—My cat jumps away when we try to pet her along her back. Is she suddenly neurotic?—B.T.

DEAR B.T.—Don't jump to conclusions. It could be a physical cause—anything from kidney trouble to a slipped disc in the spine. So have a veterinary checkup first. After that, you can look for other reasons. It may be something very simple—an idiosyncrasy or a hypersensitivity.

SELF-MUTILATION

drug therapy (cats)

DEAR DR. FOX—My nine-year-old neutered male Siamese has been diagnosed as having a hormonal imbalance. He is pulling his hair out on his side and his skin is turning black. The treatment (Ovoban) cleared it up for a while, but it started again. I really don't want a Siamese with bald sides and black skin. —A.F.W.

DEAR A.F.W.—An emotional as well as a hormonal problem can underlie the bizarre behavior of self-mutilation in cats. If no emotional cause can be identified and corrected, then your veterinarian should put your cat on Valium, which helps reduce anxiety, and if this does not prove effective along with hormonal replacement, another psychoactive drug such as Librium or Chlorpromazine may be the answer. Fortunately, a variety of compulsive and obsessive behavior problems in cats respond well to such therapy.

possible causes (birds)

DEAR DR. FOX—Six months ago we purchased a cockatoo for $700 from a local pet shop. At the time of purchase, the bird's plumage was not as it should be, but we were told this was due to molting and would soon be back to normal. Not so! The bird's feather-plucking has become a severe problem. We see no evidence of mites or lice, his cage is cleaned often, and we supplement his feed with vitamins. Can you help?—E.L.

DEAR E.L.—Cage birds lose their feathers for many reasons. Cockatoos, particularly, will become denuded when they're emotionally disturbed by the presence of a cat, restriction in a small cage, boredom, or lack of exercise and play objects. You must enrich your bird's environment as much as possible, giving it various materials to tear, shred, and generally manipulate. Such materials may help redirect the bird away from its feathers. But the sad fact is that self-mutilation is not uncommon in emotionally disturbed cage birds, especially those that are caught in the wild and never adjust to permanent imprisonment.

DEAR DR. FOX—Like one of your readers, I had a bird who kept tearing out its feathers. I found out why—the bird needed a mate. My bird was close to death. Mating was the best thing I could have done, because it just came back to life and has never pulled another feather in three years.—MRS. J.F.

DEAR MRS. J.F.—Thank you for the personal insights. I have insisted for years that when people keep social animals, like parrots, cockatiels, and parakeets, in solitary confinement, deprived of all contact with their own kind, problems can arise.

Frustration and boredom can lead to feather-pulling and gradual loss of condition. While many birds adapt to solitary confinement and bond with their human surrogates, others don't adapt so well, and the end result is inhumane.

possible causes (cats)

DEAR DR. FOX—We are always finding clumps of fur on the floor that our cat has pulled off his back. We have taken Trigger to several vets; some say it's fleas and others say it's allergies. But we know he has no fleas. Any suggestions?—J.W.

DEAR J.W.—There are several reasons why felines pull out their fur. It can be a neurotic form of self-mutilation triggered by some emotional stress such as being left alone for extended periods, losing a mate, etc. Some cats pull out their fur because of a hormonal imbalance that develops some time after being neutered. Hormone replacement therapy often works wonders. Also, too much of one kind of food or one particular brand isn't good for a cat—or anyone. So your cat's problem can be one of many things (and not just fleas or allergy). This means you must start from scratch and check out your cat's emotional life, diet, and overall physical condition. A few days on a mild tranquilizer could be the answer if the problem turns out to be primarily psychosomatic.

possible causes (dogs)

DEAR DR. FOX—How do I stop my poodle from biting her hair and pulling it out? She actually leaves raw spots. The doctor's salve did no good. After a short time, she started again.—V.H.

DEAR V.H.—Dogs will self-mutilate—in other words, lick and chew themselves excessively—when they have a skin irritation or allergy. Sometimes this allergy is caused by a contact dermatitis linked with pollen or with the saliva of fleas. Just one flea can trigger such behavior. The animal itches all over, and in order to alleviate the itch it just starts chewing on one part of its body as though greater pain will make the itch go away.

Some dogs will self-mutilate when they are bored or frustrated from being left alone for extended periods of time, when they're under emotional stress produced by strangers in the house, or even by the birth of a new child. If you can rule out all such psychological factors in the dog's environment, I suggest that you work with your veterinarian to identify a possible allergy or hypersensitivity. Light tranquilization and a so-called Elizabethan collar (a wide paper ruff) around the dog's neck may help break the vicious cycle.

DEAR DR. FOX—I thought I had my Samoyed cured of the habit of licking her legs, but I left her in a kennel for three weeks, and on my return her legs were pink again from the acidity in her saliva. I have tried putting dry hairspray on her, which she dislikes. Anything I can do to break this habit?—*K.D.*

DEAR K.D.—Find out when your dog starts to lick herself. Judging from her condition after three weeks in the kennel, I would bet that she mutilates herself when left alone for any length of time. Samoyeds are active, companionable dogs and do not do well when abandoned for extended periods. A companion dog (or cat) may be what she needs to compensate for losing you when you go out.

DEAR DR. FOX—Our Doberman licks the top of his paw until it is raw and bleeding. He is frequently bandaged and medicated, but a short time later he has the bandage off. What can I do?—*M.A.D.*

DEAR M.A.D.—Dobermans seem to be especially prone to self-mutilation. Some chew or lick one side of their flanks or a front paw until it is raw and bleeding. Your vet or dog trainer might try using a shock-collar to inhibit this behavior, or try applying bitter apple as a deterrent. Boredom and frustration can trigger self-mutilation. Is your dog left alone frequently? Taking the dog with you whenever possible will help, and a small dose of tranquilizer medication may give the foot a chance to heal and thus break the vicious cycle.

AGGRESSION

aggressive sex play (cats)

DEAR DR. FOX—I have two altered cats who fight day and night. The young male cat won't leave the older female alone. He bites her neck, jumps on her back, and exhibits sexual attraction to her even though he has been altered. What does this mean? And how can this behavior be stopped?—*C.A.*

DEAR C.A.—When cats fight day and night, the best and kindest solution is to find a home for one of them. As cats mature, or as their social relationship

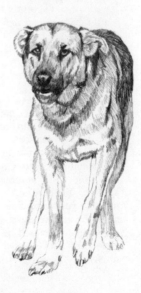

changes (and neutering can cause that), they often become unfriendly and aggressive. But, first, are you sure your cats aren't just playing roughly?

Treatment with a hormone such as Ovoban may help calm the male so that he pesters the other cat less. Have your veterinarian give that a try. You may also try giving the cat a mild tranquilizer before you make the final irrevocable decision of separating them for good. But be prepared, since your options are slim.

aggressive sex play (ducks)

DEAR DR. FOX—I have two Peking ducks—one male, one female. Whenever I bring them water, the male will mate with the female and pull her feathers out. He has pulled almost all the feathers out of the back of her head and neck. What can I do?—V.C.

DEAR V.C.—The excitement of your presence and of being given fresh water so arouses your drake (male) that he discharges his pent-up energies in a sexual and aggressive way toward the female. If they are in a small enclosure, things would be improved if the female had somewhere to escape. Another solution is to divide the pen in half and keep the birds separated until the duck has regrown her feathers. Give the drake a cabbage or tussock of grass to "attack." With time, he may grow out of this behavior, which is in part triggered by your exciting presence.

aggressive when let loose (dogs)

DEAR DR. FOX—We have a five-year-old mixed breed who's very gentle and marvelous with our kids. We usually chain her in the yard, but if the kids accidentally let her out, she becomes very aggressive toward people and other dogs, runs away, and doesn't come back till hours later. What can we do with her?—P.A.

DEAR P.A.—Well, as the story goes, there's no use closing the barn door after the horse has bolted. Your dog, like all dogs, should have gone through basic obedience training earlier in life so she would have learned to obey and you would have learned to control her. However, it's not entirely true that older dogs can't learn new tricks, so sign up for obedience school at once. Also, I know that I'd certainly run if I ever got loose from a chain, so why don't you take your dog for a long walk on the leash at least twice a day, instead of chaining her? She'll be much happier. If that's too much trouble for you, perhaps you shouldn't own a dog.

attack games (cats)

DEAR DR. FOX—My neutered Tom is a year-and-a-half old and is leash-trained to the clothesline. He spends time indoors, but often clings to our hands and bites at our scalp and hair. We are at a loss to know why. Any suggestions? —A.W.C.

DEAR A.W.C.—Cats frequently get carried away when they play, literally hallucinating that they are killing prey or fighting a rival. Give your cat a towel to chase and "kill," or some other suitable toy that you can jiggle and appropriately animate. You may even want to wear gloves and a thick-sleeved jacket when playing with your feisty feline. Pets need outlets for their natural instinctual drives, and the more we can understand their behavior and accommodate their needs, the happier they will be. His behavior could also have sexual overtones—he's giving you "love bites," or affectionate, infantile implications—he wants to nurse!

attack games (dogs)

DEAR DR. FOX—For no reason at all, our poodle will suddenly bite our feet—and draw blood. Why would he do this to us? We're only walking from one place to another, not bothering him. Also, how do we get him to quit wetting everywhere in the house?—*C.S.*

DEAR C.S.—Sounds like you have a minimonster on your hands, and I bet one that's been rather overindulged. His foot fetish is probably a misplaced play pattern of chasing and attacking would-be prey. Disciplinary training should have stopped it before it got to the bloody stage. Alternative games, such as fetch-and-carry and tug-of-war with a towel, should help fulfill this attacking instinct.

Wetting in the house can mean many things. Some possibilities are that he's marking his territory, that he wants out, or that he's angry at you for leaving him alone in the house. Which is it, C.S.?

DEAR DR. FOX—When my eleven-month-old Chihuahua gets into his box, he starts to bark and fight his box inside and out. What shall I do? He keeps us up all night.—*FRUSTRATED*

DEAR FRUSTRATED—Perhaps because Chihuahuas are so small, they need to act out being tough. I suggest you play with your puppy for a good hour before his bedtime so that he'll be exhausted and won't want to play by himself. As he matures, your pet's extreme playfulness will tend to wane somewhat. Let's hope he's not so precocious as to be expressing his frustration at not being allowed to sleep with you.

bad reaction to children (dogs)

DEAR DR. FOX—Our Great Dane, Snert, whom we've had since a pup, gets along great with us and other adults, but always barks and growls at children. (Years ago, he was teased by the kids next door.) In a dog fight two years ago, he killed another dog. We are expecting twins in March and want your opinion on how he will get along with them. Any advice?—*E.B.*

DEAR E.B.—If children were educated to respect animals and treat them humanely, the world would be a better place, and you wouldn't have a problem dog on your hands. You would be wise to find a good home for your dog. He may take to your twins, but your hands will be full enough coping with them, and you'll have him to watch, too. And later, when other kids come around to play, there could be trouble.

A good animal trainer might be able to help, but considering your dog's past experience and propensity, he's no longer reliable. I, myself, would not keep him. Support your local humane society and push for humane education in schools. A humane-education curriculum guide for teachers, by the way, is now available. Write to The Humane Society of the United States, 2100 L St. N. W., Washington, D.C. 20037.

DEAR DR. FOX—My thirteen-month-old cocker spaniel, Miller, doesn't like children. In fact, he tries to bite them when he sees them. I am single with no children, but he gets crazy even when he sees a child in the distance. How can I get him used to children without taking the chance he'll attack? I do hope to marry and have children of my own, and I want a pet that everyone loves, not fears. To me, this problem is intolerable! Please, help.—*M.L.*

DEAR M.L.—In the 1950s cocker spaniels got a bad reputation for hysteria. It was a result of sloppy mass breeding because the breed was so popular. Now this problem is coming back as cockers once more gain national popularity. Children either overexcite cockers or make then fearful, and they go bananas. You should consider obedience school. Also, expose your dog gradually to children —keep him muzzled, of course—so that he gets desensitized. Light tranquilization may help, too. And have him neutered. Be prepared, however, to have him euthanized, since "cocker hysteria" is difficult to treat.

biting (cats)

DEAR DR. FOX—When I whistle, and my cat is close to where I'm sitting, she will curl up beside me and purr. But if I'm lying down, she'll come and bite me. Any explanations?—D.D.

DEAR D.D.—When you're sitting up, you're like a warm chair or sofa for your cat. But when you're lying down, you're more accessible for play and less threatening. Try going down on all fours and playing chase or hide-and-seek. I interpret your cat's biting you as play, so you may wish to solicit her to play by lying down. Then sit up and dangle a ball on a string for her to strike at and/or attack instead of you. She could also be giving you an affectionate "love bite."

It is surprising to me how many people don't realize just how much cats enjoy playing. For more tips, read my book for young readers *What Is Your Cat Saying?*

DEAR DR. FOX—Our female calico, only four-months old, is a beauty, but she bites! She'll bite us when we're sitting in a chair reading the paper and she'll bite visiting strangers. We have to warn everyone. The rest of the time she chews papers, magazines, or furniture. We have been told that calicos are nasty cats. Is this true?—E.W.

DEAR E.W.—You do not have a nasty cat, just a naturally playful cat. Every young female cat wants somebody to play with, especially in the evenings, which is cat crazy-time. I would advise you to get some suitable playthings for her to chase and "kill," such as a stuffed mouse, squeaky toy, ball of wool on a string, etc. Why not play with the animal yourself? How about a frisky game of hide-and-seek? Another remedy, if you do not want to play "cat" yourself, is to purchase a kitten of the opposite sex. Two cats are much healthier and happier than one because they satisfy each other's behavioral and emotional needs more completely than their loving owners ever can.

biting (dogs)

DEAR DR. FOX—We own a female unspayed French poodle who came into our home three years ago after she had been abandoned on the expressway. She turned out to be beautiful in appearance and temperament. Ten months ago, an abandoned silver-gray French poodle wandered up on the porch. He bore all the marks of abuse, starvation, and neglect. He is affectionate and a good watchdog, but a biter, and has bitten everyone in the house for no apparent reason. He is also standoffish with strangers. If someone accidentally stands over him, he growls. What should I do.?—S.K.

DEAR S.K.—A choke-chain is an effective punishment. Put one on, attach a leash, and any and every time the dog readies to attack, shout "No," pull him up so his front legs are off the floor, and shake the leash for thirty seconds. Sounds brutal, but it often works. Also, have you tried obedience training? His behavior could have been the reason why he was abandoned in the first place. The love and care you have given him obviously haven't changed him one iota. If all fails, I suggest neutering, but euthanasia may be the ultimate solution before someone is badly bitten. However, if he is biting out of fear, be patient, cautious, and keep on loving him.

DEAR DR. FOX—Do you have any suggestions for curing our year-old miniature poodle of his nipping habit? Admittedly, the dog is spoiled, as the problem is particularly acute when he feels he's being ignored. He has been through two obedience courses and also was castrated at nine months, which did lessen his hostilities somewhat.—*E.E.C.*

DEAR E.E.C.—You have two alternatives. One is to ignore your dog compeletely. And the other is to bite your dog back when he nips hard for attention. This second measure means you must assert your dominance—not by biting your dog literally, but by snapping verbally, seizing his muzzle and the scruff of his neck, and giving him a firm shake. The other alternative—to ignore your animal—is based on the probability that when you respond to your dog's nip, you are teaching or conditioning him to nip you every time he wants attention or to get his own way. So you have two choices, and between times, have fun with your dog—on your own terms, please!

biting (parrots)

DEAR DR. FOX—Our parrot squawks whenever he wants attention. If he doesn't get it, he screams and flaps his wings in a fit of rage. He's also so insanely jealous of affection between my husband and me that he's taken to biting. What can we do short of getting rid of him?—*B.B.*

DEAR B.B.—The problems of having and being a parrot are difficult. They really belong in the wild, but of course, that's no solution for you and yours. First, don't reward the parrot's squawking with attention—it sounds like he has conditioned you! Try him on a T-bar or suitable perch with a tether on one leg. He may prefer that to being cooped up in a cage. If that fails, a companion of the opposite sex may do the trick. Parrots, being sociable and playful, do best with a cage mate. Keep them apart for a few days and introduce with caution. Chances are Polly will coo contentedly and wouldn't even want a cracker.

biting when touched (cats)

DEAR DR. FOX—My cat has started to bite me whenever I pet her, especially if I pet her too long. Do you know how I can train her not to do this? Once she bit my finger and drew blood!—*J.B.K.*

DEAR J.B.K.—Have your animal doctor examine your cat. She may have a sensitive area on her body that hurts when you touch it. Many cats and dogs have been punished inappropriately for snapping or biting defensively when, in fact, they were in considerable pain (as from a sore ear, slipped disc or bite abscess). If your cat has no physical problem, then look for some psychological quirk. Some cats can't tolerate too much contact. My new book *The Healing Touch* will give you more insights.

DEAR DR. FOX—Our tomcat was a perfect kitten for our preschooler four years ago. Now we have another child, and the tomcat is a monster! He acts like he wants attention, but when we pet him, he grabs with both paws and bites hard, usually breaking the skin. The children are afraid to play outdoors when he's around because he will actually grab them around the legs or jump up at them. What's wrong with our cat?—*P.L.F.*

DEAR P.L.F.—If he's still a tomcat, I would *de-tom* him. His male sex hormones may be making him more aggressive and domineering, and castration should help calm him down. Some neutered male cats still behave roughly and respond well when played with roughly (use gloves and a thick jacket). If it's aggression and not rough play, though, a squirt with a water pistol, preceded by a loud "No," and giving the cat its own blanket or fluffy toy may suffice. Male cats give love-bites, too, which can hurt. It's best not to get in the position where he's likely to bite you; if he does, slap his nose firmly and he'll get the hint.

biting when touched (dogs)

DEAR DR. FOX—Our dog has always loved to be petted. But lately, on a few different occasions, he has suddenly turned on my two boys and bitten them when they petted him! And they absolutely didn't tease or torment him! We've had this mutt since he was a puppy and love him, but we're worried now that this behavior might get worse. I have forbidden the children to pet him, but then he snuggles up to them and seems to look for petting.—MRS. J.M.

DEAR MRS. J.M.—Dogs who haven't been teased or otherwise abused, and still snap when being petted, should first have a physical exam. A sore, infected ear or a spinal injury could hurt badly when the animal is being petted, and so it snaps to protect itself. If your vet rules out a physical basis, then you may have to take a good hard look at your dog—much as you love him—and see if he hasn't been overindulged. Spoiled and socially maladjusted dogs will bite to assert dominance. Obedience training is then in order.

chasing cars (dogs)

DEAR DR. FOX—When we first got our German shepherd, he was nine months old and so timid he wouldn't get into a car unless he was physically lifted in, and wouldn't go in or out of a door. He overcame these fears, but now he's a car chaser. He also won't come to me or my husband when he's outside. As soon as the door is opened, Soccer takes off in the other direction. These habits are driving us up the wall. He's hyper, too.—N. & O.W.

DEAR N. & O.W.—You have a dog full of life who is obviously spoiled rotten and has yet to learn who's boss. Obedience school is a must, so you can learn to discipline him properly and he will learn to respect and obey you. There's no quick cure.

Meanwhile, keep him off the road. I've seen drivers deliberately try to hit dogs that chase their cars. A wire clothesline with Soccer attached to it by a chain will give him some running leeway and help if you can't fence him in.

DEAR DR. FOX—What can we do to keep two dogs from chasing cars? Both have been hit but still continue to chase.—T.M.

DEAR T.M.—Keep your dogs indoors. If they have to be outdoors, keep them on running lines or safely confined in a pen or well-fenced yard. Car-chasing dogs usually stop only when they have been killed or crippled. You could try aversion training, using a long leash and choke-chain collar; each time the dog goes after a car, you pull him off his feet. Some dogs soon learn not to chase cars. An alternative is to have a friend drive by with an assistant in the car who dumps a bucket of water onto your car-chasing dogs. A few repetitions may suffice. However, such conditioning procedures may not last long, and if that happens your best bet may well be to keep your dogs constantly restrained.

chasing joggers (dogs)

DEAR DR. FOX—My small dog is a mixed breed with an annoying habit: he chases joggers. Do you have any suggestions on how I can stop him from doing this?—*W.G. McW.*

DEAR *W.G. McW.*—Keep your dog on a leash, or try aversive training with a choke-chain collar and a twenty-foot leash. When your dog starts to chase a jogger, shout "No!" and pull sharply on the training leash to jerk the chain. Don't pull too hard or you may injure him. Your dog should soon learn that joggers are not fair game.

Now a word for joggers—when you meet a dog off the leash, stop running. Say "Hi," don't stare (that's a challenge), and walk slowly away after the dog has sniffed you. If the dog growls, stand still and don't run. Back away slowly and take a different route home.

DEAR DR. FOX—Our four-year-old neutered male Doberman growls and acts vicious whenever he sees a jogger or another dog. Needless to say, he's not popular in the neighborhood and causes me much anxiety. He lives in the house, has a beautiful backyard in which to play, an Irish setter playmate, and plenty of care, and he even sleeps on our bed. Why is he so neurotic?—*M.W.*

DEAR *M.W.*—Doberman pinschers need to be properly handled or they will react protectively toward you when joggers, strangers, or other dogs come by. Many people forget this important rule when they own a protective breed. In general, such breeds do not need to be attack-trained. But they do need to be obedience-trained at a school to control erratic behavior and to know when they should behave defensively and when they should behave in a friendly fashion. This is a great responsibility, and irresponsible owners have given the Doberman pinscher a bad reputation.

feeling threatened (dogs)

DEAR DR. FOX—My two-year-old cocker spaniel likes to sit underneath the coffee table. When I approach the sofa to sit down and read, he barks and tries to bite me. It isn't until I am finally settled that he comes out, asking to be petted. I have had to keep him out of the room to avoid these confrontations. Is he jealous of my reading and not paying attention to him?—*H.L.V.*

DEAR *H.L.V.*—Your interpretation is correct—to a point. But it's not jealousy. Some cocker spaniels become hysterical and go into a bizarre, ragelike reaction if they feel cornered and threatened, which is what is occurring when he gets under the table and you approach the sofa. Try moving the coffee table well away from the sofa so he can crawl under and not feel threatened by your proximity. He may also respond to a two- or three-week period of tranquilizer medication.

"killer animal" myth

DEAR DR. FOX—I've just finished reading a book (soon to be a movie) called *Killer Dogs*, which reminded me of *Jaws*. What do you think about books like this?—*H.R.*

DEAR *H.R.*—Such books are trite tripe and a waste of time and money. There are too many TV shows, movies, and books about "killer animals"—rats, rabbits, sharks, dogs, pigs—you name it. They demean animals and create negative myths about them. What is needed is more understanding and compassion. Instead of creating fictional "killer dogs," the people who produce such trash should quake before some of our own creations like pollutants and nuclear reactors.

protective behavior (dogs)

DEAR DR. FOX—I have a small dog that is part spitz-part terrier, as well as a beautiful German shepherd, and they dearly love each other. We have a huge fenced-in yard for them, and every time a dog comes by, the spitz jumps the fence and starts a fight, no matter what size the other dog is. Of course, the German shepherd climbs over to help his buddy, and they have almost killed a couple of dogs. I don't want to chain my spitz. What can I do?—*S.S.*

DEAR S.S.—Breeders knew years ago that it could be dangerous to have a large, volatile dog around, so the larger dogs were, as a rule, bred to be easygoing. Smaller dogs, however, who could not do so much harm to people, were bred to be more aggressive. Combine this terrier temperament with a dog's natural territorial instinct to threaten or attack a dog who trespasses, then add the packing-instinct (where one dog follows another), and you have trouble. Put up a higher fence or keep your terrier on a running line away from the fence. Other dogs clearly need protection from your canine "terrierist."

DEAR DR. FOX—My husband is a doctor, and sometimes he works nights. He wants to get two Doberman pinschers to protect me and our baby son while he is away. However, our friends are warning us that all Dobermans eventually turn on their owners. Is this true?—*E.R.*

DEAR E.R.—*Any* dog who comes from an emotionally unstable line or who hasn't been properly raised from puppyhood could "turn" on its master or other member of the household. Dobermans are just as likely or unlikely to "turn" as are most other breeds. So what to do? Get the Dobe to basic obedience school. A well-bred Doberman will be naturally protective; it just needs to learn to be controlled, and its owner needs to learn how to control it.

DEAR DR. FOX—I'm a twelve-year-old girl. Recently my dog, Brandy, has been attacking my older brother when he comes home late at night. During the day Gary (my brother) and Brandy get along so well it's impossible to think the dog could turn on him. Gary loves and takes care of him more than anyone in the family. My parents say that if Brandy doesn't straighten up, they'll put him away. I told them that if that happens, I'll never speak to them again. (We are a very close family.) Oh, please, Dr. Fox, tell me the cause of Brandy's behavior, because if he dies, I don't think I could live any longer.—*DESPERATE*

DEAR DESPERATE—I congratulate you for seeking professional help by writing to me. Only too often, parents and other pet owners give up too soon when they have a pet problem that doesn't fix itself and get rid of their pet without finding professional help.

First, I suggest that when your brother comes home late, have him call out to your pooch in a friendly voice before he opens the door. Second, your brother and your dog should go see a good dog trainer (or pet therapist) along with the rest of your family. Your local humane society or veterinarian may be able to help you find such professional help. Unfortunately, there aren't enough "doggy social workers" to go around.

protective behavior (rabbits)

DEAR DR. FOX—My rabbit, Buzzy, is four months old and has suddenly started to attack me. I feed and water him every day and always give him carrots. He was brought up in a rabbit-house, but I let him out recently and now he'll only go in again for a couple of minutes. I have scratches on my hands, neck, and arms, and also a bite from trying to control Buzzy. What should I do?—*TROU-BLED*

DEAR TROUBLED—Buzzy is turning into a territorial tough guy. When maturing, rabbits—especially bucks—often become less cuddly and act aggressively when their cage or hutch is approached and "invaded." Don't discipline him physically, or else he will just fight more. Say, "No, bad Buzzy!" and try to stress positive behavior. How do you do that? You hold out a carrot for him, and coax him to feed from your hand. That way he'll come to see you as the loving provider. Don't put food down for him until after he has been good, otherwise you will be rewarding his aggressive behavior. With time and appropriate handling, he should grow out of his adolescent buck-bravado. Incidentally, wear a long-sleeved jacket and gloves when handling Buzzy.

same-sex tensions (cats)

DEAR DR. FOX—Is it natural for two tomcats in a home to fight all the time?—*CAT LOVER*

DEAR CAT LOVER—Tomcats that have not been neutered will often fight with each other as adults. Fighting declines once they work out which one is boss. But even then, one or both may mark parts of the house with their urine—as a way of declaring their territory. You should consider having both cats neutered. If they don't improve after three to four months following surgery, it might then be advisable to find a good home for one of them. Two toms often can mean one tom too many.

same-sex tensions (dogs)

DEAR DR. FOX—I have two large Labradors who dislike each other so much they will fight to kill. When my son attempted to stop them, he got bitten in the ankle. A year ago, I had one altered, hoping that would change things, but they still fight if they're together. Is there anything I can do?—*MRS. R.H.*

DEAR MRS. R.H.—Many people who own more than one dog of the same sex have the same problem. When there are two dogs, they want to kill each other, and if there are three, it ends up with two picking on one. I am told by older vets that in the past this was not a problem, so perhaps some dog breeds are becoming more aggressive. Another possibility is that owners today are not assuming the dominant role to effectively police and inhibit rivalry and fighting in their dogs.

Dogs, especially of the same sex, will often fight until they settle which one is dominant, after which the relationship is tense but peaceful. However, this is unlikely in many breeds of dogs, and if left to it some dogs will fight to the kill. This may well be the case with your dogs, and I, for one, would not risk letting them work it out for themselves. Generally, the only solution when you have two fighters in the home is to find another home for one of them.

struggle for dominance (cats)

DEAR DR. FOX—Every time my cat doesn't get the food he wants (or sometimes for no reason at all), he attacks my eight-year-old brother and scratches him up a bit. My brother won't fight back. What should we do? I am afraid my parents will have the cat put to sleep.—*B.D.D.*

DEAR B.D.D.—Your brother must learn to be dominant over your surly feline family member. Tell him to wave around a rolled-up newspaper or occasionally use a water pistol—they will build up the confidence he needs. If your cat doesn't go outdoors, you could have him declawed. That's a better alternative than having him destroyed.

Cats rarely bite, preferring to swipe out when angry or frustrated. He will still vent his spleen by lashing out and will be satisfied that he's made his point, but he won't be able to scratch anyone up.

DEAR DR. FOX—Our male cat attacks me if I pet him, but he doesn't attack anyone else in the family. Yet I am the only one who feeds him. I never hit or abuse him, and still he won't let me touch him. What makes him hate me?—A CAT FRIEND

DEAR CAT FRIEND—You must feel quite rejected by the cat who swats the hand that feeds him. I would not go so far as to say the cat "hates" you. My guess is that he thinks of you as the "top cat" in the home because you feed him and seem to control everything. He's letting you know that you can't be top cat all the time. While you are the one that decides when, where, and what he may eat, for example, he may well want to feel he has some control over you in return, and so won't let you pet him. My advice is to ignore him. Chances are he'll eventually come to you to be petted. If not, no matter—at least you understand why he's being so standoffish.

struggle for dominance (dogs)

DEAR DR. FOX—We have a very large two-year-old German shepherd who is extremely defensive. He will not let us put on or take off a choke collar and usually prefers not to have anyone touch him. Our vet tells us that he could be trained by a professional, but there are none in this area. Should we have him put away to protect ourselves and others?—S.B.

DEAR S.B.—Your dog could be "head shy," a consequence of early improper handling or inadequate socialization. It is imperative that large dogs be brought up to regard their owner as leader and to be obedient and submissive. Your dog is reaching full maturity now, and he could become a "delinquent," dominating the family and always getting his own way through intimidation. You can't allow that to happen. Find him a good home with an experienced handler, or do your best to find an obedience school for both of you. Delinquents—canine or human—can be dangerous when crossed and are a menace to society. Neutering may help, since as male dogs reach sexual maturity, they often become more assertive, seeking "top dog" position in the home.

sudden personality changes (cats)

DEAR DR. FOX—Recently, for no reason at all, when he was sitting on my lap, my beautiful three-year-old cat suddenly attacked my arm and lacerated my hand, with such force that it swelled up and the whole arm turned black and blue. What can I do to prevent another incident like this?—P.C.

DEAR P.C.—Some cats have a Jekyll-and-Hyde reaction when being petted, switching from placid friendliness to wild aggression. Then, when the tantrum is over, they act as though nothing happened. Some cats do this when their stomach is being touched; others will react when some other area of their body is touched. It's important for you to learn which is the "trigger" area, and avoid touching it. Many cats seem to need this kind of spontaneous discharge because they're understimulated. So give your cat some furry toys to kill and chase—throw them for him to catch and even retrieve, and attach one to a string for you to pull so he can hunt and kill.

If your cat hasn't yet been neutered, this too might help. And if you were wearing a perfume containing civet cat musk, that could well have triggered the attack. So be careful how you smell.

sudden personality changes (dogs)

DEAR DR. FOX—The majority of the time our Shetland sheepdog is affectionate and friendly. But at times he appears to have a dual personality. If he's startled or if you just step on his foot he gets nervous and will suddenly turn vicious and bite with no warning. Then, just as quickly, he'll be trying to make up to you—sometimes you can actually see the realization cross his face of what he's doing. We got him from the pet shop when he was four months old. So is it possible he underwent some sort of emotional-physical trauma during that time?—*D.W.*

DEAR D.W.—Your dog has an unstable temperament rather than a dual personality. He has little inhibition when it comes to behaving aggressively. While indeed prior emotional trauma could underlie this problem, in my experience traumatized dogs usually manifest more fear than overt aggression. I would therefore advise you to assert your dominance over the dog, and consider taking him to obedience school. This may not help, however, if he is hysterical by nature. Euthanasia may be the sad solution if very careful handling doesn't prevent his outbreaks.

DEAR DR. FOX—My pedigreed, high-strung cocker spaniel always barks when people arrive at our house. Then she calms down and acts friendly, but when they get ready to leave, she acts terrible, growling and snarling at them. What makes her so friendly one minute and vicious the next?—*MRS. W.H.*

DEAR MRS. W.H.—Many dogs act up just this way when guests are ready to leave, and my advice is simply to put your dog into another room before farewell rituals are exchanged. We can't be sure why dogs act this way. Perhaps they get jealous when their owner interacts with the departing visitors by kissing or handshaking. Or they may behave aggressively because they feel that the visitors' leaving is a sign of submission. Such behavior does seem schizoid.

Try ignoring your dog when next people visit. Enlist your friends' help and stand up together three or four times way before they are due to leave. This may break the dog's possibly conditioned reaction sufficiently that he will eventually be able to bid people good-bye like a normal pooch.

NURSING BEHAVIOR

drooling (cats)

DEAR DR. FOX—My cat slobbers so much that we hate to pick him up, because we end up wet! Is this normal?—*J.D.*

DEAR J.D.—Many cats slobber a good deal when they're being petted. It's regression—behaving like a kitten and making nursing movements when petted. This is not unnatural, so don't punish your cat. Excessive drooling and smelly, sometimes even bloody, salivation mean your cat has gingivitis, infected gums. This is an all-too-common problem that cat owners easily overlook until the cat is so sick that its mouth is too sore for the cat to eat comfortably.

kneading (cats)

DEAR DR. FOX—Could you explain why there's a difference among our three cats? Seven-year-old Puck is a "kneader," and every night he will come to bed with us and knead his paws against my arm, often until he falls asleep. If I stretch out on the couch, he is there in a flash, digging right in. Ariel curls up in my lap and kneads against my stomach, once or twice a week. Poppy has *never* been a kneader. However, he is extremely affectionate. Does kneading behavior have anything to do with the way the kitten was nursed?—J.N.

DEAR J.N.—Just like people, felines have very different temperaments or personalities, which are a combined product of genetic lineage (parental traits being inherited) and of early experiences in life. There are sex differences, too: male humans and cats tend to be more assertive and aggressive, thanks to the male sex hormone. Your two cats who like to "nurse" on you before going to sleep are behaving quite normally. But as you correctly surmise, such behavior can stem from early separation from the mother. Traumatic weaning affects cats and people alike, and pets abandoned in infancy often bear the scars into mataurity. My own dog Benji is a throwaway pet from the St. Louis Humane Society, and even though he's been with us for seven years now, he still has a fit whenever he sees us going out. He doesn't want to be abandoned again.

nursing on blanket (dogs)

DEAR DR. FOX—I have a ten-month-old small mongrel who I took from his mother after six weeks. He keeps sucking on a bedspread or blanket. We can see his mouth moving as though he were nursing. Why does he do this, and is there a cure?—MRS. R.H.

DEAR MRS. R.H.—Sometimes pups aren't quite ready to be completely weaned at six weeks. Others, although ready, seem to suffer from maternal separation and often develop a habit of using a towel or blanket as a surrogate mother to nurse on and cuddle into. Your dog has a not uncommon oral vice (like many humans, too).

Don't think he's crazy, and don't take his fetish away, or else he may suffer and develop more serious problems. Often, it's best to give such a pet his very own blanket, and just replace it with a new one as needed.

nursing on companion animal (cats)

DEAR DR. FOX—My vet is at a loss with the problem of my two Siamese cats. When I got my female she was six weeks old, and she and my five-month-old male got along great. But she started to nurse on him, and to my surprise he let her and actually enjoyed it. He is now nine months old and has been neutered, and she is going on six months (has adult teeth) and is about to be spayed. But this strange behavior still continues. Her nursing is so loud that it wakes me out of my sleep, and he purrs away with content. I have used bitters and other unpleasant-tasting things, but it doesn't help.—B.S.

DEAR B.S.—It is not unusual for cats to nurse on each other. In fact, it's a sign of affection, even if it sometimes seems to be neurotic. Let your cats enjoy each other, and don't worry. If your male "nurse" gets sore, he'll let his lady cat know. Don't go out of your way to frustrate her oral cravings, because she could turn into a chewer—nibbling and sucking on your woolen clothes, drapes, and carpets. Siamese have expensive habits.

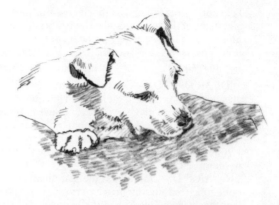

nursing on owner (cats)

DEAR DR. FOX—Fritz, my two-year-old tabby, must think I'm his mama. Whenever I lie down, he comes over to lick my earlobes, all the while purring away. Sometimes I think he does it to let me know he's hungry, because right after he "nurses" (that's what the vet calls it) he goes past his food dish and rubs up against it.—*CONFUSED HUMAN*

DEAR CONFUSED HUMAN—I'm glad you wrote about your "problem." Many cat owners find it too embarrassing to mention or concede they have a neurotic cat. Actually, it's quite natural for some adult cats to "regress" and act like little kittens—nursing while they are being petted. Some cats not only knead with their feet as though massaging their mother's nipples, they also drool. Cats that have been weaned too soon or who have been bottle-nursed are very prone to show this nursing behavior as adults. My answer is, live with it. If you really can't stand it, brush Fritz instead of petting him. Give him less tender loving care in your arms.

nursing on themselves (cats)

DEAR DR. FOX—We have a kitten who is about three months old. He has an annoying habit of sucking on the end of his tail. We've put tape and even hot sauce on it, but nothing makes him stop.—*MRS. D.T.*

DEAR MRS. D.T.—I think what your kitten does is cute and adds to its character. A soggy tip of tail makes quite a conversation piece. It is amazing how we dislike those things that might reflect negatively on us.

I'm sure no one would think ill of you for owning a tail-chomping cat. Indeed, they could become fashionable. Your kitten enjoys sucking his tail (he was probably weaned too soon)—so let him be. No more Tabasco and Band-Aids. With time, he may grow out of it.

nursing on themselves (dogs)

DEAR DR. FOX—I have an eleven-year-old cockapoo who is trying to nurse herself. She has a tumor near one nipple about the size of a quarter, which is lumpy and puffed. She has had puppies twice several years ago. How can I stop her from trying to nurse herself? Should the tumor be removed?—*MRS. M.C.*

DEAR MRS. M.C.—Your dog seems to have two problems that may be interrelated. The tumor may need to be removed and your dog spayed, which may help stop further tumor growth. Her self-nursing may be triggered by the irritation and shape of the tumor, or else she has begun this self-nursing because of a hormonal imbalance (spaying may help), or because she simply enjoys self-stimulation. If the latter is the case, let her be, but in the interim, have her examined by a veterinarian.

DEAR DR. FOX—Our four-month-old Doberman is healthy and affectionate and has never lacked for love and attention. But she will bunch her soft bed blanket or a towel into her mouth and suck or nurse, kneading her paws just as a pup will do when suckling the mother. This occurs particularly during the evenings. At times she will also take her rear quarter in her mouth and suck on that. Her mother suffered from an infection when the litter was born, and the puppies never nursed.—B.D.

DEAR B.D.—Sucking on the rear quarters or flank is a definite Doberman quirk, triggered often by anxiety or frustration. Some suck their sides so frequently that they become blemished. Dobermans and other kinds of dogs will make a "nipple" out of a blanket as a comforter. All the cases I have encountered have the same background as yours: mother-deprived, bottle-raised. I wonder how Dr. Sigmund Freud would have interpreted such orality.

nursing on wool (cats)

DEAR DR. FOX—HELP!!! Our cat is literally eating us out of house and home! We have massive holes in our wool blankets and in nine wool sweaters, two wool blazers, and three wool sports coats. If he's in the yard and you pick him up, he closes his eyes and attacks the sweater you have on.—L.D.

DEAR L.D.—You have one of those Siamese afflicted with "nursitis"—it often goes with the breed. Punishment generally intensifies the problem, so that's out. Boredom is often a factor, so a kitten for company may do the trick, plus an aquarium of fish and a bird-feeder by a window where the cat can look out ("feline TV"). The ultimate solution is to give the cat something of its own to chew on, such as a large towel, but in that case stay on the alert for constipation and/or, more serious, intestinal blockage.

pacifiers (cats)

DEAR DR. FOX—My nine-month-old cat seems to need a pacifier. Is there anything I can do to make him stop?—L.H.

DEAR L.H.—Some cats enjoy a pacifier, so why deny it to them? Why don't you just give your cat his own blanket of similar material so that he can tent it up to make a "nipple" to chomp on? Kittens that have been weaned too early or that have been bottle-raised will often seek substitute pacifiers when they get older. It's better than smoking.

shredding paper (cats)

DEAR DR. FOX—My one-year-old spayed Persian cat was born and raised indoors. My problem is that he loves paper towels and toilet paper and will shred them if I don't lock them away. He also paws and sucks on my hand towel. What's with him?—MRS. P.C.

DEAR MRS. P.C.—He needs something to nurse on. The feel, the texture, and possibly the odor triggers his needy, quite natural, kittenish behavior. We all like to regress sometimes, and this is a regressive feline form of self-indulgence.

Try giving him a wad of rolled-up newspapers or a wool blanket rolled up to serve as a mother surrogate. This kind of behavior seems more prevalent in kittens weaned too early in life. Kittens should stay with their mothers until at least eight weeks of age. A companion cat may help yours mature and cope better with the ennui of home life.

LICKING AND CHEWING

aluminum cans (dogs)

DR. DEAR FOX—My Labrador retriever is crazy about aluminum cans. She pulls them out of the garbage and chews on them. She has another dog to play with, so she can't be bored. Is she missing some vitamin? Please help. I'm so tired of picking up aluminum pieces all over the yard.—N.F.

DEAR N.F.—Your dog has acquired a penchant for aluminum cans because they prove so much fun to chew. Reminds me of those human macho types who make a big deal about crushing a beer can with two fingers—it's a game. She probably like the crunching sounds her teeth make. However, you'll have to discourage her, since I've seen more than one dog with lacerated gums and tongue from ripping into aluminum cans. Simply store them in an inaccessible place rather than the garbage pail, and then take them to a recycling plant. If you can train your retriever to retrieve aluminum cans *whole* (by giving her a treat or other reward), then you will be doing a service to your community. Our parks are being ruined by mindless litterbugs who leave trails of cans everywhere.

bedding (dogs)

DEAR DR. FOX—I have a black-and-tan dachshund who will not stop chewing holes in the pads I put in his basket. I have put in everything from bedspreads to shag rugs, and Schnappsie gradually chews them too. Now I am thinking of using newspapers. He also seems to be more nervous than our other dogs, although he's been treated the same way.—M.O.M.

DEAR M.O.M.—Schnappsie's excessive oral behavior may be a form of play and response to boredom or a reaction to anxiety or conflict. They are probably all related to his temperament. I suggest you initiate some play therapy—encourage him to "kill" an old towel or sheet and try to get him to have a tug-of-war. A rawhide chew toy could also help reduce some of his compulsive oral behavior. He may chew more when he's jealous of your attentions to the other dogs. So be discreet. As for his basket, I would stick to using newspapers.

cage bars (gerbils)

DEAR DR. FOX—I read in a book that gerbils aren't nocturnal, but they sure don't mind keeping me awake every night. They have a cage with bars around it, and they chew on them all night. Also, one of them seems to be overweight. How can I put it on a diet?—S.P.

DEAR S.P.—Give your gerbils some pieces of bark or dead tree branches to gnaw on. Such material will keep their teeth trim and make less noise than when your pets chew on metal cage bars. Some gerbils enjoy an activity wheel, and this may help your overweight one get back into shape. As gerbils age they often become overweight, and a lack of physical activity is a contributing factor, just as it is with people.

cage bars (hamsters)

DEAR DR. FOX—Is it normal for a hamster to bite on the metal bars of his cage? Does he want to get my attention so I will let him out? When I turn on the lights, he always bites on the bars. How can I stop him?—L.D.

DEAR L.D.—You have conditioned your hamster to wake up and expect attention when you switch on the light. This excitement is in part expressed by him chewing on the cage bars.

The attention you give then reinforces his bar-chewing, and so the cycle goes on. However, hamsters do need a hard piece of wood or a bone to gnaw on in their cages. This helps them keep their teeth trim. All hamster and gerbil owners should provide such items for their pets to prevent overgrown teeth and subsequent serious complications.

car seats (dogs)

DEAR DR. FOX—Our seventeen-year-old dog has the habit of licking the top and back section of the front seat of the car. How can we stop her from doing this? Especially since we now have a new car.—H.E.

DEAR H.E.—Anxiety can be expressed in many different ways. Instead of licking, your dog could also have developed a habit of panting excessively, whining, jumping to and fro, or even chewing her paws whenever she went for a car ride.

Considering her age, I would let licking dogs lick. Get some plastic seat covers or try to desensitize her by simply sitting in the car with her. With the engine switched off, go nowhere for the first week. Then switch on the engine for ten or fifteen minutes a day for a subsequent week in the car together. During the third week, drive slowly around the block. Such treatment has helped many dogs overcome excitement and anxiety associated with a ride in the car.

carpet (rabbits)

DEAR DR. FOX—My three-and-a-half-year-old rabbit has been trained to use the litter box and is a wonderful, clean house pet. The only problem is that she loves to eat my carpet and has consumed most of the fringe on a large area rug. I've added new fringe, but it's time consuming, and there comes a time when you can do only so much repairing. I've put down pepper and sprayed with bitter apple, but nothing helps. Can you?—MRS. C.L.

DEAR MRS. C.L.—You certainly have a smart bunny—housebroken and all. But rabbits will be rabbits, and a carpet could be like a meadow to him—something to nibble and dig up. So far as I can see, it's up to you—either no rabbit or no carpet. Or else choose some other floor material that will suit you both. Be sure to give him a mineral block and a hunk of wood to chew on, as well.

carrying objects around (dogs)

DEAR DR. FOX—Our Labrador retriever is the ideal pup—friendly, frisky, and quiet—except that she chews or tries to carry such items as logs, rocks, and dog dishes in her mouth. We have unsuccessfully tried many methods to break this habit. Any ideas?—J.F.W.

DEAR J.F.W.—The only way to stop a Labrador retriever from carrying things in its mouth is to make it into something that is not a Labrador retriever. That, of course, is impossible. Your dog is following her natural instincts, which have been intensified through selective breeding. Provided she does not damage her teeth or wear them down by chewing on things that she carries, do not worry about her oral behavior.

You should, however, be careful about her carrying small objects, like rocks or golf balls; they could cause intestinal damage if swallowed. If you can't control this last aspect, you might resort to a shock collar to desensitize her from carrying things, although I personally would never use such a device except for deeply ingrained behaviors. You should give her suitable toys, such as an old shoe or a knotted towel, to carry. These will distract her from going after possible hazardous objects.

cloth (cats)

DEAR DR. FOX—Rudy, our mixed-breed cat, chews and swallows chunks of potholders and washcloths. We have to keep doors closed at night so that he cannot get to them. Can you tell us the probable cause and solution to our problem? Incidentally, Rudy has been declawed, and we never let him out.—*J.M.S.*

DEAR J.M.S.—Many cats, especially Siamese, chew on various cloth materials, possibly out of boredom or as a need to obtain more roughage in the diet. Rudy would do better with a little fresh grass (or home-grown wheat), which he would eat if he could get outdoors. Boredom does seem to be related to this vice in some cats; it is common in active but understimulated cats confined indoors. Also, cats who are weaned too early often become chewers of wool or cloth.

cloth (dogs)

DEAR DR. FOX—My seven-year-old Chihuahua licks the bed sheets, the furniture covers, the shag carpets, and the kitchen and bathroom rugs. Why?— *MRS. F.D.*

DEAR MRS. F.D.—Provided your dog is on a good-quality balanced diet that includes some fresh, lightly cooked meat or fish, I doubt that she has any nutritional problem causing her licking. I have consulted with many pet owners who have nonproblem lickers just like yours. This behavior is more prevalent in females and in dogs that have a hyper temperament.

But in order to be sure that this is simply a neurotic obsession, have your veterinarian examine your dog. A bone stuck between teeth or tonsillitis can cause similar reactions. If there is no organic cause, get your pet some raw beef bones to chew and live with it. Also make sure all polishes and other household chemicals you use are nontoxic.

electrical cords (cats)

DEAR DR. FOX—My Siamese cat gets into many things, but her habit of chewing on electrical cords worries me the most. Since I work, she is alone all day and has the run of the house.—*B.B.*

DEAR B.B.—Siamese cats are especially oral, and this behavior could be a sign of boredom and frustration at being left alone for extended periods. A companion cat may be the answer, specifically a kitten of the opposite sex. As a protective measure, you should also coat all extension cords with Tabasco or hot pepper sauce, and provide your cat with a length of telephone extension cable to chew on. In addition to being nontoxic, the cable won't break and can't be swallowed. It's certainly a lot safer than a live wire!

electrical cords (rabbits)

DEAR DR. FOX—Is it dangerous for a rabbit to eat the needles and bottom branches of a Christmas tree? Also, what about icicles? Last year she enjoyed them both. She also seems to enjoy chewing electrical cords.—*M.Mc.*

DEAR M.Mc.—Christmas trees are not poisonous unless they've recently been sprayed with an insecticide or fire-retardant. I see no reason why your rabbit shouldn't be allowed to nibble on pine needles. Icicles, though usually not toxic in small amounts, should be kept out of your rabbit's reach. As for electrical cords—they are a no-no. Many pets have been severely burned and some killed by biting into electrical cords. Furthermore, a damaged cord could electrocute you or cause a house fire. Coating them with Tabasco or hot pepper sauce or threading them through brass curtain rods should frustrate that habit.

everything! (dogs)

DEAR DR. FOX—Our Airedale constantly eats foreign objects—wood, cloth, paper—even the bulbs from the Christmas tree. The vet gave him Pet Tabs to correct a possible diet deficiency, but they had no effect. He is an otherwise healthy and strong dog. Can you help?—*J.C.*

DEAR J.C.—Some dogs never seem to grow out of their puppy behavior and have to chew, taste, and even swallow anything they find. This vice is called pica, and it can lead to serious internal problems, including bowel obstruction or perforation from sharp, penetrating material.

Give your dog his very own safe toys to play with and chew on. Then after he has played with them a few days and identifies them as his own, set these toys and some "no-no's" on the floor. Use a choke chain and snap him correctively any time he takes anything into his mouth that isn't his. Shout "No" before you correct him. If he's not a real dimwit, he should learn with time.

DEAR DR. FOX—My poodle licks the woodwork, paneling, upholstery, aluminum doors, windows, anything she can reach. I have asked the vet about it, but he just shrugs it off. I'm afraid she'll get a sliver in her tongue. She has already received a shock from licking the wall socket, but that didn't deter her. Why all this licking?—*L.B.*

DEAR L.B.—This is a bizarre neurotic trait that is not all that uncommon. Boredom and a lack of regular exercise and play may be a factor. Encourage her to chew some rawhide strips. On the other hand, irritation in the mouth and throat can lead to excessive licking in order to relieve the discomfort. So have your dog's teeth, gums, and tonsils checked by your vet for infection. As a last resort, coat her favorite licking spots with jalapeño pepper juice or Tabasco sauce, or muzzle her for a few days to break the habit.

lotions (cats)

DEAR DR. FOX—My orange, short-haired cat, whom I treasure very much, enjoys licking lotions and powders off of my body. Can you please tell me if this is safe for him? Tiger is indoors except when I take him outside on his leash, and he's getting heavy. How much is a six-year-old cat supposed to weigh?—*MS. P.U.*

DEAR MS. P.U.—Some cats do get quite fat with an adipose skin fold in their groins that looks almost like a hernia. More exercise (a companion kitten might help) and a restricted diet are in order. As for body powders and creams, don't let your cat get carried away, simply because some chemicals may be harmful.

Odors seem to turn cats on, and we don't know why. But we do know that many protein-enriched creams and shampoos contain byproducts from slaughtered farm animals, and these may be attractive to both cats and dogs. For aesthetic reasons, I would stick to vegetable-based cosmetics.

paper (birds)

DEAR DR. FOX—My canary eats the newspaper on the bottom of his cage. Will this harm him?—*M.H.*

DEAR *M.H.*—Many birds will shred and chew on newspaper as a source of amusement. They need such materials to enrich their bland cage environment and to provide themselves with something to play with and manipulate. If you are certain that your canary is actually eating newspaper in quantity, give him some hay instead, but remove that too if he eats too much of it.

Eating bulk cellulose can upset the bird's nutritional balance because when he feels full, he won't eat more nutritious foods. Your bird may simply need more toys (that he can't swallow), more exercise, and some fresh greens and fruit to play with in addition to his regular seed.

paper (dogs)

DEAR DR. FOX—My dog has a habit of eating paper napkins. He also likes to eat paper bags and rags. Since he's well fed, we can't understand why he does this. One of my friends says my dog must have worms, which make him crave paper. Is that true?—*L.B.*

DEAR *L.B.*—Not so strange a habit; I've heard of people who eat newspapers, notably one lady in England who enjoys hers with salt and vinegar! Paper napkins won't harm your dog. He probably enjoys shredding them, and a little roughage will do his system good. It's a myth that worms make dogs eat unusual things. You should encourage your dog to enjoy other chewy objects that may be more satisfying, such as a large beef knucklebone or a hard, large dog biscuit.

people (birds)

DEAR DR. FOX—One of my budgerigars is always nibbling on my hands and fingers. If I take him out of the cage, he bites my hand and does nothing else. And if I put my hand into the cage, he jumps on it and starts to bite it. It hurts a lot, but he pays no attention to my orders. Help!—*S.C.*

DEAR *S.C.*—Your budgie is nibbling on your fingers probably because he is feeling playful and perhaps also wants to preen you, which is friendly social behavior. Some birds get carried away and nibble too much and too hard, and can be very difficult to retrain. Give him plenty of exercise, don't feed him from your hand, and try this trick: get two or three rubber thimbles to go on your fingers. Your bird will be attracted and can then play with your fingers to his beak's content.

people (cats)

DEAR DR. FOX—Do you find it peculiar that my young tomcat chews on my fingertips when I pet him? Thomas is a shy cat who refuses to come in the house, never picks fights with my other toms, and runs away from other people. Is this behavior strange or not?—*N.H.D.*

DEAR *N.H.D.*—It is unusual for a cat to chew fingertips while being petted. Some will rub their lips on your hand to mark you with their scent and then sometimes give a chomp or two. Sounds like your cat is getting a little too carried away. But no matter, if he doesn't break the skin.

As for his shy behavior, you said it yourself—he's young and not fully mature yet. Give him a few more months and you'll be complaining to me about his spraying, caterwauling, and going out to fight as soon as he heals from the last fight.

people (dogs)

DEAR DR. FOX—We gave our grandson a cockapoo. She is a loving and adorable dog, except for one fault—anyone she likes, she licks constantly. Can she be trained out of this habit?—F.H.

DEAR F.H.—I know just what you mean. My own mutt, Benji, often goes on a licking binge, and it is an obnoxious habit. But humans created it by making dogs subservient and dependent. Licking is submissive canine kissing. What we have done is turn the wolf into a puppy—a licking, simpering, infantalizing ball of fluffy dependence. Don't reinforce the habit by responding when the dog licks you, and transfer some of the discipline she understands to this situation. Say "No" firmly and consistently when she licks. She'll get the idea in time.

DEAR DR. FOX—My six-year-old husky-shepherd mix and my one-year-old daughter are best of friends. Our dog licks our baby all day long, from head to toe. Although I don't encourage licking on the mouth, I don't see the harm in this. My mother-in-law and sister are appalled and insist that the dog has terrible germs that will spread to the baby. Is there any truth in their claim?—J.S.

DEAR J.S.—You and your relatives are both half-right. A dog's saliva actually has healing qualities. But, like human saliva, it can be a transmission source of infection.

While human saliva and sneezes over your baby are more worrisome than canine saliva, I think you should be prudent and allow your dog to give only a few licks every day. Teach your child to wash her hands and face well always before eating.

plaster and cement (cats)

DEAR DR. FOX—Here is a dilly. My nine-year-old cat breaks his meal to go down to the cellar to lick the cement blocks. Then he comes back and finishes the meal. He's been doing this for years. Is he crazy—or what?—M.K.

DEAR M.K.—That is a dilly! Indeed, often I wonder about the possibility of some commercial catfoods not containing all the right ingredients for certain cats. Not all cats (like people) have exactly the same nutrient requirements. Your cat may be showing what's called nutritional wisdom—instinctively correcting for a salt or other mineral deficiency in his diet. Or he could simply have a "vice" and like the taste or the alkalinity of the cement. My neighbor's cat enjoys licking plastic wrapping. You're lucky your cat is none the worse for his addiction, so that you don't have the problem of weaning him off it.

plastics and glue (cats)

DEAR DR. FOX—My cat, Orion, a brown tabby, has some bizarre habits that I worry about. He licks glue from envelopes. He also licks and chomps on color photos. These, too, I have to keep hidden. He'll eat them all up if I don't stop him. I worry about his ingesting such materials.—S.C.

DEAR S.C.—One of my own cats is just as "bizarre" as your cat. He also enjoys licking various materials such as photographs, plastics, and glue from envelopes. Plastic has a sweet flavor that cats find attractive. Other materials, such as glue and certain photographic materials, contain animal products from slaughterhouses that are probably attractive to certain felines. Just hide your photos and envelopes and stop worrying if there's an occasional raid on them.

DEAR DR. FOX—My two-year-old cat often chews on plastic bags. Does that mean she is lacking something in her diet?—LINDY

DEAR LINDY—My Abyssinian cat likes to lick plastic bags too, and I wish I knew why. Cats develop odd oral cravings; some will lick plaster or cement or chew on blankets and brooms. More roughage in the diet, such as fresh grass or sprouted wheat, helps in some instances, but nothing has helped my Sam.

Plastic is a petroleum product and may contain harmful chemicals. I would advise you to keep all plastics away from your cat. I try to do this with Sam. I'm sorry I don't have a more definitive answer.

puppies' oral habits

DEAR DR. FOX—Our two-month-old puppy will not stop chewing things. We've tried everything. What shall we do?—T.M.B.

DEAR T.M.B.—It's natural for pups to chew things, especially when they, like babies, are teething. So let him chew, but please, you must protect him from any objects that might injure him, splinter when chewed, etc. Keep electrical extension cords hidden away or unplugged. Bitter apple or Tabasco sauce protects table and chair legs.

Try to keep the pup in one room that is safe and give him his own toys to chew on, such as an old shoe, a sock, or a raw beef bone. Rawhides cured in the United States are safe, but don't buy small pieces that could be swallowed whole, causing internal complications.

themselves (dogs)

DEAR DR. FOX—I have a little six-year-old terrier-cross dog. She has developed an annoying habit that my veterinarian considers neurotic, since she is otherwise healthy. She will lick for extended periods of time, her tongue darting in and out of her mouth rapidly, curling up toward her nose. She does this when she's inactive and when I'm petting her. The behavior started last summer, after we got a Labrador puppy.—M.M.

DEAR M.M.—Considering that you can pinpoint the sudden appearance of this neurotic activity with getting a new puppy, I would interpret your dog's behavior as a reaction to the latter—apprehension, excitement, or jealousy.

Once a habit like this develops, it is difficult to correct. The "hard" approach is negative conditioning (a loud "No!" and a quick squirt with a plant mister each time the dog licks). A "softer" approach is to give the dog a tranquilizer or anxiety-reducing drug for several days.

A third option is to live with it, since your dog has found her own outlet for her frustration or jealousy. But in any case, pile on the love and attention.

tobacco (dogs)

DEAR DR. FOX—Perhaps you can psychoanalyze my toy poodle, Mitzy Pooh. I smoke and Mitzy Pooh chews tobacco. She goes around getting butts out of ashtrays in my living room and bedroom, and even opens my cigarette pouches with her teeth to get a "fix." At times, she can chew a whole package to bits. She mainly chews on filter tips, and often throws up as a result. I can't break her of the habit, and after two years I am ready to give up.—M.D.M.

DEAR M.D.M.—Nicotine is poisonous to dogs and can cause convulsions and respiratory paralysis, so I hope you smoke low-nicotine cigarettes. I have learned through my column that many dogs become addicted to cigarettes. I use the word *addicted* because they so obviously crave chewing on a butt or nicotine-loaded filter tip. Perhaps you should try to give up smoking for your dog's sake, or at least stick to a brand that is nicotine-free. I hope your dog won't suffer from withdrawal symptoms and get as snappy as I did when I gave up the addictive weed.

woodwork (dogs)

DEAR DR. FOX—My peekapoo dog has started chewing on the paneling frame around the doors of my kitchen and has chewed the arm of our leather recliner. I painted these things with Tabasco sauce, which worked only for a short time. It all started when we placed him in the kitchen, because he was having the run of the house while we were at work. Any ideas?—*A.L.*

DEAR A.L.—You are the main cause of your dog's problem, I'm afraid. If you were at home your dog wouldn't be bored, lonely, and frustrated. Leave a radio on and give your dog plenty of chew toys to play with. Bitter apple or pepper juice on the woodwork may inhibit further chewing. Can a neighbor come in during the day and take your dog for a walk?

If all else fails, a training crate may work. Buy a large holding cage and put your dog in there while you're gone, along with toys, water, and a blanket. This is a cruel deprivation, but better than having the dog put to sleep, unless you want to find it a good home where it won't be abandoned all day.

FALSE PREGNANCY

DEAR DR. FOX—About every two or three months, my three-year-old Chihuahua gets hold of this small blue rubber toy, plays with it, and walks around day and night with it in her mouth. She won't go to bed without it, won't take time to eat because she won't put it down, and fights with my other dogs when they get near her. She takes it up on the davenport, licks it, and tries to cover it. Does she think she is a mother?—*M.E.*

DEAR M.E.—It's not at all unusual for a female dog to treat some toy as though it were a puppy. Chalk it up to maternal instinct, imaginative play, or fetishism—who knows? However, dogs who are having a fake pregnancy will often use a slipper or toy as a pup substitute. Their hormonal state brings on this need, and they satisfy it by finding a substitute object.

Recurrent false pregnancies can lead to uterine infections and breast cancer. If you don't get her spayed, you should not allow her to have a substitute puppy toy, because this can help prolong the false pregnancy. Spaying eliminates this problem totally, which is essentially hormonal psychosis; it may well be distressing for a dog to feel intensely maternal and yet have no pups to care for.

16

Phobias

DEAR DR. FOX—My cockapoo is the smartest dog I've ever had. The problem is she barks at jet planes. She barks at them whether the vapor trail is a faint trace in the sky or an illuminated arch running from east to west.

She seems to think it's her worst enemy. She frantically races around the yard, barking, keeping a careful watch on the "thing" in the sky. I've been tempted to donate her to the Armed Forces, but whether they could teach her to spy on the sky silently is uncertain. The only way I can stop her is to put a hose on her. Have you encountered this problem before?—*MRS. H.H.*

DEAR MRS. H.H.—You certainly do seem to have an intelligent dog. The trouble is, intelligence and sensitivity usually go hand in hand, which means that more intelligent dogs are more susceptible to emotional traumatization than less-aware pooches.

Perhaps your dog once heard a jet go through the sound barrier, and the sonic boom (which will make mink shed their fur) triggered a phobia to the sight (and sound) of high-flying jets and their vapor trails. You either have to live with it or take her indoors when she gets "spooked." As a last resort (for the neighbors' sake) try your "water cure," but please, not in winter. I heard of one pooch who behaved just like yours a few days after it had its first plane ride—another bright dog who knows what planes are all about!

DEAR DR. FOX—When my adorable boxer was about nine months old, he chased a fast-traveling Volkswagen and was nearly hit. Ever since, if a Volks-

281

wagen appears, he reacts aggressively. He seems to hate them with a passion, and I must restrain him on a leash with all the resistance I can muster. He loves riding in our station wagon, and accepts all other cars. How do I make him get over his attitude?—H.R.S.

DEAR H.R.S.—I would think twice about breaking your boxer of his aversion to Volkswagens. Many dogs would do much better if, once hit by a car and able to survive, they took extra subsequent precautions. It is bizarre that your dog should be so specific in his phobia.

That's a new one in my books, although I have heard of dogs becoming terrified of one particular breed after being beaten by one as a pup. If you insist on breaking this phobia, then—considering its intensity—he will need a mild tranquilizer, which his veterinarian can prescribe, before you attempt to desensitize him.

Have him tranquilized and sit in a Volkswagen (engine off) the first time. A few days later, switch the engine on and walk him around the car. Next session, have him ride in it, and, finally, have someone slowly drive the car past and around him. Good luck!

certain noises (dogs)

DEAR DR. FOX—My miniature poodle is afraid of certain noises like the pop of a toaster or the sound of frying food, but perfectly at ease with the sounds of saws and other machines in my husband's basement workshop. Can you explain this?—E.W.

DEAR E.W.—Your dog has most likely developed sound shyness—a phobia to sudden or loud noises that originated with some physical trauma. For example, you might have accidentally trodden on him or alarmed him with a sudden movement as you went to reach the toaster when it popped. And just as you were conditioned to reach for it when it popped, he was conditioned thereafter to fear it. My advice is to ignore your dog—the less fuss, the less you are reinforcing or rewarding him with attention when he's scared.

certain people (dogs)

DEAR DR. FOX—The elderly dog next door is quite afraid of my brother. Every time he sees him, he shivers and growls. Do dogs have heart attacks? I worry that this one will.—V.J.

DEAR V.J.—Dogs do have heart attacks, but I doubt that your brother will scare the old dog to death. This animal may once have been teased or mistreated by children in the past. My advice: Don't try to make friends. Just ignore him and get by as quickly as you and your brother can. The less you both hang around, the less distressed the dog will be. I appreciate your concern. Some older dogs can't see or hear too well, and that's probably scary for them, too.

certain smells (dogs)

DEAR DR. FOX—I recently read in your column that a dog's fear of the smell of lamb cooking may be a reaction to how the sheep was slaughtered. Isn't it possible that dogs who react this way have in their background a strong herding instinct associated with sheep? The smell of the lamb cooking must trigger this association.—MRS. Y.S.

DEAR MRS. Y.S.—You offer a thoughtful theory. We know little about the smell world of animals, which may be a million times more sensitive in dogs than ours. It's possible that some dogs may smell fear in the meat, since fear-related hormones are present in minute traces. There could also be a simpler explanation: some pooches may develop a conditioned fear reaction after being trodden on or burned while someone was in the kitchen cooking a certain kind of meat.

firecrackers (dogs)

DEAR DR. FOX—Is there a cure for dogs afraid of firecrackers? Neighborhood children delight in shooting them year round. My dog is so frightened he refuses to go into the yard.—*H.C.*

DEAR H.C.—Tranquilizers. For many dogs this is the only answer. Also, keep a radio or phonograph turned on as loud as you can tolerate; it will act as a sound screen for your dog. If you behave in a calm and collected fashion and don't fret and fuss over your dog when he's scared, that will help too. Anxiety is contagious, and anxious owners adversely affect their pets.

gunshots (dogs)

DEAR DR. FOX—My four-year-old beagle has always been an excellent hunter. He is also a family pet, and we have made fools of hunters who claim a house pet won't hunt. Two years ago he was hit by a car, and the vet placed pins in his pelvis and hip. Because of this we only hunt with him half days. In the past, he would be wild with anticipation when he saw us getting the guns out of their case. Now he's gun-shy, and I am baffled. He still delights in chasing rabbits and other game, but if we take a gun along he'll run home when a shot is fired. Incidentally, my son and I have recently gotten muzzle-loading rifles. What do you think?—*E.M.*

DEAR E.M.—I think the muzzle-loading rifles could well be too much for your beagle, especially since they smoke and spark and the black powder stinks. It's also possible that he was particularly sore from his old injury the day you and your son first took him out and fired the muzzle-loader, and this could have set up a negative reaction or phobia.

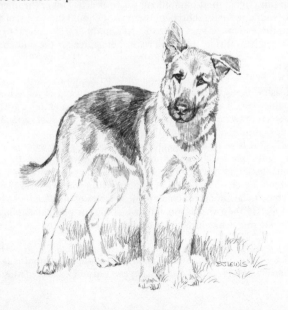

DEAR DR. FOX—My husband's dog has a fear of thunder and gunshots (which are a regular thing out here where we live, since there is always some kind of hunting season going on). He starts out by whining, and then it's nonstop barking for two hours in the morning and then again at dusk. My husband owned the dog before we were married and never reprimanded him, only petted and soothed him, which made him bark more. Now we have finally tried punishment and even spraying him with water, but nothing stops this infernal barking when he hears any kind of shooting or thunder. Please help my sanity and my marriage.— L.S.

DEAR L.S.—Since reassurance, petting, and discipline have failed, desensitization therapy is needed. An experienced trainer can do this for you, or you can give it a try yourself. Have your vet give you a prescription for a tranquilizer such as Valium that reduces anxiety (yes, animals have emotions like ours, that's why these human drugs work on them). Lightly medicate the dog. Then set off firecrackers at intervals, out of sight of the dog and about thirty feet or so away. Soothe the dog and reward him with morsels of meat or whatever he likes best. About ten ten-minute sessions over a couple of weeks should help. Increase the medication if needed. Similar treatment can be given by firing blanks near a dog who's gun-shy.

leaving house (dogs)

DEAR DR. FOX—For the past year, my dog has been petrified of noises in the street; she'll stand there shaking and refuse to move. Now she won't go out at all. What's up, doc?—T.B.

DEAR T.B.—Your young dog has a phobia about going outside, and such reactions arc not uncommon in sensitive dogs. Being frightened by children, alarmed by traffic, or psychologically traumatized by a car backfiring or a police siren can result in a dog developing agoraphobia. I suggest that you have your veterinarian prescribe a mild tranquilizer for your dog. Under this medication, you can take your dog out for short periods, and she should show signs of improvement within three to four weeks. If she doesn't, another technique is to keep her hungry and feed her outside. That will make her appreciate the outdoors.

leaving owner (dogs)

DEAR DR. FOX—I have a seven-year-old dachshund who will no longer go out on the leash with my helper. I have to go part of the way and yell at him to "get the heck up the road." I am nearly seventy–five years old, and he's a great watchdog, but he's very strong and can pull me down the road if he sees a rabbit, a cat, or another dog coming. Can you help?—MRS. G.B.

DEAR MRS. G.B.—Your helper should try to make the experience of leaving you and the house pleasurable. He should encourage your dog with a piece of meat or a suitable tidbit that your dog really enjoys eating. Do not distress yourself too much about the dog being anxious about leaving you. Just reassure the dog that you're going to be OK and encourage the person walking the dog to be gentle and reassuring. He then should quickly overcome his phobia. A choke-chain collar on the dog may make him easier for you to control.

men (dogs)

DEAR DR. FOX—We acquired a Canaan dog about three months ago from a well-respected kennel. He is two-and-a-half years old and was raised mostly in the kennel. He has taken to my wife and two children, but not to me. He appears to be man-shy and will cower and/or run if any man gets too close.

The breeder said that she and her daughter were with the dog constantly, and that her husband had little contact with it. Could that explain it? How can I make him accept me? Should we both go to obedience training?—*S.R.G.*

DEAR S.R.G.—I do not advise obedience school. Clearly, your dog was not adequately socialized to men earlier in life. This fear of men will be difficult to eliminate. I advise you to hand-feed him, groom him, and taking regular walks with him on the leash. If possible, encourage the dog to play with you, especially tug-of-war with an old towel. Such play therapy can be extremely effective. Good luck.

nonsocialized behavior (cats)

DEAR DR. FOX—About a month ago we received a four-year-old Siamese cat named Sammy. The animal was dropped off in our living room. He jumped out of his box, ran down into our basement, and has not been seen since. We know he's there because when the house is completely quiet, he apparently eats his food and uses the litter box. We've turned the cellar upside down looking for him. How do we get him out?—*M.D.*

DEAR M.D.—Nothing worse—or more pathetic—than a closet cat. Poor, shell-shocked creature. Call your local humane society and see if you can borrow a Have-a-Heart box trap. Get the cat used to eating in the trap for a while before you set it. When caught, he will be wild, so you should make up your mind what you plan to do with him then. It will require an experienced cat handler or veterinarian to resocialize your cat. Treatment with Valium (in his food) may help reduce his anxiety level and help him adjust.

psychotic behavior (cats)

DEAR DR. FOX—My stray poodle-afghan, now two years old, developed this strange problem when he was six months old. He kept biting and barking at his left leg above the paw and acted like he was in pain. I took him to three different vets, but no prescription worked. Now he leaves the leg alone but is hallucinating.

He looks up in the air, sniffs, pants, and then barks. He is always looking up. He backs into things still looking up. The vet quiets him with Valium, but Valium is expensive. Will he hallucinate the rest of his life? I love him dearly.—*R.M.*

DEAR R.M.—Some dogs, such as yours, develop bizarre, psychoticlike symptoms. If a regular veterinary examination fails to pinpoint any specific cause, I suggest you take your dog to the nearest veterinary school and have the specialists run some tests on him before you make the final, irreversible and responsible decision of having him put to sleep. Clearly, in his psychotic state he is suffering, and if you can't find a suitable psychoactive drug that you can afford and that will control his bizarre behavior, I see no point in prolonging his life. An all-natural, fresh, homemade diet may help—bleach in bread and too much wheat in commercial dog food have been known to cause hysteria and epilepsy.

storms (dogs)

DEAR DR. FOX—Our German shepherd is well behaved and healthy, but during an electrical storm he goes bananas and jumps on the bed and in the shower. We tried tying him outside, but he broke several choke chains and has even jumped a six-foot fence. What's with him?—*L.C.*

DEAR L.C.—Some dogs go out of control when a storm is coming; they can feel it just as some people and children do, most likely because of the changed electrical charge in the air. Before a storm, there are more positive ions, and a negative ionizer in the room may help. Some dogs need to be tranquilized. Others who are more upset by the noise can be desensitized by repeated exposure to a tape recording of a thunderstorm. This may be your best solution.

strangers (cats)

DEAR DR. FOX—Our young, cuddly cat started to fear strangers just recently—those in the house and even those walking outside. He simply panics, and for no apparent reason slinks from one hiding place to another, howling. He trembles for hours after the visitor leaves. Once he threw himself against the windows repeatedly just at the sight of a stranger. He lives indoors and has had no traumatic experience. Can you suggest any reason for this behavior?—*S.B.*

DEAR S.B.—Believe it or not, this kind of temperament change often occurs in cats and for two reasons. First, they are naturally that way—that is, they have an inherent shyness or wildness that doesn't begin to surface until they have outgrown kittenhood. Also, since many cats never get out to meet strangers while they're growing up, they become terrified when strangers visit. This can be aggravated if the cat has a shy temperament to begin with. My advice is, don't force your cat to be friendly. When you have visitors, put your cat in a quiet room where he will feel safe. Buy a long leash and harness, and try taking your cat outside—first into a quiet backyard—to get him used to new things. This way he might become desensitized and slowly lose his fear.

strangers (dogs)

DEAR DR. FOX—Our Shetland sheepdog frightens easily. Confronted by a stranger or anything unfamiliar, he becomes uncontrollable, will not obey commands, and will even attempt to bite members of the family who try to restrain him. Have you any advice for calming him down?—*K.K.*

DEAR K.K.—Many Shetland sheepdogs suffer from this problem—as do a number of purebred dogs. You will have to live with it or with a tranquilized dog (see your vet for a prescription). Or you will have to have the dog locked up when you have visitors. Fear of strangers—xenophobia—may be related to earlier trauma, but more often it is linked with an unstable temperament. Frequently this is a byproduct of improper breeding and is a strike in favor of mongrel dogs. The less purebred, the fewer temperament problems.

Afterword:
Wildlife Conservation
and Careers in Animal Care

helping nature along

DEAR DR. FOX—While walking along the water's edge at the beach, I came across a baby loggerhead turtle about the size of the palm of my hand. It was being battered by the surf breaking on the beach, but it was alive with a soft shell and seemed to be trying to move into the water. I placed him in shallow water, but the next wave rolled him back up on the beach. Rather than leave him as a meal for a seagull, I took him out to a depth of about four feet and released him. Was this a good idea?—D.P.C.

DEAR D.P.C.—Humans are remarkable in the way they can worry over such things as the fate of a little sea turtle. Yes, it was the right thing to take the little creature out of the tide edge so that it could get into deeper, safer water. But its chances of survival are slim. That's why turtles lay so many eggs. Today, more than ever, with destruction of their "nesting" grounds (beaches where the eggs are laid and buried in the sand) and pollution, turtles need our help to survive.

DEAR DR. FOX—I recently came across two monarch butterflies whose wings were severely damaged on the side. I felt bad, so I took them in and am now feeding them honey once a day. In spite of this, one of the butterflies seems to have lost some of his vigor, which makes me wonder whether I am really being much help to them. Is this wing damage just a natural prelude to the end of their life cycle?—C.E.E.

DEAR C.E.E.—It was nice of you to take in the injured monarch butterflies and give them some refreshment. These beautiful creatures migrate all the way to

Mexico and South America and may get killed or get so torn up that they are unable to make the trip. If they aren't in top shape, they won't make it, so your being a Good Samaritan may be of limited value. Perhaps you could help better by joining a conservation organization or environmental protection group to halt the use of certain insecticides that wipe out butterflies.

Late one fall, a bee landed on my hand. It seemed weak, uncoordinated, and hungry, so I gave it some honey and water. Within minutes it became more active, then flew away. If we take time out, it's easy to understand even bees' needs.

training for career in animal care

DEAR DR. FOX—I am in my junior year of college, with a biology/zoology major. I have taken various biology classes as well as introductory psychology and sociology, always relating them to my experiences with animals. Animals have been my life, and I am drawn to veterinary studies. But I am very curious about a future in animal psychology. Is it a limited field?—L.S.

DEAR L.S.—It's very rewarding to get so very many letters from students interested in careers with animals. Yes—jobs for people trained in animal behavior are difficult to obtain, but since there is growing interest in farm-animal welfare today, there may well be more jobs opening up for trained people. Knowledge in applied animal behavior can also lead you to a job in a zoo as a curator or educator, to college positions, and, of course, to state and federal wildlife departments. You could also work as an educator or investigator or scientist for a local or national humane or conservation organization. If you have writing ability, a background in animal behavior is invaluable in writing magazine articles and/or preparing documentaries for television. Some animal behaviorists are finding a niche as counselors for pets with behavior problems. Do check out an excellent book, *Careers with Animals*, published by The Humane Society of the United States, 2100 L St. N.W., Washington, D.C. 20037 (price: $6.95).

DEAR DR. FOX—I am interested in finding a career that involves working with animals. I love animals and should have been a veterinarian, but instead I'm a mental health counselor. Where can I learn to be an animal psychologist? Or can you suggest any other careers with animals? I am a forty-four-year-old woman.—P.W.

DEAR P.W.—You are rather "old" to be accepted by veterinary school, I am sorry to say. Being a woman may also be held against you, although most veterinary schools are improving in their attitudes toward women. With your back-

---

WHALE OF AN IDEA

At the recent international conference to discuss the ethics of killing cetaceans—the family name for whales, dolphins, and porpoises—scientists presented evidence that the structure of cetaceans' brains suggests that they have the potential for intelligence equal to or greater than humans.

Previously, the emphasis was on the factor of endangerment of species, but now scientists are also concerned about the inhumanity of killing creatures who are sensitive and self-aware.

ground, you might fit well into a newly developing veterinary area called pet-facilitated co-therapy. This is the term given to a growing field that uses pets for psychologically beneficial purposes for the elderly, for prison inmates, and for emotionally disturbed children.

The therapeutic value of people keeping pets is now being investigated with considerable enthusiasm both in the United States and in Europe, and such studies and clinical use include mental health workers, clinical psychologists, and others.

wildlife protection

DEAR DR. FOX—I enjoy your column very much, but I wish you would include more about wildlife conservation and endangered species.—*R.F.*

DEAR R.F.—If I received more letters about such topics, I would certainly answer them in my column. In my recent books *Returning to Eden* and *One Earth, One Mind*, the crises of wildlife, environment, and unethical exploitation of animals are discussed in depth. In dismantling the Environmental Protection Agency, the present administration is being perceived by many as discounting such critical issues as pollution control and water and air quality. It is more important today than ever before for concerned citizens to support local and national environmental, wildlife protection, and humane organizations.

WILDLIFE NEWS

The Atlantic striped bass, a valuable sport and commercial fish, has been drastically declining in numbers over the past decade. U.S. Fish and Wildlife Service biologists now suspect that traces of arsenic and various chemicals may be responsible. Tests show that the fish had weakened backbones, a condition scientists believe to be caused by toxic chemicals. Also, several species of fish in the Great Lakes are dying from cancer, with industrial and agrichemical pollutants being primary suspects.

DEAR DR. FOX—The Endangered Species Act is up for reauthorization this year, and some persons are advocating dropping plants and invertebrates from protected status. In your opinion, is it important to retain these for protection?—*C.S.*

DEAR C.S.—Former Interior Secretary James Watt was a key figure behind attempts to gut the Endangered Species Act. He and his ilk see this act as standing in the way of "progress," which is, essentially, greater corporate profits through exploitation of the environment. Regardless of sound ecological principles, the rights of wild species, and the concerns expressed by the public, the Reagan administration holds the reins of power and is blind to the "ecocidal" direction it is taking. This will only hasten the demise of our civilization.

However, we still have a democracy—so use your vote to get rid of state and federal senators and congressional representatives who do not stand behind protecting all plant and animal species under the act. Lobby them and join local and national groups such as Friends of the Earth and The Humane Society of the United States, who are fighting to preserve the act and protect our nation's heritage. Ecological balance and economic stability are as synonymous as environmental quality and human health. Caring for all living things and for the environment is enlightened self-interest.

Index

ABOUT THE AUTHOR

Dr. Michael W. Fox, D.Sc., Ph.D., B.Vet.Med., M.R.C.V.S., a strong animal rights advocate, is Director of the Institute of Animal Problems of the Humane Society of the United States. He is also Scientific Director of the Humane Society. The author of almost thirty books, both scientific and popular—including *Love is a Happy Cat, The Healing Touch, Understanding Your Cat,* and *Understanding Your Dog*—Dr. Fox is also a regular columnist for *McCall's* Magazine and United Feature Syndicate. He lives in Washington, D.C., with his wife, Deborah, a dog and two cats.

ABOUT THE ILLUSTRATOR

B. J. Lewis's artwork has appeared in various wildlife magazines and in *National Geographic*. She has also illustrated Dr. Fox's *The Way of the Dolphin*, a children's novel. She lives in Shingle Springs, California, with a menagerie that includes horses, dogs, cats, chickens, geese, and an Amazon parrot.